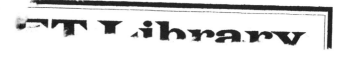

For Churchill Livingstone:

Publisher: Michael Parkinson
Project Editor: Janice Urquhart
Copy Editor: Teresa Brady
Indexer: Helen McKillop
Production Controller: Nancy Arnott
Design Direction: Erik Bigland

Mothers, Babies and Health in Later Life

D. J. P. Barker BSc MD PhD FRCP FRCOG FFPHM
Director and Professor of Clinical Epidemiology,
Medical Research Council Environmental Epidemiology Unit,
University of Southampton; Honorary Consultant Physician,
Southampton University Hospitals Trust, UK

SECOND EDITION

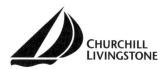

CHURCHILL
LIVINGSTONE

EDINBURGH LONDON NEW YORK PHILADELPHIA SAN FRANCISCO SYDNEY
TORONTO 1998

CHURCHILL LIVINGSTONE
A Division of Harcourt Brace and Company Limited

Robert Stevenson House
1–3 Baxter's Place
Leith Walk
Edinburgh
EH1 3AF

Formerly published by BMJ Publishing Group as *Mothers, Babies and Disease in Later Life*

🕭 is a registered trade mark of Harcourt Brace and Company Limited

First published 1994
Second edition 1998
ISBN 0 443 06165 3

British Library of Cataloguing in Publication Data
A catalogue record for this book is available from the British Library.

Library of Congress Cataloging in Publication Data
A catalog record for this book is available from the Library of Congress.

Medical knowledge is constantly changing. As new information becomes available, changes in treatment, procedures, equipment and the use of drugs become necessary. The authors and the publishers have, as far as it is possible, taken care to ensure that the information given in this text is accurate and up to date. However, readers are strongly advised to confirm that the information, especially with regard to drug usage, complies with current legislation and standards of practice.

The
publisher's
policy is to use
paper manufactured
from sustainable forests

Printed by Bell and Bain Ltd, Glasgow

Preface

This book describes how the nourishment a baby receives from its mother, and its exposure to infection after birth, determine its susceptibility to disease in later life. Its theme is that improving the nutrition and health of girls and young women, and of mothers during pregnancy and lactation, will improve the health of their children throughout their lives.

Geographical studies first suggested that if a baby is undernourished it becomes susceptible to coronary heart disease and stroke in adult life, and Chapter 1 reviews these studies. Chapter 2 attempts a comprehensive review of the many animal studies which have shown that undernutrition in early life permanently `programs' the body's structure and metabolism. Chapters 3 to 6 describe studies in humans which show that impaired growth in the womb and during infancy is followed by coronary heart disease, hypertension, non-insulin dependent diabetes, raised serum cholesterol and abnormal blood clotting in later life. Chapter 7 describes how poor lung growth before birth and respiratory infection in childhood may determine susceptibility to chronic bronchitis. Chapter 8 outlines the complex processes by which a mother nourishes her baby. Chapter 9 illustrates how other infections in early childhood may be linked to later disease. Chapter 10 describes how the poor health of people who are in lower socio-economic groups, or who live in impoverished places, can be linked to past neglect of the welfare of mothers and babies. Chapter 11 discusses strategies for the future, and suggests that further research into the nutrition of mothers and their babies may lead to better prevention of disease in future generations and to better treatment of disease in generations already born.

The influences which determine the fetus' demand for nutrients and the mother's ability to supply it are complex and many studies in the past have been too simplistic to be useful. It may be some years before we know how to improve fetal nutrition. Meanwhile it is important that people who were undernourished in the womb, and therefore had low birthweight or were thin or stunted at birth, avoid becoming overweight as children and adults; for it not only increases their own risk of coronary heart disease but, acting through the women, it increases the risk in the next generation as well. Chapter 11 offers a new explanation for the epidemics of coronary heart disease which regularly occur when populations escape from chronic malnutrition. These epidemics are not driven by the introduction of harmful influences such as cigarette smoking, though these may contribute. Rather they occur because while children and adults can become well nourished within a few years it takes several generations to optimise nutrient delivery to the fetus through the placenta. In this interim period the fetus that is undernourished because of a restricted placental supply is imperilled by the metabolic environment which the well nourished mother provides and by the metabolic consequences if it itself becomes overweight in later life.

In this book I have referred extensively to the work of my colleagues in the MRC Environmental Epidemiology Unit at the University of Southampton, and it is a pleasure to thank and acknowledge them. Clive Osmond, senior statistician in the Unit, played a central role in developing our research and I am grateful for his intellectual input and for his constant good humour during twelve years of collaboration. Cyrus Cooper, Caroline Fall, Keith Godfrey, Hazel Inskip, Catherine Law, Christopher Martyn, David Phillips and Sian Robinson direct major programmes of research within our common theme. David Coggon has been an invaluable adviser on methodology and analysis. Avan Aihie-Sayer, Janis Baird, Adrian Bull, Phillipa Clark, Janet Cresswell, Elaine Dennison, Seif Shaheen, Alistair Shiell and Claudia Stein, have all made important scientific contributions. Paul Winter our computer manager, with Vanessa Cox and Graham Wield have devised novel methods for handling and analysing the data. Brian Pannett successfully searched the country for old maternity and infant welfare records. Mary Barker, Sarah Duggleby, Catharine Gale, Julia Hammond and many others in the Unit have helped with the fieldwork, data analysis and administrative support, and I am grateful to them all. Our studies were possible because of the vision of doctors and nurses who compiled detailed records on mothers and babies many years ago, and because of the willingness of the men, women, and children who were those babies to take part in our surveys. Without the help of the staff at the NHS Central Register in Southport it would not have been possible to trace people from birth to adult life.

Our work has given us the opportunity to collaborate with clinicians and epidemiologists in several countries. In India Dr Anand Pandit, Dr Chittaranjan Yajnik and Dr Kuros Coyaji at the King Edward Memorial Hospital, Pune; Dr Shobha Rao at the Agharkar Research Institute, Pune; Dr K Kumaran at the Holdsworth Memorial Hospital, Mysore; Dr P Raghupathy and Dr Joseph Richard at the Christian Medical College, Vellore; Dr Srinath Reddy (All India Institute of Medical Sciences) and Dr Santosh Bhargava in Delhi; and Dr Ramesh Potdar in Bombay. These are founder members of SNEHA, the Indian Society for Natal Effects on Health in Adults. We collaborate in China with Professor Kong-Lai and Dr Mi Jie, at the Peking Union Medical College, Beijing: in Finland with Dr Johan Eriksson and Dr Tom Forsen at the National Public Health Institute, Helsinki: in Holland with Dr Jan van der Meulen, Tessa Roseboom and Anita Ravelli at the Amsterdam Medical Centre, Amsterdam: and in Jamaica, with Professor Terrence Forrester at the Tropical Metabolism Research Unit, Kingston.

The epidemiological findings described in this book pose questions which can only be answered by people working in other areas of medical research. Professor Nick Hales, at the University of Cambridge, Professor Peter Gluckman and Dr Jane Harding at the University of Auckland, New Zealand, Professor Jeffrey Robinson and Dr Julie Owens at the University of Adelaide, Australia, Professor John Challis at the University of Toronto, Canada, Dr Jonathan Seckl at the University of Edinburgh, Scotland and my colleagues Professor Alan Jackson and Mr Tim Wheeler at the University of Southampton, have from an early stage developed the epidemiological findings through experimental and clinical research.

The MRC has taken a lead in developing research into the maternal and fetal origins of adult disease and I am grateful to the staff at MRC Head Office in London who have enabled this. The Dunhill Medical Trust and Wessex Medical Trust have never failed to give financial support at times of special need. Other support has come from the British Heart Foundation, the Wellcome Trust, Wellbeing and Children Nationwide.

The development of a new field of research is greatly helped by the interest of a major journal. The *BMJ* published many of the earlier papers on programming and adult disease, and later published the first edition of this book. It is a pleasure to acknowledge the help of the editor Dr Richard Smith and his colleagues.

This book was typed by Lin White and edited by Shirley Simmonds. Sue McIntosh and Karen Drake checked the references. The book would not have been written without the help of my wife, Jan, who also made the embroidery for the book cover.

D J P Barker
Southampton, 1997

Contents

1. Clues from geography   1

2. Programming the baby   13

3. From birth to death   43

4. Blood pressure   63

5. Cholesterol and blood clotting   81

6. Non-insulin-dependent diabetes and obesity   97

7. Fetal growth, childhood respiratory infection and chronic bronchitis   117

8. The undernourished baby   129

9. Childhood infections and disease in later life   151

10. Preventing chronic disease: lessons from the past   167

11. Preventing chronic disease: the future   181

Index   213

Clues from geography

The three babies in Figure 1.1 were born in the same hospital in England. Each was born after an uncomplicated pregnancy and delivery, and their birth-weights were within the normal range. Yet the findings which will be described in this book suggest that the baby on the left, the smallest one, will be more susceptible to coronary heart disease, stroke, diabetes and chronic bronchitis as an adult, and is destined to have a shorter, less healthy life.

The thesis of this book is that a baby's nourishment before birth, and during infancy, and its exposure to infection during early childhood, influence the diseases it will develop in later life. Chapters 3 to 7 examine the long-term effects of nutrition in utero; Chapter 8 reviews the control of nutrition and growth in utero; Chapter 9 examines the long-term effects of infection, and

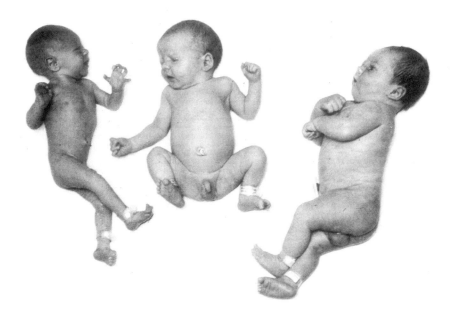

Fig. 1.1 Three newborn babies.

Chapters 10 and 11 discuss the implications of these observations for the prevention of disease.

CORONARY HEART DISEASE

At the start of this century the incidence of coronary heart disease rose steeply; it rapidly became the most common cause of death in Western countries. Its incidence is now rising in other parts of the world to which Western influences are extending, such as India, China, Eastern Europe and Russia. As such rapid increases in incidence over a short time cannot be the result of changes in gene frequency, attention has been directed at the environment, in particular the lifestyles of men and women in industrialised countries.

Given that the other major heart disorder in adult life, chronic rheumatic heart disease, was already known to be caused by events in childhood, it may seem surprising that adults rather than children were the early focus of research into coronary heart disease. Perhaps discovery of the powerful effects of cigarette smoking on lung cancer directed attention in this way. Whatever the reason, 40 years of research into adult lifestyle have met with limited success in explaining the origins of coronary heart disease: obesity and cigarette smoking have been implicated, and evidence on dietary fat has accumulated to the point where a public health policy of reduced intake is prudent, though unproven: preliminary evidence points to a role for psycho-social stress.[1] Much, however, remains unexplained.

A recent review of trials of a wide range of lifestyle interventions, including exercise, weight loss, smoking cessation and dietary changes, shows that their effects in reducing the incidence of coronary heart disease are small, less than 8% reductions at best, and statistically insignificant.[2] The limited insights provided by research into the links between lifestyle and coronary heart disease has led the British Heart Foundation to conclude that:

we shall probably never have proof that a particular lifestyle factor or item of diet is important and those who demand proof before any action are condemning us to wait forever.

Physicians are familiar with the need to advise patients in circumstances where there is only limited knowledge. If knowledge subsequently advances the advice can be changed. Unfortunately formulation of public health policies to prevent coronary heart disease, policies based on the best available advice, has simultaneously created a scientific orthodoxy. This states that the disease results from the 'unhealthy' lifestyles of westernised adults together with a contribution from genetic inheritance. Such a view of coronary heart disease, however, leaves its changing incidence and geography largely unexplained, and offers little insight into why, within westernised communities, one person develops the disease while another does not. The effectiveness of preventative measures based on this view of the disease is being questioned.[3]

In many Western countries the steep rise of coronary heart disease has been followed by a fall; in the USA,[4] this has been of the order of one-quarter over 20 years. No parallel changes in adult lifestyle seem to explain it. In Britain there were large changes in lifestyle during the Second World War, especially in diet.

Government food policy led to major and widespread changes in diet, so that fat and sugar consumption fell sharply and fibre consumption rose.[5, 6] Death rates from coronary heart disease in middle-aged men and women, however, continued to rise throughout the war and the period of post-war rationing.[7]

The geography of coronary heart disease in Britain is paradoxical. Rates are twice as high in the poorer areas of the country, and in lower income groups.[8] The steep rise of the disease in Britain and other Western countries was associated with rising prosperity,[9, 10] so why should its rates be lowest in the most prosperous places, such as London and the home counties, and in the highest income groups?[11, 12] Biochemical and physiological measurements in adult life, including serum cholesterol and blood pressure, have been shown to be linked to coronary heart disease.[13] Yet, even when combined with these biological risk factors, adult lifestyle has limited ability to predict coronary heart disease.[14] Rose[15] has pointed out that, for a man falling into the lowest risk groups for cigarette smoking, serum cholesterol concentrations, blood pressure and pre-existing symptoms of coronary heart disease, the most common cause of death is coronary heart disease.

It is, perhaps, surprising that it was geographical studies that gave the early clue that answers to these paradoxes may come from events in utero. Nevertheless, the first indication that coronary heart disease might be linked to impaired fetal growth came from the demonstration that differences in rates of death from coronary heart disease in different parts of England and Wales paralleled previous differences in death rates among newborn babies.[16] In the past most deaths among newborn babies were associated with low birthweight. In these early studies the death certificates for all people who had died in England and Wales during 1968–78 were used to calculate coronary heart disease rates for men and women in each of the 1366 local authority areas.[17] Death rates were expressed as standardised mortality ratios which take into account differences in the age and sex distribution of populations in different areas, and are calculated so that the national average is 100. Figure 1.2 shows how the concentration of low mortality from coronary heart disease in the south and east contrasts with the high mortality in the northern industrial towns, and the poorer rural areas in the north and west. This contrast is seen in men and women, with the exception of north Wales where mortality among women is low.[17]

Figure 1.3 shows infant mortality (deaths under 1 year of age) in England and Wales in the early years of the century. The distribution is surprisingly similar to that of coronary heart disease today. To compare the distribution more formally, the country was divided into the 212 areas used by the Registrar General, comprising each large town (county borough), the London boroughs, the smaller towns in each county combined together, and the rural areas in each county combined. The scattergrams in Figure 1.4 confirm the similarity of the current distribution of coronary heart disease and the distribution of infant mortality in the years 1921–25. The correlation coefficient for this relationship is 0.69 in men and 0.73 in women. In separate analyses for men and women living in large towns, small towns or rural areas, the correlation coefficients ranged from 0.65 to 0.75.[16] Analyses based on infant mortality in an earlier period (1911 onwards) gave similar results.

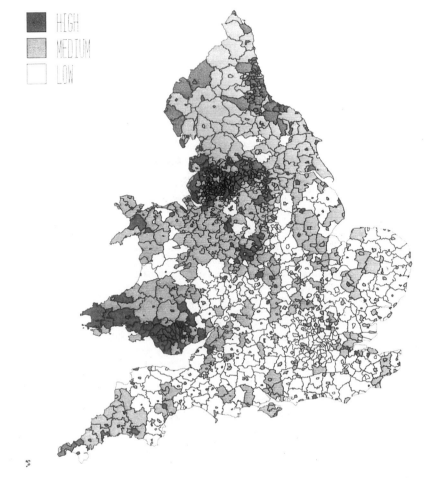

Fig. 1.2 Standardised mortality ratios (SMR) for coronary heart disease in England and Wales among men aged 35–74 years during 1968–78.

Of the 23 common causes of adult death other than coronary heart disease, only chronic bronchitis, stomach cancer and chronic rheumatic heart disease had a similarly close geographical relationship with past infant mortality. Such a relationship with infant mortality would be expected for these diseases, because they are linked to poor social conditions, and their rates, like those of infant mortality, have declined during this century. It is, however, paradoxical that coronary heart disease is related to infant mortality because the rates have increased during this century.

One possible explanation of Figure 1.4 is that the poor social conditions which caused infant deaths in the past are in some way linked to adult lifestyles which cause death from coronary heart disease. The nature of such a link is not, however, apparent. Differences in cigarette smoking do not appear to follow those of past infant mortality because the distribution of deaths from lung cancer is strikingly different from that of past infant mortality. Therefore it cannot be argued that the social conditions giving rise to infant death led to higher cigarette smoking in later life and hence to raised heart disease rates. Similarly, differences in dietary fat consumption do not have the same geographical dis-

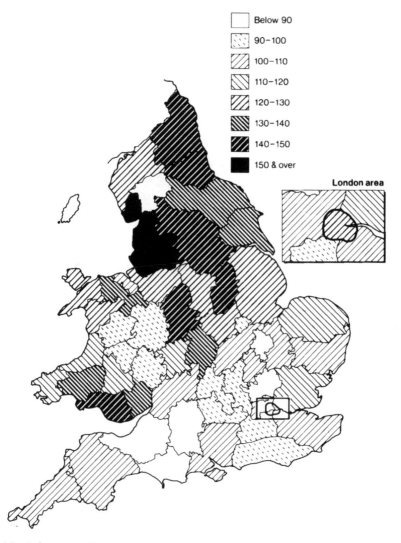

Below 90

90–100

100–110

110–120

120–130

130–140

140–150

150 & over

London area

Fig. 1.3 Infant mortality rates per 1000 births in England and Wales during 1901–10.

tribution as past infant mortality.[18] The close geographical similarity between past infant mortality and current mortality from coronary heart disease is most readily reconciled with their opposing time trends through the hypothesis that adverse environmental influences in utero and during infancy, associated with poor living standards, directly increase susceptibility to the disease.

THE ENVIRONMENT DURING CHILDHOOD

Findings from other studies support the general hypothesis that coronary heart disease is linked to adverse influences in early life. Forsdahl[19] reported that arteriosclerotic heart disease correlated with past infant mortality in the 20 counties of Norway, and he was the first to suggest that a poor standard of living in childhood and adolescence was a risk factor in heart disease. Another

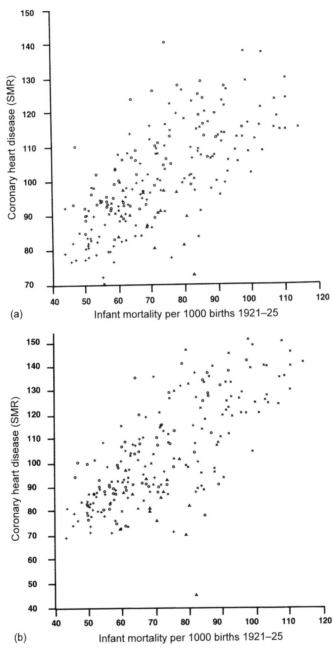

Fig. 1.4 Standardised mortality ratios (SMR) for coronary heart disease in (a) men and (b) women during 1968–78 and infant mortality during 1921–25 in England and Wales. Δ, London boroughs; X, county boroughs; O, urban districts; +, rural districts.

study compared east and west Finland and came to similar conclusions: that poor living conditions in childhood, with bad housing and recurrent exposure to infection, increased the later risk of coronary heart disease.[20] In 17 states of the USA, mortality from coronary heart disease was shown to be related to infant mortality resulting from diarrhoeal disease, which again suggested that the disease is associated with poor living conditions in early childhood.[21]

Other observations which suggest that influences in childhood are linked to coronary heart disease include those made by Rose.[22] He reported that siblings of patients with coronary heart disease had stillbirth and infant mortality rates that were twice as high as those of controls. He concluded that 'ischaemic heart disease tends to occur in individuals who come from a constitutionally weaker stock', a conclusion foreshadowing what is known today. The study of London civil servants by Marmot et al[23] showed that death rates were higher in those who were shorter in stature, and who may therefore have had a worse environment in early life. Among long-term employees of the Bell System Company in the USA, men whose parents had been in 'white collar' occupations had a lower incidence of coronary heart disease than those from 'blue collar' families.[24]

THE ENVIRONMENT IN UTERO

The size of the geographical study in England and Wales, based on almost one million deaths from coronary heart disease, together with the remarkably complete and detailed infant mortality records, made it possible to examine whether coronary heart disease was associated with specific causes of infant death and hence with particular aspects of the early environment. Infant deaths were divided into neonatal (deaths in the first month after birth) and postneonatal (deaths from 1 month to 1 year). They were also divided into five causes, using a classification devised 50 years ago for an extensive analysis of the social causes of infant mortality:[25] congenital, bronchitis and pneumonia, infectious diseases, diarrhoea and 'other'.

The distributions of neonatal and postneonatal mortality throughout England and Wales were broadly similar. Nevertheless there were areas where the rate of one was high while the other was low. The 15 boroughs of London were important in this respect. London had low neonatal but high postneonatal mortality. Possible reasons for this are examined in Chapter 10. The 212 local authority groups in the country were ordered according to the neonatal mortality rates during 1911–25 and divided into five groups according to the level of mortality.[26] Neonatal mortality rose from 30 per 1000 births in group 1 to 44 in group 5. Five groups with increasing postneonatal mortality were derived in the same way, mortality rising from 32 per 1000 in group 1 to 73 in group 5. In this way the relationship of neonatal and postneonatal mortality to adult mortality could be examined within a grid of 25 cells (Table 1.1). Areas with low neonatal but high postneonatal mortality were mainly in London, although they included the towns of Chester and Great Yarmouth. Areas with high neonatal but low postneonatal mortalities were scattered through the north and west, including the rural areas of Anglesey, Northumberland and Staffordshire.

Table 1.1 compares death rates from stroke, coronary heart disease, and chronic bronchitis. Within any of the five bands of postneonatal mortality, standardised mortality ratios for stroke increase sharply with increasing neonatal mortality. There is no independent trend in stroke mortality with postneonatal mortality. Mortality from coronary heart disease has similar but separate trends with neonatal and postneonatal mortality. Mortality from

Table 1.1 Standardised mortality ratios (SMR) from stroke, coronary heart disease, and chronic bronchitis (ages 35–74, both sexes, 1968–78) in the 212 areas of England and Wales grouped by neonatal and postneonatal mortality (1911–25)

Neonatal mortality		Postneonatal mortality				
		1 (lowest)	2	3	4	5 (highest)
Stroke	1 (lowest)	85	81	79	78	79
	2	86	90	98	74	76
	3	102	100	104	104	104
	4	—	108	110	115	117
	5 (highest)	124	—	121	123	117
Coronary heart disease	1 (lowest)	84	89	91	88	98
	2	85	93	95	88	91
	3	86	94	99	106	113
	4	—	98	109	111	115
	5 (highest)	83	—	114	119	116
Chronic bronchitis	1 (lowest)	67	78	106	115	161
	2	64	84	85	104	126
	3	69	65	89	88	151
	4	—	91	99	120	142
	5 (highest)	41	—	108	123	144

chronic bronchitis shows a steep increase with increasing postneonatal mortality, but no independent trend with neonatal mortality.

Seventy years ago most neonatal deaths occurred within a week of birth, and depended on adverse intrauterine rather than postnatal influences.[27] Of such deaths, 80% were certified to be the result of 'congenital' causes, which also correlate geographically with stroke and coronary heart disease. The link between neonatal mortality and coronary heart disease and stroke therefore suggests that early influences predisposing to cardiovascular disease act during prenatal life. Postneonatal deaths were the result of respiratory infection, diarrhoea and other infections, reflecting inadequate housing, overcrowding, and other adverse influences in the environment after birth. The association between chronic bronchitis and respiratory infection in infancy is discussed in Chapter 7.

MATERNAL NUTRITION AND HEALTH

The relationship between cardiovascular disease and the intrauterine environment can be explored further by examining maternal mortality which, geographically, was closely related to neonatal mortality. In Britain maternal mortality remained at a disturbingly high level from the late 19th century until the mid-1930s:[28] 'A deep, dark and continuous stream of mortality'. In the early part of this century the geographical distribution of maternal mortality in Britain was similar to that of neonatal mortality.[29]

Maternal mortality tends to be highest in rural, sparsely populated counties, and in industrial districts, notably those associated with the textile industries in Lancashire and Yorkshire, and with coal mining; and tends to be lowest in the South of England, in districts in and around London, and in certain large towns, such as Birmingham, Manchester and Liverpool.[29]

Two early reports analysed the causes of maternal mortality,[29, 30] grouping deaths into those caused by puerperal fever (around 40%) and those caused by 'other complications of pregnancy and parturition'. Most of these 'other' deaths resulted from toxaemia, haemorrhage or accidents of childbirth.

Figure 1.5 shows that the geographical distribution of stroke correlates close-ly with past maternal deaths from these 'other causes',[31] the correlation coeffi-cient being 0.65. The relationship occurs in both sexes and is specific. Among other causes of death, only coronary heart disease correlates as closely with past maternal mortality. As expected from Table 1.1, maternal mortality is unrelated to chronic bronchitis.

In his analysis of infant mortality in Britain, Woolf[25] stated that much of the variation in neonatal mortality depended on variations in poverty, as measured by the percentage of unemployed men in the lower socioeconomic groups. He attributed this to the adverse effects of poverty on maternal nutrition and lac-tation. Campbell's[29, 32] earlier analyses had also identified poor health and physique of mothers as a major cause of maternal mortality. She attributed them to poor nutrition, rickets in infancy and industrial employment of girls. Baird[33, 34] also related the large geographical differences in perinatal mortality in Britain to differences in the physique and health of women. He concluded that the poor living standards which accompanied industrialisation or eco-nomic depression adversely affected the development of young girls, and impaired their subsequent reproductive efficiency.

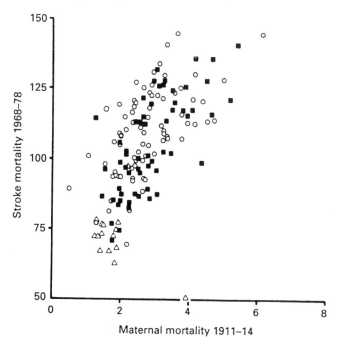

Fig. 1.5 Standardised mortality ratios (SMR) for stroke in men and women aged 55–74 years during 1968–78, and maternal mortality (per 1000 births) from 'other causes' (see text) during 1911–14. △ ,London boroughs; O, county boroughs; ■, administrative counties.

> Hypothesis
>
> An interpretation of the analyses described here is that poor nutrition, health and development among girls and young women are the origin of high death rates from cardiovascular disease in the next generation. They prejudice the ability of mothers to nourish their babies in utero and during infancy. The fetus responds to undernutrition with permanent changes in its physiology, metabolism and structure, and these lead to coronary heart disease and stroke in adult life.

MIGRANTS

If the environment in utero and during infancy influences the development of cardiovascular disease, a person's risk of that disease is likely to be related to his or her place of birth. This can be explored by examining disease rates in people who migrate from their place of birth, because the effects of the environment in early life can be distinguished from those encountered later on. In England and Wales, where variations in maternal and neonatal mortality suggest differences in maternal nutrition from place to place, disease in migrants can be analysed using data from death certificates. Place of birth is recorded on death certificates, although it is not routinely coded. For a trial period during 1969–72, however, the Office of Population Censuses and Surveys (OPCS) did code the place of birth. During this time there were almost two million deaths in England and Wales among people who had been born there. Of these people half had migrated to another part of the country during their lives.

Using these data, Osmond and colleagues[35, 36] related numbers of deaths from coronary heart disease and stroke, expressed as a proportion of all deaths, to place of birth and place of death. The results showed that a person's risk of dying from coronary heart disease or stroke was predicted by place of birth, independently of place of death. Part of the increased risk among people born in many northern counties and industrial towns, and in Wales, persisted whether or not they had moved to other areas of the country. The low risk of cardiovascular disease, especially stroke, among people born in and around London went with them when they moved.

Other evidence from migrants comes from studies of the 'stroke belt' in the USA. For the past 50 years, despite the continuing decline in stroke rates, there has been a consistent geographic variation in death rates from stroke in the USA.[37] The highest rates are in the south-east, in an area known as the 'stroke belt', that includes the coastal plain region of North Carolina, South Carolina and southern Georgia.[38] Interestingly these areas have among the highest perinatal mortality rates in the USA today. The analysis of Lackland et al of all recent deaths in South Carolina showed that the proportional mortality for stroke was some 25% lower among people born outside the south east – a difference that was considerably larger in blacks than whites.[39] Conversely an analysis of deaths in New York City found that the higher rates of coronary heart disease and stroke in blacks were largely explained by high rates among blacks who were born in the southern states but migrated to the north.[40]

The findings from migrant studies are necessarily inconclusive. People who migrate from the place where they were born differ from those who remain, in physique, mental attributes and health. Lack of information on age at migration makes it impossible to pinpoint the critical stage in early life when susceptibility to disease is acquired. Nevertheless these observations from the USA and Britain are consistent with the hypothesis that the intrauterine environment influences the development of cardiovascular disease.

Summary

The suggestion that events in childhood influence the pathogenesis of cardiovascular disease is not new. The implication of the geographical studies described in this chapter is, however, that the search for environmental causes of cardiovascular disease should not focus on the environment of children, their diets, homes, and illnesses, but rather should focus on babies, for whom mothers are the dominant environmental influence. This is a new point of departure for cardiovascular research.

References

1 Marmot MG, Bosma H, Hemingway H, Brunner E, Stansfeld S. Contribution of job control and other risk factors to social variations in coronary heart disease incidence. *Lancet* 1997; **350**: 235–239.

2 Ebrahim S, Davey Smith G. *Health promotion in older people for the prevention of coronary heart disease and stroke*. London: Health Education Authority, 1996.

3 Ebrahim S, Davey Smith G. Systematic review of randomised controlled trials of multiple risk factor interventions for preventing coronary heart disease. *Br Med J* 1997; **314**: 1666–1674.

4 Pisa Z, Uemura K. Trends of mortality from ischaemic heart disease and other cardiovascular diseases in 27 countries, 1968–1977. *World Health Stat Q* 1982; **35**: 11–47.

5 Greaves JP, Hollingsworth DF. Trends in food consumption in the United Kingdom. *World Rev Nutr Diet* 1966; **6**: 34–89.

6 Southgate DAT, Bingham S, Robertson J. Dietary fibre in the British diet. *Nature* 1978; **274**: 51–52.

7 Barker DJP, Osmond C. Diet and coronary heart disease in England and Wales during and after the second world war. *J Epidemiol Community Health* 1986; **40**: 37–44.

8 Registrar General. *Registar General's statistical review of England and Wales. Part 1. Tables, Medical*. London: HMSO, 1911 and following years.

9 Ryle JA, Russell WT. The natural history of coronary disease. A clinical and epidemiological study. *Br Heart J* 1949; **11**: 370–389.

10 Morris JN. Recent history of coronary disease. *Lancet* 1951; **i**: 1–7.

11 Gardner MJ, Crawford MD, Morris JN. Patterns of mortality in middle and early old age in the county boroughs of England and Wales. *Br J Prev Soc Med* 1969; **23**: 133–140.

12 Office of Population Censuses and Surveys. *Registrar General's decennial supplement, occupational mortality, England and Wales 1970–72*. London: HMSO, 1978.

13 Keys A. *Seven countries*. Cambridge, MA: Harvard University Press, 1980.

14 Rose G, Marmot MG. Social class and coronary heart disease. *Br Heart J* 1981; **45**: 13–19.

15 Rose G. Sick individuals and sick populations. *Int J Epidemiol* 1985; **14**: 32–38.

16 Barker DJP, Osmond C. Infant mortality, childhood nutrition and ischaemic heart disease in England and Wales. *Lancet* 1986; **1**: 1077–1081.

17 Gardner MJ, Winter PD, Barker DJP. *Atlas of mortality from selected diseases in England and Wales, 1968–78*. Chichester: John Wiley, 1984.

18 Office of Population Censuses and Surveys. *The dietary and nutritional survey of British adults*. London: HMSO, 1990.

19 Forsdahl A. Are poor living conditions in childhood and adolescence an important risk factor for arteriosclerotic heart disease? *Br J Prev Soc Med* 1977; **31**: 91–95.

20 Notkola V. *Living conditions in childhood and coronary heart disease in adulthood*. Helsinki: Finnish Society of Sciences and Letters, 1985.

21 Buck C, Simpson H. Infant diarrhoea and subsequent mortality from heart disease and cancer. *J Epidemiol Community Health* 1982; **36**: 27–30.

22 Rose G. Familial patterns in ischaemic heart disease. *Br J Prev Soc Med* 1964; **18**: 75–80.

23 Marmot MG, Shipley MJ, Rose G. Inequalities in death – specific explanations of a general pattern? *Lancet* 1984; **i**: 1003–1006.

24 Hinkle LE. Coronary heart disease and sudden death in actively employed American men. *Bull N Y Acad Med* 1973; **49**: 467–474.

25 Woolf B. Studies on infant mortality: part II, social aetiology of stillbirths and infant deaths in county boroughs of England and Wales. *Br J Social Med* 1947; **2**: 73–125.

26 Barker DJP, Osmond C, Law CM. The intrauterine and early postnatal origins of cardiovascular disease and chronic bronchitis. *J Epidemiol Community Health* 1989; **43**: 237–240.

27 Local Government Board. *Thirty-ninth annual report 1909–10. Supplement on infant and child mortality*. London: HMSO, 1910.

28 Loudon I. Deaths in childhood from the eighteenth century to 1935. *Medical History* 1986; **30**: 1–41.

29 Campbell JM. *Maternal mortality*. (Ministry of Health Reports on Public Health and Medical Subjects, No. 25) London: HMSO, 1924.

30 Local Government Board. *Forty-fourth annual report 1914–15. Supplement on maternal mortality in connection with childbearing and its relation to infant mortality*. London: HMSO, 1916.

31 Barker DJP, Osmond C. Death rates from stroke in England and Wales predicted from past maternal mortality. *Br Med J* 1987; **295**: 83–86.

32 Campbell JM, Cameron D, Jones DM. *High maternal mortality in certain areas*. (Ministry of Health Reports in Public Health and Medical Subjects, No. 68) London: HMSO, 1932.

33 Baird D. Social factors in obstetrics. *Lancet* 1949; **i**: 1079–1083.

34 Baird D. Environment and reproduction. *Br J Obstet Gynaecol* 1980; **87**: 1057–1067.

35 Osmond C, Slattery JM, Barker DJP. Mortality by place of birth. In: *Mortality and geography: a review in the mid-1980s (OPCS Series DS No 9)*. London: HMSO, 1990.

36 Osmond C, Barker DJP, Slattery JM. Risk of death from cardiovascular disease and chronic bronchitis determined by place of birth in England and Wales. *J Epidemiol Community Health* 1990; **44**: 139–141.

37 Lanska DJ, Peterson PM. Geographic variation in the decline of stroke mortality in the United States. *Stroke* 1995; **26**: 1159–1165.

38 Howard G, Evans GW, Pearce K, Howard VJ, Bell RA, Mayer EJ et al. Is the stroke belt disappearing? An analysis of racial, temporal, and age effects. *Stroke* 1995; **26**: 1153–1158.

39 Lackland DT, Egan BM, Hudson MB, Jones PJ. Dramatic effects of nativity on strokebelt mortality in blacks. *Am J Hypertens* 1996; **9**: 18A.

40 Fang J, Madhaven S, Alderman MH. The association between birthplace and mortality from cardiovascular causes among black and white residents of New York city. *N Engl J Med* 1996; **335**: 1545–1551.

2

Programming the baby

The findings described in Chapter 1 led to the hypothesis that undernutrition in utero permanently changes the body's structure, physiology, and metabolism, and leads to coronary heart disease and stroke in adult life. The principle that the nutritional, hormonal, and metabolic environment afforded by the mother may permanently 'program' the structure and physiology of her offspring was established long ago. 'Programming' describes the process whereby a stimulus or insult, at a sensitive or 'critical' period of development, has lasting or lifelong significance.[1,2] The development of the sweat glands provides an interesting example of programming.[3] In the early years of this century Japanese military expansion took their soldiers and settlers into unfamiliar climates. They found that there were wide differences in people's abilities to adapt to hot climates. Physiological studies showed that this was related to the number of functioning sweat glands. People with more functioning sweat glands cooled down faster. Rather than attributing the differences in sweat gland numbers to 'genetic effects', Japanese physiologists explored the early development of the glands. They found that at birth all humans have similar numbers of sweat glands; but none of them function. In the first 3 years after birth a proportion of the glands become functional depending on the temperature to which the child is exposed. The hotter the conditions the greater the number of sweat glands that are programmed to function. After 3 years the programming is complete and the number of sweat glands is fixed. The development of sweat glands encapsulates the essence of programming: a critical period when the system is plastic and sensitive to the environment, followed by loss of plasticity and a fixed functional capacity. The development of the eye in early childhood provides another example of programming. The young eye is usually far-sighted and uses visual information to determine whether to grow longer, in the direction of near-sightedness. Reading at an early age may cause a child's eye to grow into focus at the distance of a page, leading to short-sightedness, whereas the eyes of a child living largely outdoors may grow into focus at infinity.

There are many reasons why it may be advantageous, in evolutionary terms, for tissues to remain plastic during development. For discussion of this fascinating topic the reader is referred to the recent book by Stearns.[4] This chapter describes the extensive observations on programming in animals that may allow us to understand the observations now being made in humans.

SENSITIVE PERIODS IN DEVELOPMENT

One of the best examples of the programming phenomenon is the lifelong effect of early exposure to sex hormones on sexual physiology. A female rat injected with testosterone propionate on the 5th day after birth develops normally until puberty, but fails to ovulate or show normal patterns of female sexual behaviour thereafter.[5] Pituitary and ovarian function are normal, but the release of gonadotrophin by the hypothalamus has been irreversibly altered from the cyclical female pattern of release to the tonic male pattern. If the same injection of testosterone is given when the animal is 20 days old, it has no effect. Thus there is a critical time in which the animal's sexual physiology is plastic and can be permanently changed. Other experiments on rats have shown that neuroendocrine function can be programmed by a range of drugs.[6] Animals exposed in utero to phenobarbitone, for example, have permanently altered concentrations of gonadotrophins and sex steroids.[7]

Numerous animal experiments such as this have shown that hormones, undernutrition, and other influences that affect development during sensitive periods of early life permanently program the structure and physiology of the body's tissues and systems.[5, 8–16] The concept of sensitive periods in early life has long been familiar from experiments in which animals have been imprinted to behave abnormally.[17] Lorenz[18] showed that newly hatched goslings could be imprinted to behave as if a dog were their mother – if the first moving object they saw after hatching was a dog. Long ago Pliny described 'a goose which followed Lacydes as faithfully as a dog' and Reginald of Durham wrote of eiderducks which followed humans.

A remarkable example of programming is the effect of temperature on the sex of reptiles. If the eggs of the American alligator are incubated at 30°C all the offspring are female. If they are incubated at 33°C all the offspring are male. At temperatures between 30 and 33°C there are varying proportions of females and males. It is believed that the fundamental sex is female, and a transcription factor is required to divert growth along a male pathway. Instead of the transcription factor being controlled genetically, by a sex chromosome, it depends on the environment, specifically temperature. The temperature at which the eggs are incubated also determines postnatal growth rates, skin pigmentation, and the animal's preferred temperature: alligators will seek out an environment that has the same temperature as the one in which they were hatched.[19] Another example of programming is provided by a moth, the African army worm.[20] If the larvae are overcrowded and hence undernourished, they develop a metabolism that is more dependent on fats (triglycerides). Fats are the fuel required for long distance flights and in this way the adults are better adapted to migrate to other, less crowded places.

Many systems in the body seem to be more susceptible to programming during periods when they are growing rapidly so that their sensitive periods coincide with times of rapid cell replication[21, 22]. During the first 2 months of life, the embryonic period, the human differentiates but does not grow rapidly.

Thereafter, in the fetal period, it attains its highest growth rates. Growth slows in late gestation and continues to slow in childhood. The high growth rates of the fetus compared with the child are mostly the result of cell replication. The proportion of cells that are dividing becomes progressively less as the fetus becomes older, so that few new nerve or muscle cells, for example, appear after 30 weeks of gestation.[23]

In some animals, such as the pig, cell numbers increase most rapidly after birth rather than before, and the animal can therefore largely recover from undernutrition in utero. Humans, however, accomplish a greater proportion of their growth before birth than pigs, and the effects of intrauterine growth failure are more severe.[24] It has been calculated that the fertilised human ovum goes through some 42 rounds of cell division before birth.[25] After birth only a further five cycles of division are needed.

Tissues develop in a predetermined sequence from conception to maturity, with different organs and tissues undergoing periods of rapid cell division, and therefore being in sensitive periods, at different times. The renal nephrons, for example, are laid down during the last trimester of pregnancy whereas the pancreatic beta cells continue to differentiate during infancy.[26, 27] It follows, therefore that undernutrition at different times in gestation will program different effects.

GROWTH AND FORM OF THE BODY

The pigs in Figure 2.1 are littermates. However, they have been reared on different diets with the result that two of them are small and have different body proportions. Slowing of growth is a major adaptation to undernutrition, because if the smallest pig, given an inferior diet, had maintained the same growth trajectory as the largest it would have perished. Numerous experiments on animals, including rats, mice, sheep and pigs, have shown that, when the

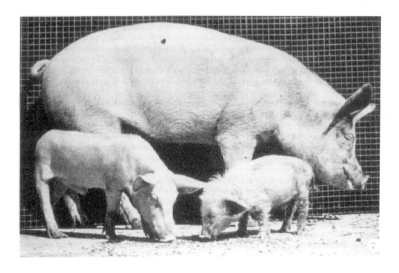

Fig 2.1 Three pigs from the same litter reared on different diets.

protein or calorie intake of the mother during pregnancy and lactation is low-ered, the offspring are smaller than they would otherwise have been.[24, 28–37] In general, the earlier in the life of an animal that undernutrition occurs, the more likely it is to have permanent effects on body weight and length.[36] Figures 2.2 and 2.3 show the results of an experiment carried out by Widdowson and McCance[38] more than 30 years ago. Rats who were undernourished from 3 to 6 weeks after birth, that is, immediately after weaning, lost weight. On resump-tion of full feeding at 6 weeks, they failed to return to the growth trajectory of the controls and remained permanently small (Fig. 2.2). By contrast, rats who were not undernourished until 9–12 weeks after birth regained their growth trajectory when full feeding was resumed, and continued to grow normally (Fig. 2.3).

Early in embryonic life, growth is regulated by the supply of nutrients and oxygen. At some point before birth, or shortly after in some species, growth begins to 'track'. Animals who are small in relation to others of the same age remain small, and vice versa. In humans tracking is demonstrated by the way in which infants grow along centile curves.[36] Once tracking is established it is no longer possible to make animals grow faster by offering them unlimited food. Their rate of growth has become 'set', homeostatically controlled by feedback systems. After a period of undernutrition they will regain their expected size. If they consume excess food they will merely become fat.

In early intrauterine life undernutrition tends to produce small but normally proportioned animals, such as the 'runt' pig, whereas at later stages of devel-opment it leads to selective organ damage.[36] During periods of undernutrition those tissues whose maturity is more advanced have a greater priority for growth and may continue to grow at the expense of other tissues.[39] For exam-ple, when rats are undernourished immediately after weaning, the weight of the brain and skeletal muscle is unaffected but the weight of the liver, kidney

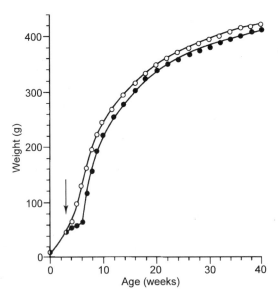

Fig 2.2   Rats undernourished at 3–6 weeks after birth remain permanently small.

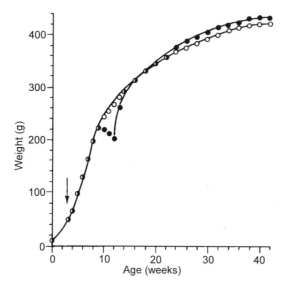

Fig 2.3 The growth of rats undernourished at 9–12 weeks after birth catches up.

and thymus is permanently reduced. When, however, undernutrition is delayed until 42 days after birth only the thymus is affected.

If growth is restricted by a reduced blood supply, rather than through undernutrition, the results are similar. If, for example, the artery supplying one horn of the rat's uterus is occluded in late gestation, the brain is spared but growth of the liver is disproportionately retarded. In general both undernutrition and uteroplacental ischaemia have the same effects on proportionate fetal growth if they occur at the same time.[40, 41] The timing of the insult is the factor that determines which tissues and systems are damaged, and hence the disproportion in size and function. The pattern of disproportion will also be influenced by the relative sensitivity of different organs. Some aspects of maturation, such as the growth of the thymus, are markedly influenced by nutrition, whereas others, such as the growth of the eye, are less sensitive.[42]

The way in which an animal's body proportions are modified by undernutrition is also related to its growth trajectory. If rats are undernourished for a brief 3-week period after weaning, those who were previously growing rapidly have different body compositions from those who were growing slowly – even if both groups of animals have the same final body weight. The bones of the fast-growing rats are longer and the testes heavier, but the livers, spleens and small intestines are lighter.[38] Similarly, in sheep the response of the fetus to maternal undernutrition in late pregnancy depends on its growth rate.[43] Slow-growing fetuses are unaffected whereas the growth of rapidly growing fetuses ceases abruptly (Fig. 2.4). One possible explanation is that slowly growing fetuses have previously encountered undernutrition in early pregnancy, and adapted to it by recruiting more placentomes. This protects them from restricted nutrition in later gestation. Again the size of the lambs at birth is similar although their body compositions differ. Placental enlargement as an adaptation to undernutrition is discussed further in Chapter 8. In humans, the growth trajectory of boys is more rapid than that of girls from early in embryonic life.[44–46] Boys may therefore be more vulnerable to undernutrition.

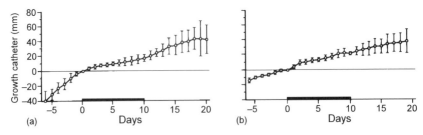

Fig 2.4 The growth of rapidly growing fetal lambs is checked by undernutrition (a) whilst slow growing fetuses are unaffected (b).

The nature of the undernutrition, as well as its timing, severity and the fetal growth trajectory, may influence body proportions. Pigs reared on very small amounts of good quality diet become small and thin. Those reared on the same diet but with unlimited amounts of carbohydrate or fat become somewhat larger. The brains of both groups of animals are disproportionately large. The bones continue to grow, whereas muscles scarcely grow at all, and the ovaries become cystic. The extra growth occurring as a result of the 'protein sparing effect' of unlimited energy leads to exaggerated enlargement of the penis and vulva.[36, 39, 47]

Small human babies are either proportionate, that is 'perfect miniatures', or disproportionate. Consistent with the findings in animals, the proportionately small baby is thought to originate through undernutrition in early gestation. The disproportionate baby is thought to result from undernutrition in later gestation. In other words, undernutrition in early gestation affects body size permanently, whereas undernutrition in late gestation has profound effects on body form. The long-term correlates of different kinds of disproportion at birth are a recurring theme of this book and are introduced in Chapter 3.

THE MECHANISMS WHICH UNDERLIE PROGRAMMING

The many permanent changes that are now known to be induced by undernutrition and other adverse influences in early life raise the question of how the memory of these events is stored and later expressed. Lucas has postulated three cellular mechanisms.[1] First, the nutrient environment may permanently alter gene expression;[48] for example, permanent changes in activity of HMG-CoA reductase (3-hydroxy-3-methylglutaryl coenzyme A reductase) and other enzymes, induced in animal experiments, are described later in this chapter. Second, early nutrition may permanently reduce cell numbers. The small but normally proportioned rat produced by undernutrition before weaning has been shown to have fewer cells in its organs and tissues.[8, 30, 33] Winick and colleagues[49] suggested that for this reason the animal does not regain its full size when adequately nourished after weaning. They argued that, as cell division cannot be restarted after the period of rapid division has come to an end, cell numbers limit ultimate body size.[50] Growth-retarded human babies have reduced numbers of cells in their organs[51] and in some instances these reduced numbers of cells can be directly linked to limitations of function. For example, reduced numbers of pancreatic beta cells may limit insulin secretion, and reduced size of the airways may limit respiratory function. In addition to reduced number of cells, the memory of early undernutrition may persist through permanent changes in organ structure. Hoet and colleagues have shown that, in the rat, protein deficiency not only lowers beta-cell mass in the pancreas but reduces the vascularisation of the islets – which may further impair insulin secretion.[52]

A third cellular mechanism of programming may be the selection of clones of cells. For example, an altered balance of the Th1 and Th2 lymphocyte subtypes characterises atopic disease. It has been suggested that this imbalance results from impairment of thymic development in late fetal life.[53] Hales and colleagues[54] have shown that undernutrition in pregnant rats changes the proportions of liver cells in the periportal and perivenous zones (p. 25).

Undernutrition may also effect permanent changes through intermediary mechanisms; the possible role of hormones as intermediaries is a recurring theme of this book. Fetal hormones are essential for normal fetal growth and development. They influence both tissue accretion and differentiation and, with the insulin-like growth factors, coordinate a precise and orderly increase in growth throughout late gestation.[55] Growth-retarded babies have an altered endocrine profile, with low insulin, insulin-like growth factor 1 and thyroid-stimulating hormone concentrations and high growth hormone and cortisol[56] (Fig. 2.5). Sensitivity to hormones may be programmed by the setting of cell receptors – structures in the cell membrane which convey the signal mediated by the hormone into the cell. Experiments suggest that membrane receptors are plastic during critical periods of maturation, and that their structure may be permanently altered. Exposure to a normal concentration of hormone seems to

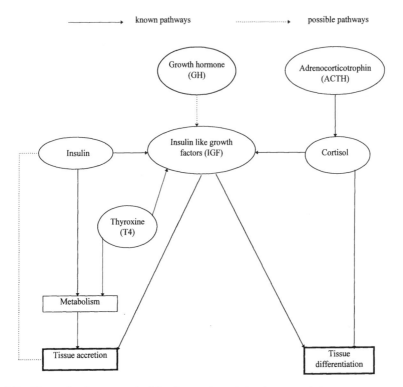

Fig 2.5 The endocrine control of fetal growth and development (after Fowden[55]).

promote receptor development, whereas exposure to other hormones that are sufficiently similar to bind to the receptor may reduce the receptor response permanently.[57, 58] A single dose of gonadotrophin hormone, which is similar in structure to thyroid-stimulating hormone (TSH), permanently changes the TSH receptors and reduces the responsiveness of the thyroid to TSH, with consequent reduction in thyroxine levels.[59]

If hormones are important as an intermediary mechanism programming disease they may act in one of two ways. Either patterns of hormone release and tissue sensitivity to hormones are programmed in utero, and over many years of postnatal life change the structure and function of the body; or transient hormonal changes in utero cause permanent changes in tissues at sensitive periods of development. Both kinds of process are known to occur in normal development. Among birds it is usually only males that sing. A male zebra finch will not sing unless it is exposed to testosterone in early life, but it also requires continued testosterone exposure in adult life.[60] The male hypothalamus is programmed by testosterone in the perinatal period and thereafter releases gonadotrophins in the tonic male pattern rather than the cyclical female one (p. 14). Hypothalamic imprinting is suspected of underlying the long-term effects of incubation temperature in reptiles, and it may prove an important mechanism in the causation of human disease.[61]

CONCLUSION

Plasticity is necessary in early development. The fetus in utero experiences continual variations in the supply of nutrients and oxygen it receives and has to adapt to them (p. 132). Whereas in adult life adaptations to environmental change are generally reversible, in fetal life they tend to be permanent. Why this should be is a fundamental question to which we have only speculative answers.

Summary

Undernutrition and other adverse influences arising in fetal life or immediately after birth have a permanent effect on the body's structure, physiology, and metabolism. The specific effects of undernutrition depend on the time in development at which it occurs. Rapidly growing fetuses and neonates are more vulnerable to undernutrition. The effects of undernutrition include altered gene expression, reduced cell numbers, imbalance between cell types, altered organ structure, and changes in the pattern of hormonal release and of tissue sensitivity to hormones.

ANIMAL PROGRAMMING EXPERIMENTS: A REVIEW

The remainder of this chapter reviews animal experiments which demonstrate programming in the different tissues and systems of the body. No review has been published recently, and the author hopes that it will prove useful as a source of reference to others working in this field. The general reader should turn to Chapter 3.

Rats, pigs and guinea pigs which are undernourished before birth stop growing at the normal chronological age and are therefore small as adults. Animals undernourished after birth, however, delay development and continue to grow beyond the normal age. In delaying development, and sexual maturation, these animals resemble humans in undernourished communities in the developing world.[36] Although some aspects of sexual maturation may be postponed by undernutrition, others seem to be protected. The experiments on pigs already cited suggest that development of the external genitalia is protected even during intense undernutrition.[39]

Undernutrition in utero seems to be associated with more rapid ageing. In rats, undernutrition in utero and up to weaning at 3 weeks after birth is followed in middle age by a more rapid progression of albuminuria and an increased activity of enzymes associated with ageing.[34] In the mouse, undernutrition during the last week of gestation leads to a reduction in peak haemoglobin and a more rapid decline in haemoglobin in later life.[62] Whereas perinatal undernutrition may be linked to more rapid ageing, numerous experiments have shown that reduced nutrient intake after weaning postpones sexual maturation, and prolongs lifespan.[63-68] These experiments, first carried out in rats by McCay and colleagues, have been repeatedly replicated. They provide a model for the study of the ageing process but the mechanisms underlying the phenomenon of dietary restriction and longevity are not understood.[69] One recent theory is that dietary restriction modulates oxidative damage. The hypothesis that ageing results from accumulation of molecular oxidative damage is based on the fact that oxygen, though necessary for the immediate survival of aerobes, is toxic in the long term.[70]

Recent experiments in rats have examined the interplay between prenatal and postnatal nutrition. A striking reduction in lifespan resulted from the combination of prenatal undernutrition, with retarded growth, and good postnatal nutrition, with accelerated growth.[71] Translated into human lifespan the reduction was the equivalent to 15 years of life beyond 60 years of age. It is not known why 'catch-up' growth is detrimental but one speculation is that fetal growth restriction leads to reduced cell numbers, and subsequent 'catch-up' growth is achieved by overgrowth of a limited cell mass.[50]

A recent theory of ageing suggests that, in terms of evolutionary benefit, there is a trade-off between allocation of energy to reproduction and repair of somatic damage. Such damage necessarily occurs as a result of extrinsic and intrinsic insults throughout life, and increases the rate of ageing. Species in which the young are exposed to high early mortality, for example from predators, may benefit from more prolific reproduction at the expense of longer survival of individuals.[72] It is postulated that fetal undernutrition leads not only to an immediate reduction in growth rate but to reduced expression of genes responsible for somatic repair. Under this hypothesis the fetus is adapting to an adverse environment, and a perceived reduced life expectancy, by diverting resources to reproduction. It thus becomes more vulnerable to somatic damage, which manifests itself in more rapid ageing.

OBESITY

Animal experiments show that early overnutrition may have permanent effects on body weight, and carbohydrate and lipid metabolism.[73–77] Rats fed enriched diets from weaning have increased fat and fat-free mass.[11] Paradoxically early undernutrition may also lead to obesity in later life. Early experiments by Stewart showed that if rats received low protein diets for 10 generations and thereafter, in the 10th generation, were given adequate protein from the 14th day of gestation they became obese. Adequate protein begun at birth or weaning had no effect. In later experiments rats whose mothers had restricted food during the first 2 weeks of pregnancy also became markedly obese.[78, 79] Depending on the strain of rat and the diet used it was either the males or the females who became obese. Guinea pigs undernourished throughout gestation similarly became centrally obese as adults (Owens J, unpublished). It has been suggested that, in humans, the numbers of adipocytes (fat-storing cells) are established in late gestation and early infancy. Rats given a reduced calorie intake during suckling have been found to have a permanently decreased number of adipocytes.[80, 81] However, observations on baboons are not consistent with this, and suggest that infant nutrition influences cell size rather than cell numbers.[76] The importance of early programming of adipocyte numbers in the development of human obesity remains unresolved.

BLOOD PRESSURE

Animal studies strongly support human studies which suggest that blood pressure is programmed in utero. Alterations in blood pressure are known to be one of the fetus' adaptive responses to hypoxia and other adverse influences.[82] Experiments in rats suggest that in some circumstances alterations in blood pressure or its control mechanisms may persist after birth. If pregnant rats are given less protein in their diets their offspring have lifelong raised blood pressure (Table 2.1),[83] even if they are fostered to normal rats immediately after birth.[84] Changes in the fetal hypothalamic–pituitary–adrenal axis are thought to underlie this,[85, 86] and these findings are described in more detail later in this chapter, under 'Glucocorticoids'(p. 29).

It has recently been shown that the blood pressures of spontaneously hypertensive rats, used as a genetic model of hypertension, are permanently lowered if they are suckled by other strains of rats for 2 weeks after birth. Analysis of the

Table 2.1 Effect of fetal exposure to low protein on systolic pressure in adult rats[83]

Maternal protein intake during pregnancy, % by weight	No. of animals	Systolic blood pressure, mm Hg
18	15	137
12	13	152
9	13	153
6	11	159
p value for trend		< 0.001

milk of spontaneously hypertensive rats shows that protein and electrolyte concentrations differ from those in other strains.[87–89] Other studies have shown that the intrauterine environment of the spontaneously hypertensive rat is different, as the amniotic fluid has high osmolality and sodium concentrations and the fetuses are underweight.[90] Altering the intrauterine environment experimentally by inducing maternal diabetes also affects blood pressure in the spontaneously hypertensive rat. In the rat blood pressure may continue to be programmed after weaning. The fatty acid content of the diet of weanling rats seems to change their systolic pressure.[91] In guinea pigs unilateral ligation of the uterine artery during pregnancy leads to reduced birthweight in the offspring and raised blood pressure after birth.[92] The mechanism underlying this is unknown, though increased circulating catecholamines have been proposed. Newborn piglets exposed to only 45 minutes of hypertension, induced by norepinephrine infusion, developed lesions in their coronary arteries. There was fragmentation and dissolution of the internal elastic lamina and disruption of the endothelium.[93] This led to the suggestion that perinatal surges in blood pressure may initiate changes in arterial structure that lead in turn to atheroma.

ORGAN GROWTH

Brain

The growth of the brain occurs in two phases. Multiplication of neuronal and glial cells is followed by the outgrowth of dendrons and axons. The extensive literature on the long-term consequences of nutritional, hormonal and other environmental influences on brain growth has been brought together in a number of recent reviews.[94–97] There is considerable evidence that early undernutrition adversely affects neurological, cognitive and emotional development. As with other tissues, undernutrition generally affects those parts of the brain that are undergoing rapid differentiation at the time, even though the brain tends to be 'spared' in relation to other organs.[10, 16, 98, 99] Hormone concentrations also influence brain development. Corticosteroids affect the rate of brain cell acquisition whereas thyroid hormones affect the timing of periods of rapid brain cell division. Gonadal hormones control the development of sexual physiology and behaviour.

Studies of visual development provide some of the best known observations on the importance of environmental stimulation in brain development.[100, 101] For example, temporary closure of the lids of one eye in kittens causes neurons in the visual cortex to become unresponsive to signals from the deprived eye, which becomes blind.

Lucas and colleagues[2, 102] have demonstrated programming in humans in a study of preterm infants randomly assigned to either a standard formula for term infants or a nutrient-enriched formula. Infants assigned to the standard formula, for only a few weeks after birth, had major deficiencies in developmental scores at 18 months of age. The deficiencies were particularly marked in motor development where the deficit was of the order of one standard deviation. The greatest deficiencies were seen in children who were small for gestation, that is, already undernourished at birth. Preliminary findings of a parallel study suggest that breast milk promotes cognitive development and protects against allergy, but restricts linear growth.[103] Although the findings in these remarkable studies cannot necessarily be generalised to normal infants, born at term, they provide important experimental support for the thesis that nutritional programming during sensitive periods in early life influences long-term health and development. Other studies of preterm infants have shown that formula foods enriched with fish oil are associated with better visual acuity.[104] This points to the possible long-term importance of lipids to brain development, perhaps an unsurprising conclusion given that lipids are an integral part of the morphology of neural cells.

Lung

In animals, a fetus deprived of calories or oxygen may develop pulmonary hypoplasia, defined by a reduction in the ratio of lung weight to body weight or a reduction in total lung DNA.[105–109] In the rat, interference with fetal growth can induce lung changes that resemble human emphysema, with persisting reduction in elastin and collagen, enlargement of air spaces, and a loss of elastic recoil.[110–114]

The timing of undernutrition determines whether its effects are permanent. In guinea pigs, whose alveolar development is largely completed before birth,[115] fetal undernutrition permanently changes alveolar morphology, whereas the changes induced by postnatal undernutrition are reversible.[116, 117] In rats, whose lungs undergo a period of rapid cell replication between 4 and 13 days after birth,[118, 119] permanent changes in alveolar structure can be induced by protein or calorie restriction in early postnatal life,[113] whereas changes induced after weaning may be reversible.[112, 117]

Physical influences are important in the regulation of lung growth.[120] An adequate amount of fluid within the airways appears to be necessary. In animals, reducing the volume of amniotic fluid[121–123] or draining lung fluid from the airways[124, 125] leads to pulmonary hypoplasia. Similarly, in humans, oligohydramnios (a lack of amniotic fluid) is associated with lung hypoplasia and narrow airways.[126, 127] The earlier the onset of the reduction in amniotic fluid volume, the more severe the degree of lung hypoplasia.[128, 129] A congenital diaphragmatic hernia allows abdominal contents to encroach on the intrathoracic space and is associated with a reduction in the number of airway branches.[130, 131] The growing chest wall is thought to provide a 'stretch' stimulus for growth of the underlying lung.[132] Abnormal chest wall growth, as a result of either compression in association with oligohydramnios,[122, 132] or skeletal deformity in kyphoscoliosis, impairs lung development.[133, 134]

In humans airway division down to the level of the terminal bronchioles is completed by week 16 of gestation.[135] Around half of the adult number of alveoli are present at birth, and cell multiplication is almost complete by 2 years of age. Lung growth in humans is described in Chapter 7.

Liver

Undernutrition of a pregnant ewe leads to marked reduction in the liver weight of the lambs. In the guinea pig moderate restriction of food intake before and during pregnancy similarly reduces the liver weight of the offspring who, in addition, become centrally obese as adults and have altered cholesterol metabolism (Owens J, unpublished).

Hales and colleagues have shown that if pregnant rats are given a low protein diet it permanently alters the activities of two enzymes that are synthesised by the liver and regulate the formation and breakdown of glycogen.[54, 71] The activity of PEPCK (phosphoenolpyruvate carboxykinase) an enzyme involved in glycogen synthesis, was doubled while that of glucokinase, an enzyme involved in glycogen breakdown, was halved. These changes can be related to changes in the morphology of the liver. PEPCK is expressed in the periportal zone while glucokinase is expressed in the perivenous zone. It is thought that undernutrition enhances replication of periportal cells and reduces that of perivenous cells. Altered zonation is likely to be linked to other important changes in hepatic function, though these are as yet unknown. Many aspects of liver function, including cholesterol synthesis and fibrinogen production are differentially expressed in the periportal and perivenous zones.[54]

Another demonstration of programming of liver enzyme activity comes from experiments in which newborn rats were exposed to high oxygen concentrations for up to 3 days. These brief exposures led to permanent reduction in activity of cytochrome P450 enzymes in the males. The functional consequences of this are not known but the authors of the report predict that it will lead to feminisation.[136]

Pancreas (See also insulin)

Much of the development of the islets of Langerhans occurs in utero.[137] The exact timing of islet formation differs between species. In rats the number of islets increases in the last 4–6 days of intrauterine life. In humans beta cell mass increases more than 130–fold between the 12th intrauterine week and the 5th postnatal month. Studies in animals show that undernutrition in utero or during early postnatal life may reduce the number of beta cells and the secretion of insulin.[13, 52, 138] The pancreatic beta cells seem highly sensitive to dietary protein. If pregnant rats are given a low protein diet the beta cell mass of the offspring is reduced, and the vascularisation of the islets is profoundly reduced.[52, 139]

Kidney

In the rat, restriction of the mother's protein intake leads to smaller kidneys, with fewer and less differentiated glomeruli and collecting tubules.[140] The number of nephrons in the rat kidney is strongly related to birthweight.[141] In humans, 60% of the normal complement of nephrons develop during the last trimester and development of the kidney ceases around week 35.[27, 142] There is a large variation in the number of nephrons at birth, and newborn babies that are thin have reduced numbers of nephrons.[27] Brenner & Chertow[143] have proposed that hypertension in humans is initiated by in utero reduction in nephron number (p. 73).

Intestine

In the rat the intestine develops rapidly in late gestation, and low maternal protein intake at this time leads to marked changes in structure, especially in the small intestine. The villi are fewer and less well differentiated.[144] The fibre content of the diet of pregnant rats also affects colonic structure.[145] Low fibre diets are associated with altered collagen crosslinkage and an increased incidence of colonic diverticulosis – a disorder that may be partly determined by age-related weakening of the colonic wall associated with increasing collagen crosslinkages.

Intrauterine growth retardation is common in pigs and is thought to arise through placental insufficiency. It is associated with reduction in the weight of the gastrointestinal tract, and in the numbers of cells in it, and also with altered patterns of enzyme maturation.[146] Pancreatic exocrine function is also impaired. The contribution of these lesions to the poor postnatal growth of runt pigs is not known. In humans growth-retarded neonates have persisting abnormalities in exocrine pancreatic function which may be linked to failure of catch-up growth.[147]

METABOLISM

Lipid metabolism

Cholesterol is an essential component of cell membranes and is a metabolic precursor of steroid hormones. It is synthesised de novo in the body and is also absorbed from the diet. With a varying supply of dietary cholesterol, the body maintains tissue concentrations by a balance between synthesis, controlled by the enzyme HMG-CoA reductase, and excretion, mainly in the bile after conversion to bile acids.[148]

There has been considerable speculation that the high cholesterol content and saturated fat content of human milk may program lipid metabolism throughout life and thereby influence the risk of cardiovascular disease. The results of early experiments gave some support to this hypothesis because animals suckled on low cholesterol-containing milk were found to have raised serum cholesterol concentrations subsequently, by reason of high activity of HMG-CoA reductase in the liver.[149, 150] However, the results of other experiments and follow-up studies of infants into childhood have failed to support the hypothesis.[148] The concentration of cholesterol in infants' food seems to have no more than a transient effect on serum cholesterol concentrations.[151–154]

Although cholesterol intake in infancy may not be important in the long term, animal experiments have unequivocally demonstrated that interference with cholesterol metabolism during development, by either changing the composition of the diet or giving cholestyramine, which increases cholesterol excretion, has permanent effects. Manipulations during gestation up-regulate cholesterol synthesis[148, 155] whereas manipulations after birth permanently change the body's capacity to excrete cholesterol in bile. The system of bile acid synthesis and excretion may be too immature in fetal life to be programmed.[156] When given to newborn guinea pigs, cholestyramine reduces the elevation of cholesterol in response to a dietary cholesterol challenge by increasing bile acid excretion.[152, 157, 158]

The age at which an animal is weaned also appears to have a long lasting influence on metabolism.[159–161] Weaning onto solid food entails a sharp fall in fat intake and a rise in carbohydrate intake. Rats that are prematurely weaned have a raised serum cholesterol in later life, which only becomes apparent after 7 months.[160, 162] Rats given a low protein diet after weaning have a significantly lower bile flow and bile acid secretion.[163]

The experiments of Mott, Lewis and colleagues on baboons have shown that breast feeding leads to a higher ratio of low density lipoprotein cholesterol to high density lipoprotein cholesterol in later life than is found in formula-fed baboons.[15, 164–166] Since in humans a high ratio is linked to coronary heart disease, this could suggest that breast feeding is associated with an unfavourable outcome. Another interpretation, however, is that breast-fed animals use cholesterol more efficiently, having an increased absorption and reduced turnover. Other experiments in baboons have suggested that it is not the ingested cholesterol which permanently changes lipid metabolism but the hormones or growth factors contained in breast milk. Thyroid hormone may be important, resetting thyroid homeostasis and hence mediating sustained differences in cholesterol and bile acid metabolism[15, 167–169]

In human infants, serum cholesterol concentrations are related to day to day intake of cholesterol and saturated fat.[170–173] From around the age of 6 months, however, cholesterol concentrations tend to 'track' so that children maintain their rank order by concentration through childhood.[174, 175] Recent studies suggest that raised serum cholesterol concentrations in humans may be programmed through failure of development of the liver in late gestation and by prolonged breast feeding. These studies are discussed in Chapter 5.

Protein metabolism

Studies of protein metabolism in both humans and rats suggest that the mother's intake of protein may program nitrogen metabolism in her children.[176–178] Children whose mothers had a low protein intake in pregnancy were found to excrete an unusually high proportion of their absorbed nitrogen.

ENDOCRINE SYSTEMS

Insulin

This hormone is of central importance to fetal growth and metabolism, and has been intensively studied in both fetal animals and humans.[179] It primarily stimulates tissue accretion (Fig. 2.5) and has little effect on tissue differentiation.[55] It stimulates growth by increasing the mitotic drive and nutrient availability for cell proliferation. It has major metabolic effects, increasing the utilisation of glucose and reducing the catabolism of amino acids. It responds to nutrient levels and acts as a signal of nutrient sufficiency, ensuring that fetal growth rates are commensurate with the nutrient supply.[180]

Much of the development of the endocrine pancreas occurs in utero.[180] In humans beta cell mass increases more than 130-fold between the 12th week of gestation and 5 months after birth. The pancreatic beta cells seem highly sensitive to dietary protein. In the rat a low protein diet during gestation reduces the beta cell mass and profoundly reduces islet vascularisation.[52] The insulin content of the islets is permanently reduced as is the activity of pancreatic glucokinase, which is the major glucose sensor in the beta cell and regulates glucose-stimulated insulin release.[71] The deficiency in insulin response to glucose which follows low protein in utero is not restored by normal feeding from birth to adulthood.[181] Low protein in the early postnatal period, however, may also impair insulin production. A low protein diet, given for only 3 weeks after weaning, permanently impairs the insulin response to glucose.[13] In the mouse undernutrition during lactation also permanently lowers serum insulin concentrations.[35]

Neither famine nor feast seem to benefit the growing pancreas. Raised plasma glucose concentrations as a consequence of maternal diabetes may also have lifelong effects on pancreatic structure and function. Remarkable experiments by van Assche & Aerts[182] have shown that changes in the glucose concentrations to which a fetus is exposed produce effects through several generations, mimicking genetic transmission. Pregnant rats were made mildly diabetic by injection of streptozotocin on the day of mating. Their female offspring had islet cell hyperplasia and beta cell degradation and developed gestational diabetes when they became pregnant; in turn their offspring developed islet cell hyperplasia, beta cell degradation, and disordered glucose metabolism as adults. The changes in the third generation were independent of the origins of the father. These findings have been replicated in other experiments using streptozotocin[183] and in experiments where rats were fed a high carbohydrate diet from days 4 to 24 after birth.[184, 185] These rats were hyperinsulinaemic and obese as adults and the offspring of the females, though fed normally, similarly became hyperinsulinaemic and obese. Other demonstrations of intergenerational effects initiated during gestation or early postnatal life have come from studies of nutrient deficiencies, drugs and hormones.[33, 184, 186] The links between insulin deficiency and resistance, acquired in utero, and non-insulin-dependent diabetes in later life are discussed in Chapter 6.

Growth hormone

In late gestation growth hormone assumes increasing importance in driving fetal growth. Babies with growth hormone deficiency are relatively short at birth, although of normal weight.[187] Limited evidence suggests that growth hormone secretion may be permanently influenced by events in early life. In particular, studies in rats have suggested that maternal dietary restriction during gestation and lactation, and transient dietary protein restriction after weaning, may permanently reduce growth hormone secretion in the offspring.[188–190]

Insulin-like growth factor 1 (IGF-1) is an important regulator of fetal growth, and is itself regulated by nutrition and growth hormone.[187] Transient starvation lowers fetal IGF-1 concentrations, which are rapidly restored by replacement of glucose or insulin.[191, 192] Growth-retarded fetal sheep, however, have low circulating IGF-1 concentrations which fail to increase in response to restoration of glucose supply. This suggests that chronic undernutrition permanently reduces IGF-1 production.[193]

In humans the growth-retarded fetus who is not growth hormone-deficient, but who shows slow postnatal growth, has elevated growth hormone concentrations and reduced IGF-1 concentrations.[194–199] These babies may therefore be resistant to growth hormone. Studies of children in England and India, however, have shown that those who had low birthweight but were tall or heavy in childhood, and whose postnatal growth therefore 'caught-up', had high plasma IGF-1 concentrations.[200] One explanation of this is that prenatal undernutrition led to persisting resistance to IGF-1, at least to its growth-promoting actions, in the lower birthweight children. A study of the 24-hour growth hormone profiles of elderly men showed that the median plasma concentrations correlated with weight at 1 year, which suggests that this aspect of the secretory profile may be programmed in early life.[201]

Glucocorticoids

In contrast to insulin, which has an important role in tissue accretion during fetal life, the main effects of cortisol are on cell differentiation.[202] Whereas tissue accretion seems to be closely related to fetal metabolism and nutrient supply, differentiation is controlled by hormones that can enter cells and alter gene transcription and/or protein processing (Fig. 2.5).[55] Cortisol triggers maturation, being responsible for a range of biochemical and cytoarchitectural changes which occur in fetal tissues towards term, in preparation for extrauterine life. The timing and magnitude of the cortisol surge in late gestation may have important long-term sequelae. Cortisol only modulates growth during late gestation and in adverse conditions when the exogenous nutrient supply is restricted. In these circumstances fetal cortisol concentrations rise and may contribute to reduced rates of tissue accretion.

Interest in the possible long-term effects of fetal exposure to glucocorticoids has been stimulated by findings that treatment of pregnant rats with low dose dexamethasone leads to persistently raised blood pressure in the offspring.[203] This observation has been replicated in pregnant sheep, in whom treatment with dexamethasone in early gestation, 22-29 days, led to persisting elevation of blood pressure in the offspring while treatment at 59-66 days was without effect.[204] Under normal conditions glucocorticoids in the maternal circulation are prevented from gaining access to the fetus by a placental enzyme, 11-β-hydroxysteroid dehydrogenase, which catalyses the rapid metabolism of cortisol and corticosterone to inactive products.[203, 205] In rats the activity of this enzyme in the placenta is lowest in neonates who have large placentas but low birthweight. As described in Chapter 4, humans who have a high ratio of placental weight to birthweight have raised blood pressure in adult life.[206]

Other studies in rats have shown that undernutrition in utero leads to lifelong elevation of blood pressure.[83] Female rats were given diets with differing protein content before mating and throughout pregnancy. Only mild protein deficiency was imposed. Normal feeding was restored after birth, and the offspring were allowed to develop normally. Those whose mothers had less protein during pregnancy persistently had raised blood pressure (Table 2.1). This was independent of the mothers' blood pressures which were not altered by the amount of protein in the diet.[207] In subsequent experiments it was shown that induction of hypertension by reduced maternal protein was abolished if fetal cortisol synthesis was inhibited.[208] This led to the hypothesis that maternal protein restriction programs lifelong changes in the fetus' hypothalamic–pituitary–adrenal axis, which in turn resets homeostatic mechanisms controlling blood pressure. Maternal protein restriction attenuates activity of 11-β-hydroxy-steroid dehydrogenase and an alternative explanation is that fetal blood pressure is altered through increased exposure to maternal glucocorticoids.[209, 210] A third possibility is that placental activity of the enzyme plays a crucial role in the development of the fetal adrenal and hence may determine patterns of glucocorticoid secretion throughout life.[85, 211]

Thyroid hormones

These hormones have an important role in cell differentiation, and may also be involved in matching fetal oxygen consumption to the oxygen supply. In newborn rats, changes in the serum concentrations of thyroid hormones may permanently change the sensitivity of the hypothalamic–pituitary axis to the hormone.[212-214] In this way the level of negative feedback between the hypothalamus and thyroid gland becomes reset. In the newborn baboon, thyroid homeostasis may likewise be reset by the thyroid hormones in the mother's milk.[166] In adult humans circulating levels of thyroxine and thyroid-stimulating hormone (TSH) are related to birthweight and infant feeding. (These findings are described in Chapter 5.) This suggests that thyroid function may be set during fetal growth and infant feeding.[215]

Sex hormones

Fifty years ago experiments in rats showed that in early life the hypophysis is plastic and able to differentiate as either male or female, depending on whether or not a testis is present.[216] Low concentrations of androgen during a sensitive perinatal phase imprint the hypothalamus so that gonadotrophin is secreted in cycles, the characteristic female pattern; high concentrations of androgens result in continuous 'tonic' secretion of gonadotrophin, the male pattern.[217] Manipulation of androgen or oestrogen concentrations during sensitive periods soon after birth changes sexual behaviour of males and females permanently, leading to reduced sexual drive and behaviour that is interpreted as homosexual.[218] In females it also changes sexual physiology, producing anovulatory sterility and polycystic ovaries.[5, 219] Remarkably, female rats may be masculinised in utero merely by the presence of male littermates sharing the same uterine horn, perhaps because masculinising hormones are carried from the males through the intrauterine vasculature.[220] Similarly female mice that were positioned in utero between two male fetuses are more aggressive and less sexually attractive to males than females that were positioned between two females.[219] A phenomenon similar to this intrauterine position effect is seen in twin lambs. The postnatal growth of the twin is influenced by the sex of its co-twin.[221] Males that had shared the uterus with a female grow more slowly than those who had shared it with another male. Similarly, among spotted hyenas females that shared a uterus with a male are more aggressive.

The effects of early exposure to androgens are not limited to sexual physiology, aggression and postnatal growth. Bjorntorp and colleagues have shown that a single dose of testosterone given to a newborn female rat leads to lifelong insulin resistance as well as other characteristics of women with a relative hyperandrogenicity, including centralisation of body fat and elevated lean body mass (Bjorntorp, personal communication). Testosterone is thought to induce insulin resistance by direct action on muscle cells.[222]

In sheep the sensitive period for androgen exposure is prenatal, rather than perinatal as in the rat. Single injections of androgens given to pregnant ewes have marked effects on the postnatal growth and body composition of the female offspring – effects which depend on the timing of the injection.[223]

IMMUNE SYSTEM

The thymus seems to be particularly sensitive to fetal and neonatal undernutrition. In the rat the size and DNA content of the thymus are permanently reduced by transient maternal undernutrition during pregnancy and early lactation.[8, 42, 224] Undernutrition also impairs development of thymic derived T lymphocytes and humoral immunity.[225–227] Reduced immune responses in animals can be produced by maternal protein-energy malnutrition[228, 229] or deficiency of specific nutrients such as iron and selenium.[224, 230] Undernutrition in one generation may affect immunity in the next two generations.[228]

In humans impaired fetal nutrition throughout gestation leads to growth-retarded babies who have low birthweight, global impairment of thymic development, and increased susceptibility to infection.[227, 231, 232] Undernutrition in late gestation may be associated with the diversion of blood and nutrients to the brain at the expense of the trunk.[233] In these babies, who tend to have disproportionately small body size at birth in relation to head size, the weight of the thymus may be severely reduced.[234, 235] In the post-term fetus there is a selective and marked wasting of the thymus.[236] A recent study has shown that middle-aged men and women who had disproportionately small body size at birth have persistently raised serum IgE concentrations.[53] It was suggested that this was due to an increase in the numbers of thymic derived TH-2 lymphocytes in relation to TH-1 lymphocytes, though this is speculative.

A recent study in the Gambia gives considerable impetus to the study of immune programming in humans.[237] There is seasonal famine in the Gambia. Men and women born in the 'hunger months' were found to have increased death rates, usually from infection, after the age of 15 years. This was attributed to reduced immune competence as a result of undernutrition in mid-gestation.

There is a considerable body of evidence which suggests that the method of infant feeding and the age at weaning influence the later occurrence of allergic disease:[227, 238–242] specifically, some studies have shown that breast feeding is associated with reduced occurrence of these diseases.[238, 243, 244] Studies in preterm infants have shown that breast milk reduces a range of allergic reactions, including eczema, but only in babies with a family history of atopy.[245]

References

1 Lucas A. Programming by early nutrition in man. In: Bock GR, Whelen J, eds. *The childhood environment and adult disease*. Chichester: John Wiley, 1991; 38–55.

2 Lucas A. Role of nutritional programming in determining adult morbidity. *Arch Dis Child* 1994; **71**: 288–290.

3 Diamond J. Pearl Harbor and the Emperor's physiologists. *Natural History* 1991; **12**: 2–7.

4 Stearns S. Evolution in health and disease. *Oxford University Press* 1998; (in press).

5 Barraclough CA. Production of anovulatory, sterile rats by single injections of testosterone propionate. *Endocrinology* 1961; **68**: 62–67.

6 Sonawane BR, Yaffe SJ. Drug exposure in utero: reproductive function in offspring. In: Kacew S, Lock S, eds. *Toxicologic and pharmacologic principles in pediatrics*. New York: Hemisphere, 1988; 41–65.

7 Yaffe SJ, Dorn LD. Effects of prenatal treatment with phenobarbital. *Dev Pharmacol Ther* 1990; **15**: 215–223.

8 Winick M, Noble A. Cellular response in rats during malnutrition at various ages. *J Nutr* 1966; **89**: 300–306.

9 Roeder LM, Chow BF. Influence of the dietary history of test animals on responses in pharmacological and nutritional studies. *Am J Clin Nutr* 1971; **24**: 947–951.

10 Osofsky HJ. Relationships between nutrition during pregnancy and subsequent infant and child development. *Obstet Gynecol Surv* 1975; **30**: 227–241.

11 Stephens DN. Growth and the development of dietary obesity in adulthood of rats which have been undernourished during development. *Br J Nutr* 1980; **44**: 215–227.

12 Hahn P. Effect of litter size on plasma cholesterol and insulin and some liver and adipose tissue enzymes in adult rodents. *J Nutr* 1984; **114**: 1231–1234.

13 Swenne I, Crace CJ, Milner RDG. Persistent impairment of insulin secretory response to glucose in adult rats after limited period of protein-calorie malnutrition early in life. *Diabetes* 1987; **36**: 454–458.

14 Hahn P. Late effects of early nutrition. In: Subbiah MTR, ed. *Atherosclerosis: a pediatric perspective*. Florida: CRC Press, 1989; 155–164.

15 Mott GE, Lewis DS, McGill HC. Programming of cholesterol metabolism by breast or formula feeding. In: Bock GR, Whelen J, eds. *The childhood environment and adult disease*. Chichester: John Wiley, 1991; 56–76.

16 Smart JL. Critical periods in brain development. In: Bock GR, Whelen J, eds. *The childhood environment and adult disease*. Chichester: John Wiley, 1991; 109–128.

17 Scott JP. Critical periods in behavioral development. Critical periods determine the direction of social, intellectual, and emotional development. *Science* 1962; **138**: 949–958.

18 Lorenz KZ. *King Solomon's ring. New light on animal ways*. London: Methuen, 1952.

19 Deeming DC, Ferguson MWJ. Physiological effects of incubation temperature on embryonic development in reptiles and birds. In: Deeming DC, Ferguson MWJ, eds. *Egg incubation: its effects on embryonic development in birds and reptiles*. Cambridge: Cambridge University Press, 1992; 147–171.

20 Gunn A, Gatehouse AG. The influence of larval phase on metabolic reserves, fecundity and life-span of the African army worm, *Spodoptera exempta* (Walker). *Bull Entomol Res* 1987; **77**: 6451–6660.

21 Widdowson EM, McCance RA. A review: new thoughts on growth. *Pediatr Res* 1975; **9**. 154–156.

22 Child CM. *Patterns and problems of development*. Chicago: Chicago University Press, 1941;

23 Tanner JM. *Foetus into man: physical growth from conception to maturity*. London: Open Books, 1978.

24 Widdowson EM. Intra-uterine growth retardation in the pig. *Biol Neonate* 1971; **19**: 329–340.

25 Milner RDG. Mechanisms of overgrowth. In: Sharp F, Fraser RB, Milner RDG, eds. *Fetal growth. Proceedings of the 20th study group of the Royal College of Obstetricians and Gynaecologists*. London: Royal College of Obstetricians and Gynaecologists, 1989; 139–148.

26 Hellerström C, Swenne I, Andersson A. Islet cell replication and diabetes. In: Lefebvre PJ, Pipeleers DG, eds. *The pathology of the endocrine pancreas in diabetes*. Heidelberg: Springer, 1988; 141–170.

27 Hinchliffe SA, Lynch MRJ, Sargent PH, Howard CV, Van Velzen D. The effect of intrauterine growth retardation on the development of renal nephrons. *Br J Obstet Gynaecol* 1992; **99**: 296–301.

28 Chow BF, Lee C-J. Effect of dietary restriction of pregnant rats on body weight gain of the offspring. *J Nutr* 1964; **82**: 10–18.

29 Dubos R, Savage D, Schaedler R. Biological Freudianism – lasting effects of early environmental influences. *Pediatrics* 1966; **38**: 789–800.

30 Winick M, Noble A. Cellular response with increased feeding in neonatal rats. *J Nutr* 1967; **91**: 179–182.

31 Blackwell B, Blackwell RQ, Yu TTS, Weng Y, Chow BF. Further studies on growth and feed utilization in progeny of underfed mother rats. *J Nutr* 1968; **97**: 79–84.

32 Zeman FJ, Stanbrough EC. Effect of maternal protein deficiency on cellular development in the fetal rat. *J Nutr* 1969; **99**: 274–282.

33 McLeod KI, Goldrick RB, Whyte HM. The effect of maternal malnutrition on the progeny in the rat: studies on growth, body composition and organ cellularity in first and second generation progeny. *Aust J Exp Biol Med Sci* 1972; **50**: 435–446.

34 Roeder LM. Effect of the level of nutrition on rates of cell proliferation and of RNA and protein syntheses in the rat. *Nutrition Reports International* 1973; **7**: 271–287.

35 Lemonnier D, Suquet J, Aubert R, Rosselin G. Long term effect of mouse neonate food intake on adult body composition, insulin and glucose serum levels. *Horm Metab Res* 1973; **5**: 223–224.

36 McCance RA, Widdowson EM. The determinants of growth and form. *Proc R Soc Lond B* 1974; **185**: 1–17.

37 Smart JL, Massey RF, Nash SC, Tonkiss J. Effects of early-life undernutrition in artificially reared rats: subsequent body and organ growth. *Br J Nutr* 1987; **58**: 245–255.

38 Widdowson EM, McCance RA. The effect of finite periods of undernutrition at different ages on the composition and subsequent development of the rat. *Proc Roy Soc Lond B* 1963; **158**: 329–342.

39 McCance RA, Widdowson EM. Nutrition and growth. *Proc Roy Soc Lond B* 1962; **156**: 326–337.

40 Wigglesworth JS. Experimental growth retardation in the foetal rat. *J Pathol Bacteriol* 1964; **88**: 1–13.

41 Roux JM, Tordet-Caridroit C, Chanez C. Studies on experimental hypotrophy in the rat. I. Chemical composition of the total body and some organs in the rat foetus. *Biol Neonate* 1970; **15**: 342–347.

42 Moment GB. The effects of rate of growth on the post-natal development of the white rat. *J Exp Zool* 1933; **65**: 359–393.

43 Harding J, Liu L, Evans P, Oliver M, Gluckman P. Intrauterine feeding of the growth retarded fetus: can we help? *Early Hum Dev* 1992; **29**: 193–197.

44 Xu KP, Yadar BR, King WA, Betteridge KJ. Sex related differences in developmental rates of bovine embryos and cultured in vivo. *Mol Reprod Dev* 1992; **31**: 249–252.

45 Garn SM, Burdi AR, Babler WJ. Male advancement in prenatal head development. *Am J Phys Anthropol* 1974; **41**: 353–359.

46 Pedersen JF. Ultrasound evidence of sexual difference in fetal size in first trimester. *Br Med J* 1980; **281**: 1253.

47 Clarke MF, Smith AH. Recovery following suppression of growth in the rat. *J Nutr* 1938; **15**: 245–256.

48 Brown SA, Rogers LK, Dunn JK, Gotto AM, Patsch W. Development of cholesterol homeostatic memory in the rat is influenced by maternal diets. *Metabolism* 1990; **39**: 468–473.

49 Winick M, Fish I, Rosso P. Cellular recovery in rat tissues after a brief period of neonatal malnutrition. *J Nutr* 1968; **95**: 623–626.

50 Pitts GC. Cellular aspects of growth and catch-up growth in the rat: A reevaluation. *Growth* 1986; **50**: 419–436.

51 Widdowson EM, Crabb DE, Milner RDG. Cellular development of some human organs before birth. *Arch Dis Child* 1972; **47**: 652–655.

52 Snoeck A, Remacle C, Reusens B, Hoet JJ. Effect of a low protein diet during pregnancy on the fetal rat endocrine pancreas. *Biol Neonate* 1990; **57**: 107–118.

53 Godfrey KM, Barker DJP, Osmond C. Disproportionate fetal growth and raised IgE concentration in adult life. *Clin Exp Allergy* 1994; **24**: 641–648.

54 Desai M, Crowther NJ, Ozanne SE, Lucas A, Hales CN. Adult glucose and lipid metabolism may be programmed during fetal life. *Biochem Soc Trans* 1995; **23**: 331–335.

55 Fowden AL. Endocrine regulation of fetal growth. *Reprod Fertil Dev* 1995; **7**: 351–363.

56 Nieto-Diaz A, Villar J, Matorras-Weinig R, Valenzuela-Ruiz P. Intrauterine growth

retardation at term: association between anthropometric and endocrine parameters. *Acta Obstet Gynecol Scand* 1996; **75**: 127–131.

57 Nagy SU, Csaba G. Dose dependence of the thyrotropin (TSH) receptor damaging effect of gonadotropin in the newborn rats. *Acta Phys Acad Scient Hung* 1980; **56**: 417–420.

58 Csaba G, Török O. Influence of insulin and biogenic amines on the division of Chang liver cells after primary exposure (imprinting) and repeated treatments. *Cytobios* 1991; **66**: 153–156.

59 Csaba G. Phylogeny and ontogeny of hormone receptors: the selection theory of receptor formation and hormonal imprinting. *Biol Rev* 1980; **55**: 47–63.

60 Gurney ME, Konishi M. Hormone-induced sexual differentiation of brain and behaviour in zebra finches. *Science* 1980; **208**: 1380–1382.

61 Deeming DC, Ferguson MWJ. The mechanism of temperature dependent sex determination in crocodilians: a hypothesis. *Am Zoologist* 1989; **29**: 973–985.

62 Kahn AJ. Embryogenic effect on post-natal changes in hemoglobin concentration with time. *Growth* 1968; **32**: 13–22.

63 McCay CM, Maynard LA, Sperling G, Barnes LL. Retarded growth, life span, ultimate body size and age changes in the albino rat after feeding diets restricted in calories. *J Nutr* 1939; **18**: 1–13.

64 Ross MH. Protein, calories and life expectancy. *Fed Proc* 1959; **18**: 1190–1207.

65 Berg BN, Simms HS. Nutrition and longevity in the rat. II. Longevity and onset of disease with different levels of food intake. *J Nutr* 1960; **71**: 255–263.

66 Comfort A. Nutrition and longevity in animals. *Proc Nutr Soc* 1960; **19**: 125–129.

67 Widdowson EM, McCance RA. Some effects of accelerating growth. I. General somatic development. *Proc Roy Soc Lond B* 1960; **152**: 188–206.

68 Ross MH. Aging, nutrition and hepatic enzyme activity patterns in the rat. *J Nutr* 1969; **97**: 565–601.

69 Yu BP. Aging and oxidative stress: modulation by dietary restriction. *Free Radical Biology and Medicine* 1996; **21**: 651–668.

70 Sohal RS, Weindruch R. Oxidative stress, caloric restriction, and aging. *Science* 1996; **273**: 59–63.

71 Hales CN, Desai M, Ozanne SE, Crowther NJ. Fishing in the stream of diabetes: from measuring insulin to the control of fetal organogenesis. *Biochem Soc Trans* 1996; **24**: 341–350.

72 Kirkwood TBL, Cremer T. Cytogerontology since 1881: a reappraisal of August Weismann and a review of modern progress. *Hum Genet* 1982; **60**: 101–121.

73 Davis RL, Hargen SM, Yeomans FM, Chow BF. Long term effects of alterations of maternal diet in mice. *Nutrition Reports International* 1973; **7**: 463–473.

74 El Habet A, Aust L, Noack R. The influence of postnatal nutrition on lipoprotein lipase activity and hormone sensitive lipolysis in vitro of rat adipose tissue. *Acta Biol Med Germ* 1979; **38**: 601–609.

75 Duff DA, Snell K. Effect of altered neonatal nutrition on the development of enzymes of lipid and carbohydrate metabolism in the rat. *J Nutr* 1982; **112**: 1057–1066.

76 Lewis DS, Bertrand HA, McMahan CA, McGill HC, Carey KD, Masoro EJ. Preweaning food intake influences the adiposity of young adult baboons. *J. Clin Invest* 1986; **78**: 899–905.

77 Davis RL, Hargen SM, Chow BF. The effect of maternal diet on the growth and metabolic patterns of progeny (mice). *Nutrition Reports International* 1972; **6**: 1–7.

78 Anguita RM, Sigulem DM, Sawaya AL. Intrauterine food restriction is associated with obesity in young rats. *J Nutr* 1993; **123**: 1421–1428.

79 Jones AP, Friedman MI. Obesity and adipocyte abnormalities in offspring of rats undernourished during pregnancy. *Science* 1982; **215**: 1518–1519.

80 Knittle JL, Hirsch J. Effect of early nutrition on the development of rat epididymal fat pads: cellularity and metabolism. *J. Clin Invest* 1968; **47**: 2091–2098.

81 Faust IM, Johnson PR, Stern JS, Hirsch J. Diet-induced adipocyte number increase in adult rats: a new model of obesity. *Am J Physiol* 1978; **235**: E279–E286.

82 Giussani DA, Spencer JAD, Hanson MA. Fetal cardiovascular reflex responses to hypoxaemia. *Fetal and Maternal Medicine Review* 1994; **6**: 17–37.

83 Langley SC, Jackson AA. Increased systolic blood pressure in adult rats induced by fetal exposure to maternal low protein diets. *Clin Sci* 1994; **86**: 217–222.

84 Woodall SM, Johnston BM, Breier BH, Gluckman PD. Chronic maternal undernutrition in the rat leads to delayed postnatal growth and elevated blood pressure of offspring. *Pediatr Res* 1996; **40**: 438–443.

85 Stewart PM, Rogerson FM, Mason JI. Type 2 11b-hydroxysteroid dehydrogenase messenger ribonucleic acid and activity in human placenta and fetal membranes: its relationship to birth weight and putative role in fetal adrenal steroidogenesis. *J Clin Endocrinol Metab* 1995; **80**: 885–890.

86 Langley-Evans S, Jackson A. Intrauterine programming of hypertension: nutrient–hormone interactions. *Nutr Rev* 1996; **54**: 163–169.

87 McCarty R, Lee JH. Maternal influences on adult blood pressure of SHRs: a single pup cross-fostering study. *Physiol Behav* 1996; **59**: 71–75.

88 McCarty R, Fields-Okotcha C. Timing of preweanling maternal effects on development of hypertension in SHR rats. *Physiol Behav* 1994; **55**: 839–844.

89 Di Nicolantionio R, Ikeda K, Yamori Y. Altered electrolyte and taurine levels in milk from nursing hypertensive rats. *Hypertens Res* 1993; **16**: 179–184.

90 Erkadius E, Di Iulio EJ, Lucente F, Bramich C, Morgan T, Di Nicolantonio R. Role of uterine factors in the development of hypertension in SHR. *Clin Exp Pharmacol Physiol* 1994; **21**: 239–242.

91 Langley-Evans SC, Clamp AG, Grimble RF, Jackson AA. Influence of dietary fats upon systolic blood pressure in the rat. *International Journal of Food Sciences and Nutrition* 1996; **47**: 417–425.

92 Persson E, Jansson T. Low birth weight is associated with elevated adult blood pressure in the chronically catheterized guinea-pig. *Acta Physiol Scand* 1992; **145**: 195–196.

93 Bolande RP, Leistikow EA, Wartmann FS, Louis TM. The effects of acute norepine-phrine-induced hypertension on the coronary arteries of newborn piglets. *Exp Mol Pathol* 1995; **63**: 87–100.

94 Winick M, Rosso P, Brasel JA. Malnutrition and cellular growth in the brain: existence of critical periods. In: [Anonymous]. *Lipids, malnutrition and the developing brain*. New York: Associated Scientific Publishers, 1972; 199–212.

95 Davies PA, Stewart AL. Low-birth-weight infants: neurological sequelae and later intelligence. *Br Med Bull* 1975; **31**: 85–91.

96 Katz HB. The influence of undernutrition on learning performance in rodents. *Nutr Abstr Rev A* 1980; **50**: 767–784.

97 Patel AJ, Balazs R, Smith RM, Kingsbury AE, Hunt A. Thyroid hormone and brain development. In: Di Benedetta C, ed. *Multidisciplinary approach to brain development*. Amsterdam: Elsevier, 1980; 261–277.

98 Davison AN, Dobbing J. Myelination as a vulnerable period in brain development. *Br Med Bull* 1966; **22**: 40–44.

99 Smart JL. Early life malnutrition and later learning ability. A critical analysis. In: Oliverio A, ed. *Genetics, environment and intelligence*. Elsevier, 1977; 215–235.

100 Boothe RG, Dobson V, Teller DY. Postnatal development of vision in human and non-human primates. *Annu Rev Neurosci* 1985; **8**: 495–545.

101 Blakemore C. Sensitive and vulnerable periods in the development of the visual system. In: Bock GR, Whelen J, eds. *The childhood environment and adult disease*. Chichester: John Wiley, 1991; 129–154.

102 Lucas A, Morley R, Cole TJ, Gore SM, Lucas PJ, Crowle P, et al. Early diet in preterm babies and developmental status at 18 months. *Lancet* 1990; **335**: 1477–1481.

103 Lucas A. Influence of neonatal nutrition on long-term outcome. In: Salle BL, Swyer PR, eds. *Nutrition of the low birthweight infant. Nestle Nutrition Workshop Series*. New York: Raven Press, 1993; **32**: 183–196.

104 Gibson RA. Early fatty acid supply and mental development. In: Boulton J, Laron Z, Rey J, eds. *Long-term consequences of early feeding*. Philadelphia: Lippincott-Raven, 1996.

105 Goswami T, Vu ML, Srivastava U. Quantitative changes in DNA, RNA and protein content of the various organs of the young of undernourished female rats. *J Nutr* 1974; **104**: 1257–1264.

106 Bassi JA, Rosso P, Moessinger AC, Blanc WA, James LS. Fetal growth retardation due to maternal tobacco smoke exposure in the rat. *Pediatr Res* 1984; **18**: 127–130.

107 Collins MH, Moessinger AC, Kleinerman J, Bassi J, Rosso P, Collins AM, et al. Fetal lung hypoplasia associated with maternal smoking: a morphometric analysis. *Pediatr Res* 1985; **19**: 408–412.

108 Lechner AJ, Winston DC, Bauman JE. Lung mechanics, cellularity, and surfactant after prenatal starvation in guinea pigs. *J Appl Physiol* 1986; **60**: 1610–1614.

109 Faridy EE, Sanii MR, Thliveris JA. Fetal lung growth: influence of maternal hypoxia and hyperoxia in rats. *Respir Physiol* 1988; **73**: 225–242.

110 O'Dell BL, Kilburn KH, McKenzie WN, Thurston RJ. The lung of the copper-deficient rat. *Am J Pathol* 1978; **91**: 413–432.

111 Das RM. The effects of intermittent starvation on lung development in suckling rats. *Am J Pathol* 1984; **117**: 326–332.

112 Sahebjami H, MacGee J. Effects of starvation on lung mechanics and biochemistry in young and old rats. *J Appl Physiol* 1985; **58**: 778–784.

113 Kalenga M, Eeckhout Y. Effects of protein deprivation from the neonatal period on lung collagen and elastin in the rat. *Pediatr Res* 1989; **26**: 125–127.

114 Matsui R, Thurlbeck WM, Fujita Y, Yu SY, Kida K. Connective tissue, mechanical, and morphometric changes in the lungs of weanling rats fed a low protein diet. *Pediatr Pulmonol* 1989; **7**: 159–166.

115 Lechner AJ, Banchero N. Advanced pulmonary development in newborn guinea pigs (*Cavia porcellus*). *Am J Anat* 1982; **163**: 235–246.

116 Lechner AJ. Perinatal age determines the severity of retarded lung development induced by starvation. *Am Rev Respir Dis* 1985; **131**: 638–643.

117 Gaultier C. Malnutrition and lung growth. *Pediatr Pulmonol* 1991; **10**: 278–286.

118 Winick M, Noble A. Quantitative changes in DNA, RNA, and protein during prenatal and postnatal growth in the rat. *Dev Biol* 1965; **12**: 451–456.

119 Burri PH, Dbaly J, Weibel ER. The postnatal growth of the rat lung. I. Morphometry. *Anat Rec* 1974; **178**: 711–730.

120 Kitterman JA. Fetal lung development. *J Dev Physiol* 1984; **6**: 67–82.

121 Moessinger AC, Bassi GA, Ballantyne G, Collins MH, James LS, Blanc WA. Experimental production of pulmonary hypoplasia following amniocentesis and oligohydramnios. *Early Hum Dev* 1983; **8**: 343–350.

122 Nakayama DK, Glick PL, Harrison MR, Villa RL, Noall R. Experimental pulmonary hypoplasia due to oligohydramnios and its reversal by relieving thoracic compression. *J Pediatr Surg* 1983; **18**: 347–353.

123 Higuchi M, Kato T, Yoshino H, Matsuda K, Gotoh K, Hirano H et al. The influence of experimentally produced oligohydramnios on lung growth and pulmonary surfactant content in fetal rabbits. *Dev Physiol* 1991; **16**: 223–227.

124 Moessinger AC, Harding R, Adamson TM, Singh M, Kiu GT. Role of lung fluid volume in growth and maturation of the fetal sheep lung. *J Clin Invest* 1990; **86**: 1270–1277.

125 Fisk NM, Parkes MJ, Moore PJ, Haidar A, Wigglesworth J, Hanson MA. Fetal breathing during chronic lung liquid loss leading to pulmonary hypoplasia. *Early Hum Dev* 1991; **27**: 53–63.

126 Wigglesworth JS, Desai R. Is fetal respiratory function a major determinant of perinatal survival? *Lancet* 1982; **i**: 264–267.

127 Wigglesworth JS, Desai R, Guerrini P. Fetal lung hypoplasia: biochemical and structural variations and their possible significance. *Arch Dis Child* 1981; **56**: 606–615.

128 Nimrod C, Varela-Gittings F, Machin G, Campbell D, Wesenberg R. The effect of very prolonged membrane rupture on fetal development. *Am J Obstet Gynecol* 1984; **148**: 540–543.

129 Roberts AB, Mitchell JM. Direct ultrasonographic measurements of fetal lung length in normal pregnancies and pregnancies complicated by prolonged rupture of membranes. *Am J Obstet Gynecol* 1990; **163**: 1560–1566.

130 Hislop A, Reid L. Persistent hypoplasia of the lung after repair of congenital diaphragmatic hernia. *Thorax* 1976; **31**: 450–455.

131 Helms P, Stocks J. Lung function in infants with congenital pulmonary hypoplasia. *J Pediatr* 1982; **101**: 918–922.

132 Thurlbeck WM. Prematurity and the developing lung. *Clinical Perinatology* 1992; **19**: 497–519.

133 Davies G, Reid L. Effect of scoliosis on growth of alveoli and pulmonary arteries and on right ventricle. *Arch Dis Child* 1971; **46**: 623–632.

134 Owage-Iraka JW, Harrison A, Warner JO. Lung function in congenital and idiopathic scoliosis. *Eur J Pediatr* 1984; **142**: 198–200.

135 Bucher U, Reid L. Development of the intrasegmental bronchial tree: the pattern of branching and development of cartilage at various stages of intra-uterine life. *Thorax* 1961; **16**: 207–218.

136 Kikkawa Y, Fujita I, Sindhu RK. Neonatal hyperoxia and cytochrome P450 imprinting in adulthood. *Pediatr Res* 1994; **35**: 255–258.

137 Van Assche FA, Aerts L. The fetal endocrine pancreas. *Contrib Gynecol Obstet* 1979; **5**: 44–57.

138 Weinkove C, Weinkove EA, Pimstone BL. Insulin release and pancreatic islet volume in malnourished rats. *S Afr Med J* 1974; **118**: 1888.

139 Berney DM, Desai M, Palmer DJ, Greenwald S, Brown A, Hales CN, et al. The effects of maternal protein deprivation on the fetal rat pancreas: major structural changes and their recuperation. *J Pathol* 1997; **183**: 109–115.

140 Zeman FJ. Effects of maternal protein restriction on the kidney of the newborn young of rats. *J Nutr* 1968; **94**: 111–116.

141 Merlet-Benichou C, Leroy B, Gilbert T, Lelievre-Pegorier M. Retard de croissance intra-utérin et déficit en néphrons (Intrauterine growth retardation and inborn nephron deficit). *Médecine/Sciences* 1993; **9**: 777–780.

142 Osathanondh V, Potter EL. Development of human kidney as shown by microdissection. III. Formation and interrelationship of collecting tubules and nephrons. *Arch Pathol* 1963; **76**: 290–302.

143 Brenner BM, Chertow GM. Congenital oligonephropathy and the etiology of adult hypertension and progressive renal injury. *Am J Kidney Dis* 1994; **23**: 171–175.

144 Shrader RE, Zeman FJ. Effect of maternal protein deprivation on morphological and enzymatic development of neonatal rat tissue. *J Nutr* 1969; **99**: 401–412.

145 Wess L, Eastwood M, Busuttil A, Edwards C, Miller A. An association between maternal diet and colonic diverticulosis in an animal model. *Gut* 1996; **39**: 423–427.

146 Xu RJ, Mellor DJ, Birtles MJ, Reynolds GW, Simpson HV. Impact of intrauterine growth retardation on the gastrointestinal tract and the pancreas in newborn pigs. *J Pediatr Gastroenterol Nutr* 1994; **18**: 231–240.

147 Williams SP, Durbin GM, Morgan MEI, Booth IW. Catch up growth and pancreatic function in growth retarded neonates. *Arch Dis Child* 1995; **73**: F158–F161.

148 Innis SM. The role of diet during development on the regulation of adult cholesterol homeostasis. *Can J Physiol Pharmacol* 1985; **63**: 557–564.

149 Reiser R, Sidelman Z. Control of serum cholesterol homeostasis by cholesterol in the milk of the suckling rat. *J Nutr* 1972; **102**: 1009–1016.

150 Reiser R, Henderson GR, O'Brien BC. Persistence of dietary suppression of 3-hydroxy-3-methylglutaryl coenzyme-A reductase during development in rats. *J Nutr* 1977; **107**: 1131–1138.

151 Kris-Etherton PM, Layman DK, York PV, Frantz ID. The influence of early nutrition on the serum cholesterol of the adult rat. *J Nutr* 1979; **109**: 1244–1257.

152 Li JR, Bale LK, Kottke BA. Effect of neonatal modulation of cholesterol homeostasis on subsequent response to cholesterol challenge in adult guinea pig. *J Clin Invest* 1980; **65**: 1060–1068.

153 Green MH, Dohner EL, Green JB. Influence of dietary fat and cholesterol on milk lipids and on cholesterol metabolism in the rat. *J Nutr* 1981; **111**: 276–286.

154 Wong WW. Early feeding and regulation of cholesterol metabolism. In: Boulton J, Laron Z, Rey J, eds. *Long-term consequences of early feeding. Nestle Nutrition Workshop Series 36*. Philadelphia: Lippincott-Raven, 1996; 123–131.

155 Innis SM. Influence of maternal cholestyramine treatment on cholesterol and bile acid metabolism in adult offspring. *J Nutr* 1983; **113**: 2464–2470.

156 Little MTE, Hahn P. Diet and metabolic development. *FASEB J* 1990; **4**: 2605–2611.

157 Hassan AS, Yunker RL, Subbiah MTR. Decreased bile acid pool in neonates of guinea pigs fed cholesterol during pregnancy. *J Nutr* 1981; **111**: 2030–2033.

158 Hassan AS, Gallon LS, Yunker RL, Subbiah MTR. Effect of enhancement of cholesterol catabolism in guinea pigs after weaning on subsequent response to dietary cholesterol. *Am J Clin Nutr* 1982; **35**: 546–550.

159 O'Brien BC, McMurray DN, Reiser R. The influence of premature weaning and the

nature of the fat in the diet during development on adult plasma lipids and adipose cellularity in pair-fed rats. *J Nutr* 1983; **113**: 602–609.

160 Angel JF, Back DW. Weaning and metabolic regulation in the rat. *Can J Physiol Pharmacol* 1985; **63**: 538–545.

161 Hahn P. Obesity and atherosclerosis as consequences of early weaning. In: Ballabriga A, Rey J, eds. *Weaning: why, what, and when?* New York: Vevey/Raven Press, 1987; 93–109.

162 Hahn P, Kirby L. Immediate and late effects of premature weaning and of feeding a high fat or high carbohydrate diet to weanling rats. *J Nutr* 1973; **103**: 690–696.

163 Villalon L, Tuchweber B, Yousef IM. Low protein diets potentiate lithocholic acid-induced cholestasis in rats. *J Nutr* 1992; **122**: 1587–1596.

164 Mott GE, Jackson EM, McMahan CA, McGill HC. Cholesterol metabolism in adult baboons is influenced by infant diet. *J Nutr* 1990; **120**: 243–251.

165 Mott GE, Lewis DS, McGill HC. Deferred effects of preweaning nutrition on lipid metabolism. *Ann N Y Acad Sci* 1991; **6**: 70–80.

166 Lewis DS, McMahan CA, Mott GE. Breast feeding and formula feeding affect differently plasma thyroid hormone concentrations in infant baboons. *Biol Neonate* 1993; **63**: 327–335.

167 Hahn HB, Spiekerman AM, Otto WR, Hossalla DE. Thyroid function tests in neonates fed human milk. *Am J Dis Child* 1983; **137**: 220–222.

168 Franklin R, O'Grady C, Carpenter L. Neonatal thyroid function: comparison between breast-fed and bottle-fed infants. *J Pediatr* 1985; **106**: 124–126.

169 Oberkotter LV, Periera GR, Paul MH, Ling H, Sasanow S, Farber M. Effect of breast-feeding vs formula feeding on circulating thyroxine levels in premature infants. *J Pediatr* 1985; **106**: 822–825.

170 Fomon SJ, Bartels DJ. Concentrations of cholesterol in serum of infants in relation to diet. *Am Med Assoc J Dis Child* 1960; **99**: 43–45.

171 Darmady JM, Fosbrooke AS, Lloyd JK. Prospective study of serum cholestrol levels during first year of life. *Br Med J* 1972; **ii**: 685–688.

172 Andersen GE, Lifschitz C, Friis-Hansen B. Dietary habits and serum lipids during first four years of life. *Acta Paediatr Scand* 1979; **68**: 165–170.

173 Van Biervliet JP, Rosseneu M, Caster H. Influence of dietary factors on the plasma lipoprotein composition and content of neonates. *Eur J Pediatr* 1986; **144**: 489–493.

174 Labarthe DR, Eissa M, Varas C. Childhood precursors of high blood pressure and elevated cholesterol. *Annu Rev Public Health* 1991; **12**: 519–541.

175 Sporik R, Johnstone JH, Cogswell JJ. Longitudinal study of cholesterol values in 68 children from birth to 11 years of age. *Arch Dis Child* 1991; **66**: 134–137.

176 Chow BF, Blackwell RQ, Blackwell BN, Hou TY, Anilane JK, Sherwin RW. Maternal nutrition and metabolism of the offspring: studies in rats and man. *Am J Public Health* 1968; **58**: 668–677.

177 Hsueh AM, Blackwell RQ, Chow BF. Effect of maternal diet in rats on feed consumption of the offspring. *J Nutr* 1970; **100**: 1157–1164.

178 Lee CJ, Chow BF. Protein metabolism in the offspring of underfed mother rats. *J Nutr* 1965; **87**: 439–443.

179 Fowden AL. The role of insulin in prenatal growth. *J Dev Physiol* 1989; **12**: 173–182.

180 Fowden AL. Pancreatic endocrinology, function and carbohydrate metabolism in the fetus. In: Albrecht E, Pepe GJ, eds. *Perinatal endocrinology, Vol. IV, Research in perinatal medicine.* 1985; 71–90.

181 Dahri S, Snoeck A, Reusens-Billen B, Remacle C, Hoet JJ. Islet function in offspring of mothers on low-protein diet during gestation. *Diabetes* 1991; **40 (suppl 2)**: 115–120.

182 Van Assche FA, Aerts L. Long-term effect of diabetes and pregnancy in the rat. *Diabetes* 1985; **34**: 116–118.

183 Oh W, Gelardi NL, Cha CJM. The cross-generation effect of neonatal macrosomia in rat pups of streptozotocin-induced diabetes. *Pediatr Res* 1991; **29**: 606–610.

184 Vadlamudi S, Kalhan SC, Patel MS. Persistence of metabolic consequences in the progeny of rats fed a HC formula in their early postnatal life. *Am J Physiol* 1995; **269**: E731–E738.

185 Laychock SG, Vadlamudi S, Patel MS. Neonatal rat dietary carbohydrate affects pancreatic islet insulin secretion in adults and progeny. *Am J Physiol* 1995; **269**: E739–E744.

186 Pollard I, Smallshaw J. Male mediated caffeine effects over two generations of rats. *J Dev Physiol* 1988; **10**: 271–281.

187 Gluckman PD, Gunn AJ, Wray A, Cutfield WS, Chatelin PG, Guilbaud O, et al. Congenital idiopathic growth hormone deficiency associated with prenatal and early postnatal growth failure. *J Pediatr* 1992; **121**: 920–923.

188 Stephan JK, Chow B, Frohman LA, Chow BF. Relationship of growth hormone to the growth retardation associated with maternal dietary restriction. *J Nutr* 1971; **101**: 1453–1458.

189 Zeman FJ, Shrader RE, Allen LH. Persistent effects of maternal protein deficiency in postnatal rats. *Nutrition Reports International* 1973; **7**: 421–436.

190 Harel Z, Tannenbaum GS. Long-term alterations in growth hormone and insulin secretion after temporary dietary protein restriction in early life in the rat. *Pediatr Res* 1995; **38**: 747–753.

191 Bassett NS, Oliver MH, Breier BH, Gluckman PD. The effect of maternal starvation on plasma insulin-like growth factor 1 concentrations in the late gestation ovine fetus. *Pediatr Res* 1990; **27**: 401–404.

192 Oliver MH, Harding JE, Breier BH, Evans PC, Gluckman PD. Glucose but not a mixed amino acid infusion regulates plasma insulin-like growth factor-1 concentrations in fetal sheep. *Pediatr Res* 1993; **34**: 62–65.

193 Owens JA. Endocrine and substrate control of fetal growth: placental and maternal influences and insulin-like growth factors. *Reprod Fertil Dev* 1991; **3**: 501–517.

194 Furuhashi N, Fukaya T, Kono H, Shinkawa O, Tachibana Y, Takahashi T, et al. Cord serum growth hormone in the human fetus. Sex difference and a negative correlation with birth weight. *Gynecol Obstet Invest* 1983; **16**: 119–124.

195 Thieriot-Prevost G, Boccara JF, Francoual C, Badoual J, Job JC. Serum insulin-like growth factor 1 and serum growth-promoting activity during the first postnatal year in infants with intrauterine growth retardation. *Pediatr Res* 1988; **24**: 380–383.

196 Deiber M, Chatelain P, Naville D, Putet G, Salle B. Functional hypersomatotropism in small for gestational age (SGA) newborn infants. *J Clin Endocrinol Metab* 1989; **68**: 232–234.

197 de Zegher F, Kimpen J, Raus J, Vanderschueren-Lodeweyckx M. Hypersomatotropism in the dysmature infant at term and preterm birth. *Biol Neonate* 1990; **58**: 188–191.

198 Leger J, Noel M, Limal JM, Czernichow P. Growth factors and intrauterine growth retardation II. Serum growth hormone, insulin-like growth factor (IGF) 1, and IGF-binding protein 3 levels in children with intrauterine growth retardation compared with normal control subjects: prospective study from birth to two years of age. *Pediatr Res* 1996; **40**: 101–107.

199 Hirano T, Chin I, Miyamoto Y, Jogamoto M, Ishikawa E. Cross-sectional assessments of growth hormone concentrations in normal neonates in the first week of life. *Acta Paediatr Scand* 1989; **356**: 126.

200 Fall CHD, Pandit AN, Law CM, Yajnik CS, Clark PM, Breier B, et al. Size at birth and plasma insulin-like growth factor-1 concentrations. *Arch Dis Child* 1995; **73**: 287–293.

201 Fall C, Hindmarsh P, Dennison E, Kellingray S, Barker DJP, Cooper C. Programming of growth hormone secretion and bone mineral density in elderly men: an hypothesis. *Clin Endocrinol Metab* 1998; (in press).

202 Silver M. Prenatal maturation, the timing of birth and how it may be regulated in domestic animals. *Exp Physiol* 1990; **75**: 285–307.

203 Edwards CRW, Benediktsson R, Lindsay RS, Seckl JR. Dysfunction of placental glucocorticoid barrier: link between fetal environment and adult hypertension? *Lancet* 1993; **341**: 355–357.

204 Dodic M, May CN, Wintour EM, Coghlan JP. An early prenatal exposure to excess glucocorticoid leads to hypertensive offspring in sheep. *Clin Sci* 1998; (in press).

205 Seckl JR. Glucocorticoids and small babies. *Q J Med* 1994; **87**: 259–262.

206 Barker DJP, Bull AR, Osmond C, Simmonds SJ. Fetal and placental size and risk of hypertension in adult life. *Br Med J* 1990; **301**: 259–262.

207 Langley-Evans SC, Phillips GJ, Jackson AA. In utero exposure to maternal low protein diets induces hypertension in weanling rats, independently of maternal blood pressure changes. *Clin Nutr* 1994; **13**: 319–324.

208 Langley-Evans SC, Phillips GJ, Gardner DS, Jackson AA. Role of glucocorticoids in programming of maternal diet-induced hypertension in the rat. *J Nutr Biochem* 1996; **7**: 173–178.

209 Langley-Evans SC, Phillips GJ, Benediktsson R, Gardner DS, Edwards CRW, Jackson AA, et al. Protein intake in pregnancy, placental glucocorticoid metabolism and the programming of hypertension in the rat. *Placenta* 1996; **17**: 169–172.

210 Langley-Evans SC. Maternal carbenoxolone treatment lowers birthweight and induces hypertension in the offspring of rats fed a protein-replete diet. *Clin Sci* 1997; **93**: 423–429.

211 Langley-Evans SC, Gardner DS, Jackson AA. Maternal protein restriction influences the programming of the rat hypothalamic-pituitary-adrenal axis. *J Nutr* 1996; **126**: 1578–1585.

212 Besa ME, Pascual-Leone AM. Effect of neonatal hyperthyroidism upon the regulation of TSH secretion in rats. *Acta Endocrinol* 1984; **105**: 31–39.

213 Walker P, Courtin F. Transient neonatal hyperthyroidism results in hypothyroidism in the adult rat. *Endocrinology* 1985; **116**: 2246–2250.

214 Pracyk JB, Seidler FJ, McCook EC, Slotkin TA. Pituitary-thyroid axis reactivity to hyper- and hypothyroidism in the perinatal period: ontogeny of regulation of regulation and long-term programming of responses. *J Dev Physiol* 1992; **18**: 105–109.

215 Phillips DIW, Barker DJP, Osmond C. Infant feeding, fetal growth and adult thyroid function. *Acta Endocrinol* 1993; **129**: 134–138.

216 Pfeiffer CA. Sexual differences of the hypophyses and their determination by the gonads. *Am J Anat* 1936; **58**: 195–225.

217 Barraclough CA, Gorski RA. Evidence that the hypothalamus is responsible for androgen-induced sterility in the female rat. *Endocrinology* 1961; **68**: 68–79.

218 Dörner G. Environment-dependent brain differentiation and fundamental processes of life. *Acta Biol Med Germ* 1974; **33**: 129–148.

219 vom Saal FS, Bronson FH. Sexual characteristics of adult female mice are correlated with their blood testosterone levels during prenatal development. *Science* 1980; **208**: 597–599.

220 Meisel RL, Ward IL. Fetal female rats are masculinized by male littermates located caudally in the uterus. *Science* 1981; **213**: 239–242.

221 Gill JW, Holst PJ, Hosking BJ, Egan AR. The intrauterine environment of twin lambs predetermines their growth characteristics. *Proceedings of the Nutrition Society of Australia* 1995; **19**: 135–138.

222 Holmang A, Larsson BM, Brzezinska Z, Bjorntorp P. Effects of short term testosterone exposure on insulin sensitivity of muscles in female rats. *Am J Physiol* 1992; **262**: E851–E855.

223 Gill JW, Hosking BJ. Acute prenatal androgen treatment increases birth weights and growth rates in lambs. *J Anim Sci* 1995; **73**: 2600–2608.

224 Kochanowski BA, Sherman AR. Decreased antibody formation in iron-deficient rat pups – effect of iron repletion. *Am J Clin Nutr* 1985; **41**: 278–284.

225 Jarrett E, Hall E. Selective suppression of IgE antibody responsiveness by maternal influence. *Nature* 1979; **280**: 145–147.

226 Kochanowski BA, Sherman AR. Cellular growth in iron-deficient rats: effect of pre- and postweaning iron repletion. *J Nutr* 1985; **115**: 279–287.

227 Chandra RK. Interactions between early nutrition and the immune system. In: Bock GR, Whelen J, eds. *The childhood environment and adult disease*. Chichester: John Wiley, 1991; 77–92.

228 Chandra RK. Antibody formation in first and second generation offspring of nutritionally deprived rats. *Science* 1975; **190**: 289–290.

229 Srivastava US, Thakur ML, Majumdar PK, Bhatnagar GM, Supakar PC. Lymphoid organ mRNA translatability in rats: effect of protein energy undernutrition in early life. *J Nutr* 1987; **117**: 242–246.

230 Mulhern SA, Taylor GL, Magruder LE, Vessey AR. Deficient levels of dietary selenium suppress the antibody response in first and second generation mice. *Nutr Res* 1985; **5**: 201–210.

231 Chandra RK. Fetal malnutrition and postnatal immunocompetence. *Am J Dis Child* 1975; **129**: 450–454.

232 Moscatelli P, Bricarelli FD, Piccinini A, Tomatis C, Dufour MA. Defective immunocompetence in foetal undernutrition. *Helv Paediatr Acta* 1976; **31**: 241–247.

233 Rudolph AM. The fetal circulation and its response to stress. *J Dev Physiol* 1984; **6**: 11–19.

234 Pauerstein CJ. *Clinical obstetrics*. New York: John Wiley, 1987.

235 Owens JA, Owens PC, Robinson JS. Experimental fetal growth retardation: metabolic and endocrine aspects. In: Gluckman PD, Johnston BM, Nathanielsz PW, eds. *Advances in fetal physiology*. Ithaca, New York: Perinatology Press, 1989; 263–286.

236 Gruenwald P. Pathology of the deprived fetus and its supply line. In: Elliott K, Knight J, eds. *Size at birth. Ciba Foundation Symposium No. 27*. Amsterdam: Elsevier, 1974; 3–19.

237 Moore SE, Cole TJ, Poskitt EME, Sonko BJ, Whitehead RG, McGregor IA, et al. Season of birth predicts mortality in rural Gambia. *Nature* 1997; **388**: 434

238 Kramer MS, Moroz B. Do breast-feeding and delayed introduction of solid foods protect against subsequent atopic eczema? *J Pediatr* 1981; **98**: 546–550.

239 Miskelly FG, Burr ML, Vaughan-Williams E, Fehily AM, Butland BK, Merrett TG. Infant feeding and allergy. *Arch Dis Child* 1988; **63**: 388–393.

240 Chandra RK. Long-term health implications of mode of infant feeding. *Nutr Res* 1989; **9**: 1–3.

241 Chandra RK, Singh G, Shridhara B. Effect of feeding whey hydrolysate, soy and conventional cow milk formulas on incidence of atopic disease in high risk infants. *Ann Allergy* 1989; **63**: 102–106.

242 Chandra RK. Long-term health consequences of early infant feeding. In: Atkinson SA, Hanson LA, Chandra RK, eds. *Breastfeeding, nutrition, infection and infant growth in developed and emerging countries*. St Johns, Newfoundland: ARTS Biomedical Publishers, 1990; 47–53.

243 Chandra RK, Puri S, Cheema PS. Predictive value of cord blood IgE in the development of atopic disease and role of breast feeding in its prevention. *Clin Allergy* 1985; **15**: 517–522.

244 Kramer MS. Does breast feeding help protect against atopic disease? Biology, methodology, and a golden jubilee of controversy. *J Pediatr* 1988; **112**: 181–190.

245 Lucas A, Brooke OG, Morley R, Cole TJ, Bamford MF. Early diet of preterm infants and development of allergic or atopic disease: randomised prospective study. *Br Med J* 1990; **300**: 837–840.

From birth to death

MARGARET BURNSIDE'S LEDGERS

To examine the hypothesis that coronary heart disease and stroke are programmed in utero has required novel epidemiological studies, since evidence
from geography and time trends can only be suggestive. To advance the
hypothesis by epidemiological methods it is necessary to use size at birth as a
marker of fetal nutrition and relate it, in groups of men and women, to the
occurrence of cardiovascular disease in later life.

Staff from the Medical Research Council (MRC) searched archives and hospital record departments throughout Britain, looking for maternity and infant
welfare records from the early years of the century. Many were found. Some
were in large collections preserved over many years; in some there were no
more than a few hundred records kept by one clinic or even one midwife. Some
were detailed and some perfunctory. Some were in archives; others were in
lofts, sheds, garages, boiler rooms, or flooded basements. The largest set of
records were those made by health visitors in the county of Hertfordshire.

In Britain, in the early years of the century, there was widespread concern
about the apparent physical deterioration of the British people. The birth rate
was declining. One in 10 babies died before they were a year old and many of
those who survived reached adult life in poor health. During 1902, reports in
the national press claimed that up to two-thirds of the young men who volun-
teered to fight in the South African war had been rejected because of unsatis-
factory physique.[1] An interdepartmental committee set up in 1903 drew a
shocking picture of the nation's children – malnourished, poorly housed,
deprived. The Medical Officer of Health for Hertfordshire, writing at around
this time, stated:

Hertfordshire does less than forty out of the fifty-five counties to perpetuate the national
stock; for England and Wales the birth-rate has for thirty-three years been steadily
declining, only two Continental countries (Belgium and France) having lower birth-rates
in 1909, while that for Japan is increasing and is now ahead of every white race but
Russia and three of the Balkan States. The new census figures show a lower rate of
increase than in any decennium of the last century. This decay must betoken the doom
of modern civilisation as it did that of Rome and Greece, unless some new moral or

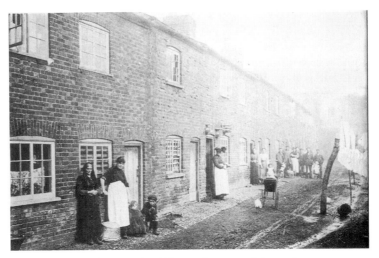

Fig. 3.1 Mothers in Hitchin, Hertfordshire at the turn of the century.

physical factor arise to defeat it. [He added] it is of national importance that the life of every infant be vigorously conserved.

Miss Ethel Margaret Burnside, the county's first ever 'Chief Health Visitor and Lady Inspector of Midwives' set up an 'army' of trained nurses to attend women in childbirth and to advise mothers on how to keep their babies healthy. From 1911 onwards when women in Hertfordshire, like those shown in Figure 3.1, had their babies, they were attended by a midwife. She recorded the birthweight and notified the birth to the county medical officer of health. The local health visitor was informed. She went to the baby's home at intervals throughout infancy and recorded its illnesses and development on a card. When the baby was 1 year old the visits ceased; the card was handed in to the county health visitor and the details carefully transferred into ledgers. Figure 3.2 shows details from one of the ledgers, with birthweight, weight at 1 year,

Weight at Birth.	Weight 1st Year.	Food.	No. of Visits.	Condition, and Remarks of Health Visitor.			
				W	r	D	T
8¼ lbs	24½ lbs	B.	11	4	-	-	4
Healthy & well developed.				Buckland School. Card to S.c			
7 lbs	18¾ lbs	B	12	h.	4.	4.	8
moved to Bury Green. L? Hadham.				Had measles, pneumonia & u			
8	20	Bot.	11	Y.	Y.	?	4
T.8. abcess in of neck opened. Ant. fontanelle still open @ 3 yrs. Abdomen very large & prom							
8½	22	B.B.	9	y	y	y	10
Healthy & normal.				Buckland School. Card .			

Fig. 3.2 Details from one of Miss Burnside's ledgers in 1917.

whether the baby was weaned at 1 year, number of teeth, and other details. From 1923 onwards the health visitors continued their visits until the child was 5 years old. Records of these visits were also entered in the ledgers. The ledgers were maintained until 1945, many years after Miss Burnside had retired. In 1986, the MRC found that those which covered the eastern part of the county had been sent to the County Record Office. Over the next 2 years those for other areas of the county came to light, preserved in local hospitals.

Surprisingly little is known about Margaret Burnside (1877–1953), whose foresight and dedication have given us the Hertfordshire records. The only known photograph of her (Figure 3.3) was taken when she was 17 years old. She was born in 1877, one of six children. Her father was rector of Hertingfordbury, a village near Hertford. After training as a nurse at St George's Hospital, London, she became Lady Inspector of Midwives for Hertfordshire in 1905. We know that she worked energetically; 'The cyclometer of my bicycle registered 2,921 miles for the year [1907]', she reported. In 1910 she was made a Queen's Nurse and the county nursing association recorded its 'high appreciation' of her 'unremitting labours'. The following year she was appointed as County Health Visitor, following the Notification of Births Act in 1907 which required such an appointment. In 1913 she persuaded the County Council to buy her a car. It was 9.5 horsepower and she called it 'little hero'.

She is remembered as a reserved but formidable woman. The Clerk to the County Council would make himself immediately available if he knew Miss Burnside was in the building and wished to see him. In 1919 she moved to London, to the newly formed Ministry of Health. Systematic observations of the growth and health of each baby born in Hertfordshire continued for another 25 years.

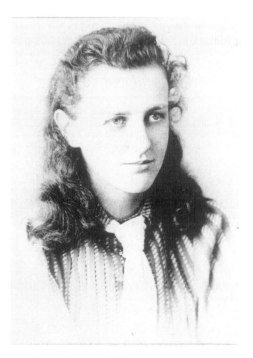

Fig. 3.3 Ethel Margaret Burnside aged 17 years.

LOW BIRTHWEIGHT AND INFANT WEIGHT AND CARDIOVASCULAR DISEASE

The Hertfordshire records made it possible, for the first time, to relate people's early growth, feeding, and illness to their health in later life. The National Health Service Central Register at Southport was used to trace 16 000 men and women born in the county from 1911 to 1930. Tracing required both the fore-name and surname, and where forenames of the Hertfordshire babies were not recorded they were found through the national index of births or local bap-tismal registers. In Britain women are more difficult to trace than men because of their change of name at marriage, and it proved impossible to trace most women born before 1923, many of whom married before the Central Register became fully operational. The study was therefore based on 10 141 men born during 1911–30 and a younger cohort of 5585 women born during 1923–30.[2, 3] Of these people 2990 men and 875 of the women had died at ages from 20 to 74 years.

Hertfordshire is in the south of England and the death rates from coronary heart disease were below the national average, the standardised mortality ratios being 79 in men and 64 in women. In men 35% of all deaths were due to coronary heart disease and Table 3.1 shows that standardised mortality ratios for both coronary heart disease and stroke fell with increasing birthweight. There were stronger and highly statistically significant trends with weight at 1 year. These did not depend on the way the infants were fed. The trends in car-diovascular disease with birthweight and weight at 1 year were reflected in falls in all-causes mortality (Table 3.1). They were specific: there were no cor-responding trends in deaths from non-cardiovascular causes.

Only 14% of the deaths among women were due to coronary heart dis-ease and, because of the smaller numbers of women, there were too few deaths

Table 3.1 Standardised mortality ratios (SMR) among 10 141 men born in Hertfordshire according to birthweight and weight at 1 year

	Cause of death, SMR		
Weight pounds (kg)	Coronary heart disease	Stroke	All causes
At birth			
≤5.5 (2.5)	110 (63)	67 (6)	99 (163)
–6.5 (2.9)	88 (147)	97 (25)	81 (390)
–7.5 (3.4)	82 (311)	85 (50)	82 (895)
–8.5 (3.9)	78 (321)	64 (41)	78 (920)
–9.5 (4.3)	62 (124)	68 (22)	71 (413)
>9.5 (4.3)	70 (67)	52 (8)	76 (209)
1 year old			
≤18 (8.2)	108 (80)	100 (12)	92 (196)
–20 (9.1)	87 (190)	89 (31)	91 (573)
–22 (10.0)	88 (369)	87 (57)	84 (1012)
–24 (10.9)	70 (251)	53 (30)	70 (724)
–26 (11.8)	64 (113)	61 (17)	74 (371)
>26 (11.8)	47 (30)	49 (5)	62 (114)
All	79 (1033)	74 (152)	79 (2990)

Figures in parentheses are numbers of deaths.

Table 3.2 Standardised mortality ratios among 5585 women born in Hertfordshire according to birthweight and weight at 1 year

| Weight pounds (kg) | Cause of death, SMR | |
	Coronary heart disease	All causes
At birthweight		
≤5.5 (2.5)	72 (7)	102 (58)
–6.5 (2.9)	84 (30)	81 (167)
–7.5 (3.4)	62 (40)	83 (311)
–8.5 (3.9)	61 (32)	76 (228)
–9.5 (4.3)	47 (9)	80 (87)
>9.5 (4.3)	36 (2)	75 (24)
1 year old		
≤18 (8.2)	91 (19)	101 (120)
–20 (9.1)	54 (27)	79 (227)
–22 (10.0)	69 (44)	73 (270)
–24 (10.9)	54 (20)	82 (175)
–26 (11.8)	64 (8)	91 (64)
>26 (11.8)	57 (2)	96 (19)
All	64 (120)	81 (875)

Figures in parentheses are numbers of deaths.

from stroke for useful analysis. Table 3.2 shows that as in men deaths from coronary heart disease fell with increasing birthweight and this was reflected in a similar trend in all-causes mortality. There were however, no trends with weight at 1 year.

Figures 3.4 and 3.5 illustrate these trends. They show premature deaths, that is deaths below the age of 65 years, from coronary heart disease in men and women. Standardised mortality ratios fell between people who had low birthweight and those who weighed 9.5 pounds (4.3 kg). Above this birthweight there was a small increase in both men and women. The trends with weight at

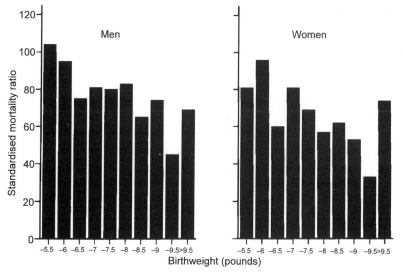

Fig. 3.4 Standardised mortality ratios for coronary heart disease below the age of 65 according to birthweight.

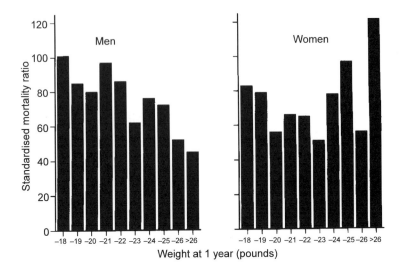

Fig. 3.5 Standardised mortality ratios for coronary heart disease below the age of 65 according to weight at 1 year.

1 year were different in the two sexes, the large fall in disease rates between men with low and high weights at 1 year contrasting with the absence of any trend in women. Among men the highest rates of coronary heart disease were in those who had below average birthweight and remained small in infancy – that is, their growth failed to catch up. Among women the highest rates were in those who had below average birthweight. Studies of men who still live in Hertfordshire have shown that failure of infant weight gain, with a low weight at 1 year, is followed by persisting short stature. While weight at 1 year is closely correlated to adult height, it is only weakly linked to adult body mass (weight/height^2), which is an index of obesity.

Birthweight and weight at 1 year are related, although not as strongly as is sometimes suggested (the correlation coefficient was 0.36 in Hertfordshire). Their combined effect on death rates from coronary heart disease in men is shown in Figure 3.6, which was derived using Cox's proportional hazards method.[4] The lines join points that have an equal risk of coronary heart disease, and the values are the risks relative to the value of 100 for those with average birthweight and weight at 1 year of age. Clearly the combination of poor prenatal and postnatal growth leads to the highest death rates from coronary heart disease. Few men with low birthweight attained the heavier weights at 1 year of age, and hence the lowest risks of coronary heart disease.

A study of deaths from coronary heart disease and stroke among 3108 men born in the Jessop Hospital, Sheffield, England, which is described on page 50, confirmed that mortality from coronary heart disease and stroke fell between those with the lowest and highest birthweights.[5] Confirmation that low birthweight is associated with coronary heart disease and stroke in women has come from the large study of 121 000 American female nurses who were recruited into a postal questionnaire study of health and lifestyle in 1976.[6,7] In 1992 they were asked to ascertain their birthweights and 70 000 were able to do so. Figure 3.7 shows that the relative risk of non-fatal coronary heart disease and stroke

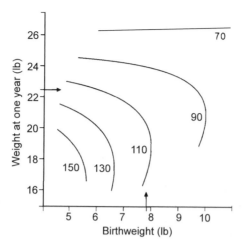

Fig. 3.6 Relative risks for coronary heart disease in men according to birthweight and weight at 1 year. Lines join points with equal risk. Arrows indicate mean weights.

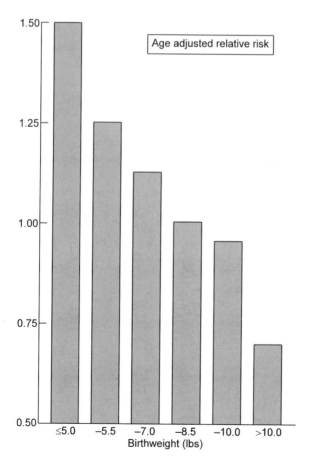

Fig. 3.7 Relative risk of non-fatal coronary heart disease and stroke according to birthweight in the American nurses study.

fell across the range of birthweight. Hypertension, non-insulin-dependent diabetes and raised serum cholesterol concentrations, which were self-reported, showed similar trends but the trends in cardiovascular disease were largely independent of these. A study among 1200 men in Caerphilly, Wales, also showed that those who had had high birthweight had lower rates of fatal and non-fatal coronary heart disease.[8] Again this association was independent of conventional coronary risk factors. Among 1300 men in Uppsala, Sweden, low birthweight was related to death from both coronary heart disease and stroke.[9]

BODY PROPORTIONS AT BIRTH AND CARDIOVASCULAR DISEASE

The Hertfordshire records and the American nurses and Caerphilly studies did not include measurements of body size at birth other than weight. The weight of a newborn baby without a measure of its length is as crude a summary of its physique as is the weight of a child or adult without a measure of height.[10] The addition of birth length allows the long thin baby to be distinguished from the short fat baby. With the addition of head circumference the baby whose body is small or stunted in relation to its head, as a result of 'sparing' of brain growth, can also be distinguished. Thinness, stunting and a small trunk reflect differing fetal adaptations to undernutrition and other influences and they have different long term consequences.

The first study linking body proportions at birth and later death rates from coronary heart disease, was carried out on a group of men and women born in the Jessop Hospital, Sheffield.[11] Since 1907 this hospital has kept unusually detailed records on each newborn baby. The baby was not only weighed but its length from crown to heel, head circumference, biparietal and other head diameters, and placental weight were recorded. Chest and abdominal circumference were later added to this list of measurements. Figure 3.8 shows one of the records from the hospital. Not only was the baby measured in detail, but external measurements of the mother's pelvis were recorded, including the conjugate diameter, that is, the distance between the symphysis pubis and the fifth lumbar vertebra, and the intercristal diameter, that is, the distance between the iliac crests. The reason why such astonishingly detailed observations were made on each baby in this and other hospitals in Europe is not known.

Stunting and thinness at birth

In Sheffield death rates for coronary heart disease were higher in men who were stunted or thin at birth.[5] The mortality ratio for coronary heart disease in men who were 18.5 inches (47 cm) or less in length was 138 compared with 98 in the remainder.[5] A study of men and women in South India (p. 58) showed a similar association with short body length at birth. In Sheffield thinness at birth, as measured by a low ponderal index (birthweight/length³), was also associated with coronary heart disease. Table 3.3 shows that among 3300 men born in Helsinki, Finland during 1924–33, death rates for coronary heart disease were

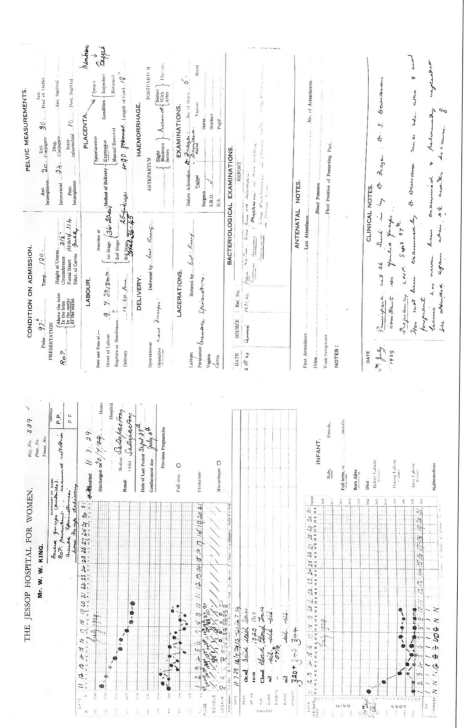

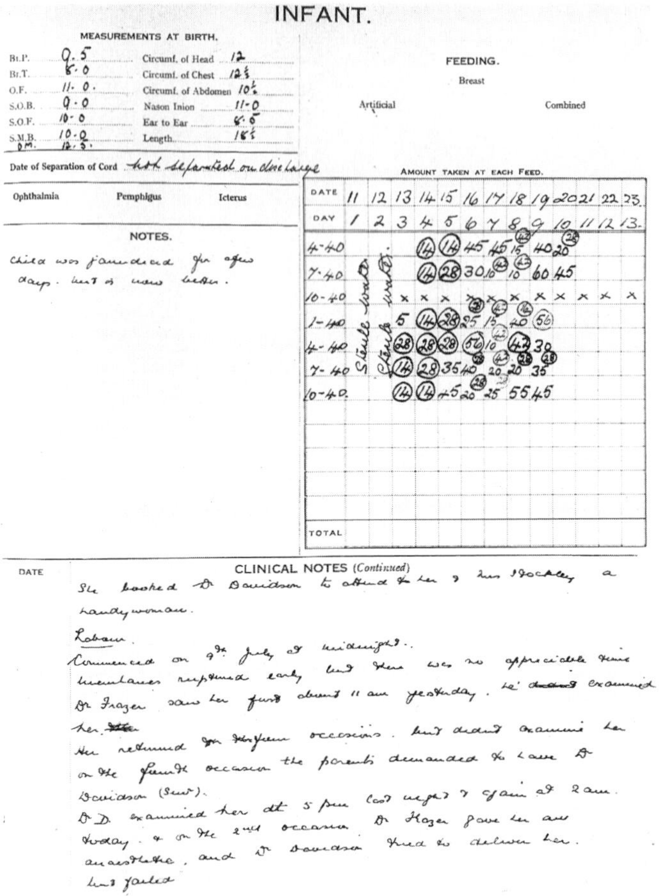
INFANT.

MEASUREMENTS AT BIRTH.

Bi.P.	9.5	Circumf. of Head	12
Bi.T.	8.0	Circumf. of Chest	12½
O.F.	11.0	Circumf. of Abdomen	10½
S.O.B.	9.0	Nason Inion	11.0
S.O.F.	10.0	Ear to Ear	6.5
S.M.B.	10.0	Length	18½
O.M.	12.5		

FEEDING. Breast Artificial Combined

Date of Separation of Cord

Ophthalmia Pemphigus Icterus

AMOUNT TAKEN AT EACH FEED.

DATE 11 12 13 14 15 16 17 18 19 20 21 22 23

DAY 1 2 3 4 5 6 7 8 9 10 11 12 13

TOTAL

NOTES.

Child was jaundiced for a few days. but is now better.

DATE CLINICAL NOTES (Continued)

Fig. 3.8 Detailed birth records kept at the Jessop Hospital, Sheffield, from 1907 onwards.

only weakly related to low birthweight,[12] but were strongly associated with thinness at birth, measured by a low ponderal index, especially in men born at term. Men who were thin at birth had death rates that were twice those of men who had a high ponderal index at birth.

A thesis of this book, which is developed in later chapters, is that babies who are thin at birth were undernourished.[13, 14] Among the consequences of this are persisting elevation of blood pressure (Chapter 4), disturbance of glucose/insulin metabolism (Chapter 6) and death from coronary heart disease. Figure 3.9 shows such a baby. Babies who are stunted at birth, and have a reduced abdominal circumference, were also undernourished.[14] Among the consequences of stunting are persisting elevation of blood pressure (Chapter 4) and disturbances of liver function with altered cholesterol metabolism and blood clotting (Chapter 5). Figure 3.10 shows such a baby. It is disproportionately short in relation to the size of its head. It also has a low birthweight in relation to its head size. These body proportions suggest that there was interruption of growth of the trunk in late gestation with relative 'sparing' of brain growth. Evidence that both thinness at birth and a low birthweight in relation

Table 3.3 Standardised mortality ratios for coronary heart disease in 3302 Finnish men

	SMR	*p* value for trend
Birthweight, kg (lb)		
≤2.5 (5.5)	84 (11)	
–3.0 (6.6)	83 (44)	
–3.5 (7.7)	99 (124)	
–4.0 (8.8)	76 (80)	
>4.0 (8.8)	66 (27)	
All	85 (286)	0.09
Term babies only: ponderal index at birth, kg/m³		
≤25	116 (59)	
–27	105 (88)	
–29	72 (64)	
>29	56 (33)	
All	86 (244)	<0.0001

Figures in parentheses are numbers of deaths

to head circumference are associated with undernutrition comes from the Dutch study of people exposed to war-time famine when they were in utero.[15] Those exposed in mid or late gestation tended to be either thin at birth or had low birthweight in relation to head circumference (Table 8.1)

The pattern of infant growth which follows reduced intrauterine growth differs according to the body proportions at birth.[16–19] Thin babies tend to catch up in weight during infancy whereas short and proportionately small babies do

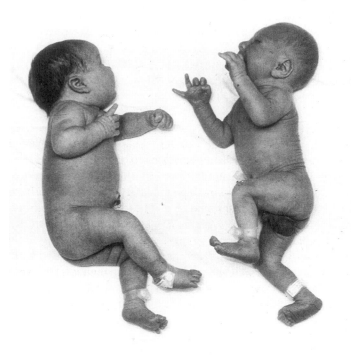

Fig. 3.9 The newborn baby on the right is thinner and has a smaller head circumference than the other baby.

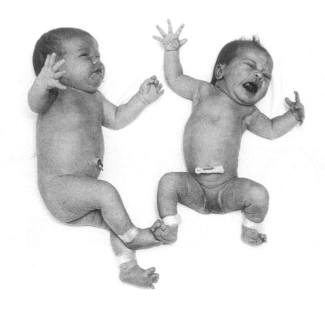

Fig. 3.10 The newborn baby on the right has a similar head circumference to the other baby but is shorter and has a smaller abdominal circumference.

not. Among men in Hertfordshire the stronger relationship of coronary heart disease to weight at 1 year than to birthweight is thought to reflect an association with shortness at birth and consequent failure of infant growth. Catch-up growth of growth-retarded babies seems to depend on two phenomena: first, the rate of catch-up during the first months of postnatal life, which is higher in industrialised than developing countries, and second, the occurrence of growth-faltering between 6 and 18 months of age, which is widespread in developing countries.[20]

Head circumference at birth

Head circumference at birth is strongly related to birthweight, and in Sheffield coronary heart disease showed similar trends with head circumference as with birthweight (Table 3.4). Standardised mortality ratios fell progressively between the men with the smallest and largest head circumferences. In Helsinki the trends were similar, though weaker. The trends in stroke, which have only been reported in Sheffield were different. There were no trends with head circumference (Table 3.4). When, however, head circumference and birthweight were analysed together, stroke was found to occur in men who had a low ratio of birthweight tó head circumference.

Length of gestation

The data from Sheffield, Uppsala and Helsinki include the length of gestation in weeks, estimated from the date of the mother's last menstrual period.[5, 9, 12] The issue of whether the associations between coronary heart disease and small

Table 3.4 Standardised mortality ratios (SMR) among men born in Sheffield, according to head circumference at birth

Head circumference inches (cm)	Cause of death, SMR		
	Coronary heart disease	Stroke	Non-cardiovascular causes
≤13 (33.0)	116 (98)	104 (15)	84 (107)
–14 (35.6)	104 (126)	89 (21)	102 (190)
14 (35.6)	90 (119)	143 (34)	106 (212)
>14 (35.6)	88 (83)	90 (16)	107 (152)
All	99 (426)	108 (86)	101 (661)

Figures in parenthesis are numbers of deaths

size at birth reflect slow intrauterine growth or premature birth can therefore be resolved. The associations of coronary heart disease with low birthweight, thinness and stunting were independent of the length of gestation and strongest in term babies. This shows that the disease is associated with low rates of fetal growth. In Sheffield, however, the disease showed a U-shaped variation with length of gestation, the highest SMRs being in men born at 37 weeks of gestation or less and in men born after 41 weeks. In Helsinki there was similarly a raised death rate in men born after term. Stroke seems unrelated to the length of gestation, though the smaller numbers of deaths makes this conclusion less secure.[5]

Placental size

In Finland raised death rates for coronary heart disease were associated with low placental weight, which in turn was strongly associated with thinness at birth. In Sheffield, however, coronary heart disease did not vary with placental weight but showed a U-shaped relation with the ratio of placental weight to birthweight, the highest mortality ratios being at either end of the distribution. The pattern of body proportions at birth which predicts death from coronary heart disease may be therefore summarised as a small head circumference, stunting or thinness, which reflect retarded fetal growth, and either low placental weight or an altered ratio of placental weight to birthweight.

The pattern for stroke is different. In Sheffield death rates for stroke were highest in men who had low placental weight at birth, particularly if the placenta was light in relation to the size of the head.[5] The standardised mortality ratio for stroke in men whose placental weight was 1.25 pounds (560 g) or less and whose head circumference was 14 inches (35.6 cm) or more was twice that in men whose placental weight was more than 1.25 pounds (560 g) and head circumference less than 14 inches (35.6 cm). The pattern of body proportions at birth which predicts death from stroke is therefore low birthweight and low placental weight in relation to normal head size at birth. One interpretation is that normal head growth, which occurs relatively early in gestation, has been followed by interrupted growth of the body in late gestation in association with inadequate growth of the placenta.

These findings suggest that influences linked to early growth have an important effect on the risk of coronary heart disease and stroke. It has been argued, however, that people whose growth was impaired in utero and during infancy may continue to be exposed to an adverse environment in childhood and adult life, and it is this later environment that produces the effects attributed to programming.[21-24] The findings in this chapter, and in later chapters, which describe the links between early growth and cardiovascular risk factors such as blood pressure, provide strong evidence that this argument cannot be sustained.

In three of the studies which have replicated the association between birthweight and coronary heart disease data on lifestyle factors, including smoking, employment, alcohol consumption and exercise were collected. In the nurses health study allowance for these factors had little effect on the association between birthweight and coronary heart disease.[6] Similar results came from the Caerphilly and Uppsala studies.[8, 9] Lifestyle factors also did not explain the association between low weight at 1 year and the prevalence of coronary heart disease in a sample of Hertfordshire men who were examined clinically.[25] The association was found within each social class and in both smokers and non-smokers. In the British Regional Heart Study of middle-aged men, low socioeconomic status during childhood increased the risk of coronary heart disease independently of socioeconomic status during adult life, though such data cannot distinguish prenatal and postnatal influences.[26] Finally in a study in South India, described on p. 58, associations between short body length at birth and prevalent coronary heart disease were independent of socioeconomic status and smoking habits.[27]

In studies of blood pressure (see Ch. 4), plasma fibrinogen and serum cholesterol concentrations (see Ch. 5), and non-insulin-dependent diabetes (see Ch. 6) the associations with size at birth are again independent of social class as an adult, cigarette smoking and alcohol consumption. Adult lifestyle, however, adds to the effects of early life. For example, the prevalence of impaired glucose tolerance is highest in people who had low birthweight but become obese as adults (Table 6.3).

The associations between small size at birth and cardiovascular disease are specific, strong and graded. They are specific in that non-cardiovascular disease is mostly unrelated to small size at birth, though chronic airways obstruction is one important exception to this. The associations are strong despite body weight being only a proxy for the changes in the body's structure, physiology, and metabolism which have been programmed in utero. Yet the relative risks associated with low birthweight are large: for example, the risk of the insulin resistance syndrome (non-insulin-dependent diabetes, hypertension, and hyperlipidaemia) is 10 times higher among men whose birthweight was 6.5 lb or less ($\leq$ 2.9 kg) than among men whose birthweight was more than 9.5 lb (> 4.3 kg).

It is reasonable to conclude that reduced growth in utero and cardiovascular disease are causally linked. This conclusion is greatly strengthened by recent animal and clinical studies which are beginning to reveal the cellular and molecular mechanisms that underlie programming.

The associations between low birthweight and cardiovascular disease raise two questions about the possible effects of the biological and social environment in childhood. First, does birthweight serve as a 'highly sensitive marker of family socioeconomic circumstances' and is it therefore a predictor of influences acting in early childhood rather than in utero which determine later susceptibility to coronary heart disease?[24-28] Second, do growth, nutrition and development in childhood modify risks established in utero?

The answer to the first question seems reasonably clear. Birthweight is not a sensitive marker of the conditions in which the mother is living and into which the baby will be born. Chapter 8 describes how the nutrition of the fetus reflects the nutrition of the mother throughout her life, including her own fetal life, and not simply what happens to her during pregnancy. Even famine during pregnancy has little effect on birthweight. Although in industrial Britain in the past poorer families had smaller babies, this did not apply in rural counties like Hertfordshire. Chapter 10 describes how the low neonatal mortality of babies born in London at the beginning of this century was consistent with the good nutritional state of the mothers, many of whom grew up in the home counties, but quite at variance with the wretched conditions under which many of them lived during pregnancy. Furthermore studies of today's children show that associations between size at birth and blood pressure and glucose tolerance (Chs 4 and 6) are not determined by the child's socio-economic circumstances after birth. Animal experiments (Ch. 2) strongly support the conclusion that undernutrition before birth has persisting effects irrespective of the living conditions of the animals after birth.

Given that events in utero have persisting effects on the structure and function of the body, are these effects modified by experiences in childhood? The evidence from animals is that they can be, though not in ways that are readily predictable. Rats undernourished in utero but fed normally after birth have much shorter lives than those undernourished throughout life (p. 21). Findings in the Helsinki study, described in Chapter 11, are similar in that men who were thin at birth but became overweight in childhood were at greatly increased risk of coronary heart disease. It is clear from the Hertfordshire study that failure of growth in infancy strongly predicts later coronary heart disease in men (Fig. 3.5). This does not result from the way the men were fed during infancy nor from their exposure to infections.[3] Rather it is thought to reflect prenatal 'settings' of hormones, including growth hormone, which control fetal growth.[14] A similar issue arises in interpreting the association between reduced leg length in childhood and later coronary heart disease, a finding based on follow-up of children who took part in the Carnegie survey of family diet and health in Britain before the Second World War.[29] Does this reflect the consequences of poor living conditions in childhood or is it the result of prenatal settings of growth hormone and the other hormones that regulate the childhood phase of growth?

Preliminary studies of adults, in which information on childhood socioeconomic conditions was obtained retrospectively, have given varying results. Among 2636 men in Finland childhood socioeconomic conditions were not related to cardiovascular mortality.[30] In the nurses study in the USA women from 'blue collar' backgrounds had a small increase in risk of death from cardiovascular disease, their relative risk being 1.13 compared with women from 'white collar' backgrounds.[31] At present we do not know whether and how a child's health, housing, family life and schooling influence its risk of later cardiovascular disease but studies now in progress in several countries should help to resolve this.

Meanwhile it is important that the debate remains open. It is ominous that Susser, in the preface to a new book on life course epidemiology writes:

But it [intrauterine programming] cannot by itself account for much of many adult disorders and, even less, for cardiovascular disease. Too much can already be attributed to other factors that accumulate over the life course . . .[32]

Is the old orthodoxy being replaced by a new one, even before the necessary research has been carried out?

INTERACTION BETWEEN FETAL GROWTH AND OBESITY IN ADULT LIFE?

In the Caerphilly study the increased risk of coronary heart disease was restricted to men who had a high body mass index.[8] The authors suggested that disease risk was therefore defined by the combination of poor growth in utero and an affluent environment in later life. An obvious objection to this is that birthweight, unaccompanied by other measures of body size at birth, or placental size, or length of gestation or infant growth is an inadequate index of fetal growth from which to draw such a conclusion. Furthermore the findings in Wales do not match those from other studies, in which small size at birth was related to coronary heart disease at all levels of body mass index.[25, 27] Chapter 6 demonstrates how the effects of low birthweight on adult onset diabetes are compounded by adult obesity; but also points out that the extent to which adult obesity is entrained by events in early life is unknown.

CORONARY HEART DISEASE AND FETAL GROWTH IN INDIA

It is a common objection to the fetal origins hypothesis that intrauterine growth retardation is common in many developing countries whereas coronary heart disease is rare.[21] An answer to this may lie in the different nature of fetal growth retardation in developing countries. This is discussed further in Chapter 11. Meanwhile studies in India have addressed the question of whether the hypothesis can contribute to an understanding of the rising epidemic of coronary heart disease in developing countries. Death rates from the disease are rising steeply in India and are expected to overtake those due to infectious disease by the year 2010.[33, 34] Already, cardiovascular deaths account for half the deaths occurring under 70 years. These high rates of coronary heart disease in India are not explained by known risk factors including obesity, raised blood pressure, smoking and raised cholesterol. Coronary heart disease in Indian populations is, however, associated with a particular metabolic profile that is known to be unfavourable. This includes impaired glucose tolerance or non-insulin-dependent diabetes, insulin resistance, raised serum triglyceride concentrations, low concentrations of high density lipoprotein cholesterol, abnormal plasma clotting factors and central obesity.[35] Coronary heart disease in India has other particular characteristics. It is more common in urban areas and among lower socioeconomic groups,[36, 37] and rates in women are similar to those in men, even though women in many parts of India do not smoke.

When people from India migrate to other countries they take their high rates of coronary heart disease with them. Indeed, the rates rise still further.[38] These observations raise the possibility that Indian people have a genetically determined susceptibility to coronary heart disease which is enhanced on exposure to a sedentary lifestyle, high energy intake and other aspects of westernisation.[39-41] The genes responsible for this have not been identified, but it is hypothesised that they conferred a survival advantage to Indian people in past times when food supplies were unreliable and physical work was demanding. The implications of this speculation are that Indian people will continue to have high rates of coronary heart disease unless they return to a more primitive way of life.[42] This conflicts, however, with experience elsewhere in the world, where epidemics of coronary heart disease have been followed by declining rates[43] which, though perhaps assisted by health education, are largely unexplained.

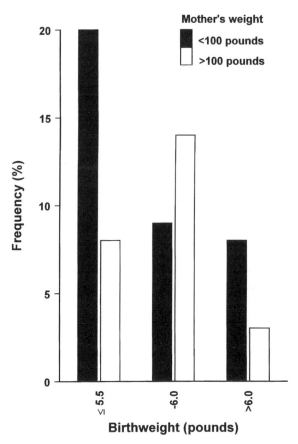

Fig. 3.11 Frequency of coronary heart disease according to mother's weight in pregnancy and birthweight in India.

The possibility that the associations between poor fetal growth and adult disease may have important implications for the epidemic of both coronary heart disease and non-insulin-dependent diabetes in India has not gone unremarked.[39] Fetal growth is known to be retarded throughout the country. The average birthweight is less than 6 pounds (2.7 kg). Until recently, however there has been no firm evidence. A recent study in South India has shown however, that, as in other countries, low birthweight and coronary heart disease are linked.[27] A total of 517 men and women who were born during 1934–53 in the Mary Calvert Holdsworth Hospital, Mysore, were traced. The occurrence of coronary heart disease and its biological risk factors was related to birthweight and body proportions at birth, which were recorded at the time. Among men and women aged 45 years and over, the prevalence of coronary heart disease fell from 15% in those who weighed 5.5 pounds (2.5 kg) or less at birth to 4% in those who weighed 7.0 pounds (3.2 kg) or more. Rates of the disease were also higher in men and women who were stunted at birth, and whose mothers had low weight in pregnancy. Figure 3.11 shows that the highest rates were in people who had low birthweight and whose mothers were thin. The average birthweight and maternal weight were both low by European standards though consistent with values from other parts of India (mean birthweight 6.2 pounds (2.8 kg), and mean maternal weight in pregnancy 103 pounds (47 kg)). Clearly these early findings in India need to be replicated and extended. Meanwhile the association between low maternal weight and coronary heart disease is further evidence that the fetal growth failure which leads to coronary heart disease is a consequence of fetal undernutrition.

CONSTRAINT OF GROWTH IN UTERO

The findings described in this chapter show that the relationship between fetal growth and cardiovascular disease is continuous. Rates of the disease fall across the range of birthweights and ponderal index and, in men, across the range of weight at 1 year. If the criteria for successful fetal growth are to include adult health and longevity, these findings reinforce the view that babies with significant intrauterine growth retardation need not necessarily be 'light for gestational age' as defined clinically.[44] Intrauterine growth retardation seems to be widespread, affecting many babies whose birthweights are within the normal range, not just those few who are recognised clinically by their unusually small size and high risk of perinatal complications and death.

The associations between cardiovascular disease and fetal growth are not adequately summarised by associations with birthweight, which is a crude summary of fetal experience. The associations with small head circumference, shortness and thinness described here suggests that coronary heart disease originates in particular patterns of altered fetal growth resulting from undernutrition at particular stages of gestation.

References

1 Acheson ED. Tenth Boyd Orr Memorial Lecture. Food policy, nutrition and government. *Proc Nutr Soc* 1986; **45**: 131–138.

Summary

In men and women small size at birth is associated with raised death rates from cardiovascular disease in later life. These associations do not depend on length of gestation and therefore reflect low rates of fetal growth. Coronary heart disease is not only associated with low birthweight but with thinness and stunting at birth, and with a small head circumference, which result from reduced fetal growth at particular stages of gestation. Stroke is associated with low birthweight and placental weight in relation to head size and may originate in restriction of placental growth. In India, where there is a rising epidemic of coronary heart disease, the disease is similarly associated with low birthweight and short body length at birth. Cardiovascular disease in men, but not women, is strongly associated with failure of weight gain in infancy, which may be a consequence of reduced linear growth in late gestation. The associations between body size in early life and later cardiovascular disease cannot be explained by confounding variables. They are strong and statistically robust and support the conclusion that cardiovascular disease originates in utero.

2 Barker DJP, Osmond C, Winter PD, Margetts B, Simmonds SJ. Weight in infancy and death from ischaemic heart disease. *Lancet* 1989; **2**: 577–580.

3 Osmond C, Barker DJP, Winter PD, Fall CHD, Simmonds SJ. Early growth and death from cardiovascular disease in women. *Br Med J* 1993; **307**: 1519–1524.

4 Cox DR. Regression models and life-tables. *J R Stat Soc Ser B* 1972; **34**: 187–220.

5 Martyn CN, Barker DJP, Osmond C. Mothers' pelvic size, fetal growth, and death from stroke and coronary heart disease in men in the UK. *Lancet* 1996; **348**: 1264–1268.

6 Rich-Edwards JW, Stampfer MJ, Manson JE, Rosner B, Hankinson SE, Colditz GA, et al. Birth weight and risk of cardiovascular disease in a cohort of women followed up since 1976. *Br Med J* 1997; **315**: 396–400.

7 Curhan GC, Chertow GM, Willett WC, Spiegelman D, Colditz GA, Manson JE, et al. Birth weight and adult hypertension and obesity in women. *Circulation* 1996; **94**: 1310–1315.

8 Frankel S, Elwood P, Sweetnam P, Yarnell J, Davey Smith G. Birthweight, body-mass index in middle age, and incident coronary heart disease. *Lancet* 1996; **348**: 1478–1480.

9 Koupilova I, Leon DA. Birthweight and mortality from ischaemic heart disease and stroke in Swedish men aged 50–74 years. *J Epidemiol Community Health* 1996; **50**: 592 (Abstract).

10 Beatie RB, Johnson P. Practical assessment of neonatal nutrition status beyond birthweight: an imperative for the 1990s. *Br J Obstet Gynaecol* 1994; **101**: 842–846.

11 Barker DJP, Osmond C, Simmonds SJ, Wield GA. The relation of small head circumference and thinness at birth to death from cardiovascular disease in adult life. *Br Med J* 1993; **306**: 422–426.

12 Forsen T, Eriksson JG, Tuomilehto J, Teramo K, Osmond C, Barker DJP. Mother's weight in pregnancy and coronary heart disease in a cohort of Finnish men: follow up study. *Br Med J* 1997; **315**: 837–840.

13 Robinson SM, Wheeler T, Hayes MC, Barker DJP, Osmond C. Fetal heart rate and intrauterine growth. *Br J Obstet Gynaecol* 1991; **98**: 1223–1227.

14 Barker DJP, Gluckman PD, Godfrey KM, Harding JE, Owens JA, Robinson JS. Fetal nutrition and cardiovascular disease in adult life. *Lancet* 1993; **341**: 938–941.

15 Ravelli ACJ, van der Meulen JHP, Michels RPJ, Osmond C, Barker DJP, Hales CN, et al. Glucose tolerance in adults after prenatal exposure to the Dutch famine. *Lancet* 1998; **351**: 173–177.

16 Villar J, Smeriglio V, Martorell R, Brown CH, Klein RE. Heterogeneous growth and mental development of intrauterine growth-retarded infants during the first 3 years of life. *Pediatrics* 1984; **74**: 783–791.

17 Tenovuo A, Kero P, Piekkala P, Korvenranta H, Sillanpaa M, Erkkola R. Growth of 519 small for gestational age infants during the first two years of life. *Acta Paediatr Scand* 1987; **76**: 636–646.

18 Holmes GE, Miller HC, Hassanein K, Lansky SB, Goggin JE. Postnatal somatic growth in infants with atypical fetal growth patterns. *Am J Dis Child* 1977; **131**: 1078–1083.

19 Karlberg J, Albertsson-Wikland K. Growth in full-term small-for-gestational-age infants: from birth to final height. *Pediatr Res* 1995; **38**: 733–739.

20 Karlberg J, Albertsson-Wikland K, Baber FM, Low LCK, Young CY. Born small for gestational age: consequences for growth. *Acta Paediatr Suppl* 1996; **417**: 8–13.

21 Kramer MS, Joseph KS. Commentary: Enigma of fetal/infant origins hypothesis. *Lancet* 1996; **348**: 1254–1255.

22 Paneth N, Susser M. Early origin of coronary heart disease (the 'Barker hypothesis'). *Br Med J* 1995; **310**: 411–412.

23 Elford J, Whincup P, Shaper AG. Early life experience and adult cardiovascular disease: longitudinal and case-control studies. *Int J Epidemiol* 1991; **20**: 833–844.

24 Ben-Shlomo Y, Davey Smith G. Deprivation in infancy or in adult life: which is more important for mortality risk? Lancet 1991; **337**: 530–534.

25 Fall CHD, Vijayakumar M, Barker DJP, Osmond C, Duggleby S. Weight in infancy and prevalence of coronary heart disease in adult life. *Br Med J* 1995; **310**: 17–19.

26 Wannamethee SG, Whincup PH, Shaper G, Walker M. Influence of fathers' social class on cardiovascular disease in middle-aged men. *Lancet* 1996; **348**: 1259–1263.

27 Stein CE, Fall CHD, Kumaran K, Osmond C, Cox V, Barker DJP. Fetal growth and coronary heart disease in South India. *Lancet* 1996; **348**: 1269–1273.

28 Bartley M, Power C, Blane D, Davey Smith G, Shipley M. Birth weight and later socioeconomic disadvantage: evidence from the 1958 British cohort study. *Br Med J* 1994; **309**: 1475–1478.

29 Gunnell DJ, Davey Smith G, Frankel SJ, Nanchahal K, Braddon FEM, Peters TJ. Childhood leg length and adult mortality – follow up of the Carnegie survey of diet and growth in prewar Britain. *J Epidemiol Community Health* 1996; **50**: 580–581.

30 Lynch JW, Kaplan GA, Cohen RD, Kauhanen J, Wilson TW, Smith NL, et al. Childhood and adult socioeconomic status as predictors of mortality in Finland. *Lancet* 1994; **343**: 524–527.

31 Gliksman MD, Kawachi I, Hunter D, Colditz GA, Manson JE, Stampfer MJ, et al. Childhood socioeconomic status and risk of cardiovascular disease in middle aged US women: a prospective study. *J Epidemiol Community Health* 1995; **49**: 10–15.

32 Susser M. Preface. In: Kuh D, Ben-Shlomo Y, eds. *A life-course approach to chronic disease epidemiology* . Oxford: Oxford University Press, 1997.

33 Chadha SL, Radhakrishnan S, Ramachandran K, Kaul U, Gopinath N. Epidemiological study of coronary heart disease in urban population of Delhi. *Indian J Med Res* 1990; **92(B)**: 424–430.

34 Bulatao RA, Stephens PW. Global estimates and projections of mortality by cause 1970–2015. Pre-working paper 1007. 1992.

35 McKeigue PM, Shah B, Marmot MG. Relation of central obesity and insulin resistance with high diabetes prevalence and cardiovascular risk in South Asians. *Lancet* 1991; **337**: 382–386.

36 Gupta R, Gupta VP, Ahluwalia NS. Educational status, coronary heart disease, and coronary risk factor prevalence in a rural population of India. *Br Med J* 1994; **309**: 1332–1336.

37 Pais P, Pogue J, Gerstein H, Zachariah E, Savitha D, Jayprakash S, et al. Risk factors for acute myocardial infarction in Indians: a case-control study. *Lancet* 1996; **348**: 358–363.

38 Singh RB, Niaz MA. Coronary risk factors in Indians. *Lancet* 1995; **346**: 778–779.

39 Bhatnagar D, Anand IS, Durrington PN, Patel DJ, Wander GS, Mackness MI, et al. Coronary risk factors in people from the Indian subcontinent living in west London and their siblings in India. *Lancet* 1995; **345**: 405–409.

40 Williams B. Westernised Asians and cardiovascular disease: Nature or nurture? *Lancet* 1995; **345**: 401–402.

41 Shaukat N, de Bono DP, Jones DR. Like father like son? Sons of patients of European or Indian origin with coronary artery disease reflect their parents' risk factor patterns. *Br Heart J* 1995; **74**: 318–323.

42 Eatan SB, Konner M, Shostak M. Stone ages in the fast lane: chronic degenerative diseases in evolutionary perspective. *Am J Med* 1988; **84**: 739–749.

43 Barker DJP. Rise and fall of western diseases. *Nature* 1989; **338**: 371–372.

44 Altman DG, Hytten FE. Intrauterine growth retardation: let's be clear about it. *Br J Obstet Gynaecol* 1989; **96**: 1127–1132.

Blood pressure

The association of reduced growth rates in fetal life and infancy with increased death rates from cardiovascular disease poses the question of what processes link the two. Raised blood pressure increases the risk of coronary heart disease and stroke, and is one obvious possible link because there is already good evidence that it originates in childhood.[1-3] The persistence of rank order of blood pressure among subjects examined at intervals – so-called 'tracking' – has been repeatedly observed in longitudinal studies of children as well as of adults.[4-8]

FETAL GROWTH AND ADULT BLOOD PRESSURE

The first suggestion that adult blood pressure may be related to fetal growth came from the study by Wadsworth and colleagues[9] of a national sample of people who were born in Britain during 1946, and followed up and examined at 36 years of age. Those with lower birthweights had higher systolic blood pressure. This observation has been confirmed in a re-analysis of the data.[10] Another early indication that low birthweight is associated with raised blood pressure came from a study of recruits in the Swedish army.[11] These observations have now been confirmed in a series of studies of adults in Europe and the USA. Figure 4.1 shows mean systolic blood pressure in a group of men and women in Hertfordshire. The pressures fall progressively between those who weighed 5.5 lb or less ($\leq$2.5 kg) at birth and those who weighed more than 8.5 lb (>3.9 kg).[12] Diastolic pressure shows similar trends. As would be expected blood pressure was higher in people who were currently obese, as measured by the body mass index (weight/height^2). However, men and women who had lower birthweight had higher systolic pressure at any level of current body mass.

Figure 4.2 shows the results of a systematic review of published papers describing the association between birthweight and blood pressure[13] – a review based on 34 studies of more than 66 000 people of all ages. Each point on the figure with its confidence interval represents a study population and the populations are ordered by their ages. The horizontal position of each population describes the change in blood pressure that was associated with a 1-kg (2.2-lb)

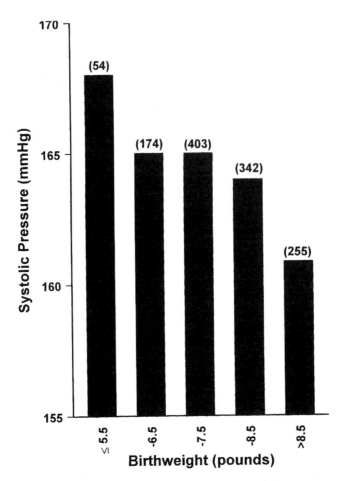

Fig. 4.1 Mean systolic pressure in 1228 men and women aged 60–71 years according to birthweight. (Figures in brackets are numbers of people).

increase in birthweight. In almost all the studies an increase in birthweight was associated with a fall in blood pressure; and there was no exception to this in the studies of adults which now total nearly 8000 men and women. These associations were not confounded by socioeconomic conditions at the time of birth or in adult life.[14] The difference in systolic pressure associated with a 1-kg difference in birthweight was around 3.5 mmHg. In clinical practice this would be a small difference but these are large differences between the mean values of populations. Available data suggest that lowering the mean systolic pressure in a population by 10 mmHg would correspond to a 30% reduction in total attributable mortality.[15]

The adult populations included in Figure 4.2 are European,[12, 16–19] but findings from 160 000 women taking part in the Nurses' Health Study in the USA were recently reported.[20] Blood pressure levels, which were self-reported, were lower than those in the European studies and the fall associated with an increase in birthweight was also smaller. Nevertheless low birthweight was associated with hypertension, the odds ratio in women with birthweights below 5 lb (2.3 kg) being 1.4 in relation to those with birthweights around the

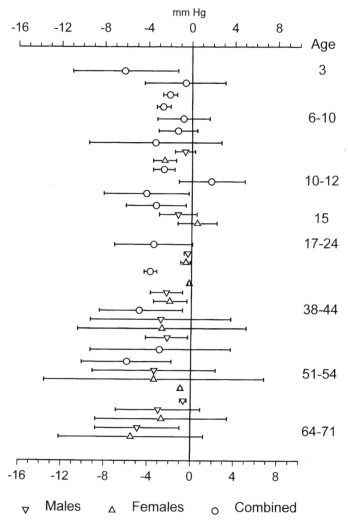

Fig. 4.2 Difference in systolic pressure (mmHg) per kg increase in birthweight (adjusted for weight in children and body mass index in adults).

average. Similarly to other studies, this association was little changed by allowing for a range of variables, including parental history of hypertension.

Two of the early studies in Britain were carried out in Sheffield and Preston. The study in Sheffield was based on the detailed records kept at the Jessop Hospital for Women (Fig. 3.8). Similarly detailed records were kept at Sharoe Green Hospital, in Preston.[21] In both studies the association between low birthweight and raised blood pressure was shown to depend on babies who were small for dates, after reduced fetal growth, rather than on babies who were born preterm. This observation was confirmed by Leon and colleagues in a study of 50-year-old men born in Uppsala, Sweden.[19] Although in these studies alcohol consumption and higher body mass were also associated with raised blood pressure, the associations between birthweight and blood pressure were independent of these factors. Nevertheless body mass remains an important influence on blood pressure and, in humans and animals, the highest pressures are found in people who were small at birth but become over-weight as adults.[22]

As an alternative to a direct intrauterine influence on blood pressure, Ounsted and colleagues have postulated that the accelerated growth of healthy babies of low birthweight during the first 6 months after birth might, of itself, acceler-ate the rise in blood pressure, and the resultant above average values might per-sist.[23] Infant growth was recorded in the Hertfordshire data. Weight gain in infancy was not related to later blood pressure after making allowances for birthweight and current body size.[12] This suggests that high blood pressure is initiated pre- rather than postnatally. Table 4.1 shows findings from the Swedish study mentioned above.[19] The association between low birthweight and raised systolic and diastolic pressure was stronger in men who are above the median adult height. The authors conclude that low birthweight in tall men reflects a greater intrauterine impairment of growth potential than it does in short men. Again the suggestion is that it is the prenatal growth failure rather than the accelerated postnatal growth which initiates raised blood pressure.

As has already been discussed in Chapter 3, birthweight is a crude measure of fetal growth that does not distinguish stunting and thinness, differences in head size, or variations in the balance of fetal and placental size. In the Sheffield and Preston studies blood pressure in middle life could be related to body pro-portions at birth, as well as to birthweight. To examine the links between body proportions at birth and later blood pressure babies born preterm are excluded, because body proportions change during gestation. Analyses of the Preston data define two groups of babies who develop raised blood pressures.[24, 25] The first group are thin with a low ponderal index (birthweight/ length³) and a below average head circumference (see Fig. 3.9). The second have a short crown–heel length in relation to their head circumference, and therefore a high head circumference to length ratio (Fig. 3.10). Short babies tend to be fat and may have above average birthweight.

The Preston analyses revealed a difficulty that occurs when there are both thin and short babies in a study sample. Thin babies tend to have a low head circumference to length ratio, and short babies tend to have a high ponderal index. The trends of raised blood pressure with low ponderal index and a high head circumference to length ratio therefore oppose each other. Table 4.2 shows that in Preston there was no trend in blood pressure with ponderal index. Thin babies, however, had below average placental weight, whereas short babies

Table 4.1 Mean systolic pressure (mmHg) among 50-year-old men in Uppsala, Sweden, according to birthweight and current height

| Height (cms*) at age 50 | Birthweight, kg (lb) | | | | |
	<3.25 (7.2 lb)	–3.75 (8.2 lb)	–4.25 (9.3 lb)	≥4.25 (9.3 lb)	All
≤176	133 (196)	135 (284)	130 (179)	137 (43)	133 (702)
>176	137 (110)	135 (233)	133 (212)	129 (76)	134 (631)

Figures in parentheses are numbers of men.
* 176 cm = 5 ft 9 in.

Table 4.2 Mean systolic pressure (mmHg) of men and women aged 46–54, born after 38 completed weeks of gestation, according to ponderal index at birth and placental weight

Placental weight, g (lb)	Ponderal index, kg/m³					p value for trend
	≤20.8	–22.9	–25.5	>25.5	All	
≤568 (1.25)	154	147	142	141	147	0.0001
	(53)	(54)	(42)	(25)	(174)	
>568 (1.25)	148	149	152	154	152	0.02
	(27)	(27)	(48)	(50)	(152)	
All	152	148	147	150	149	
	(80)	(81)	(90)	(75)	(326)	

Figures in parentheses are numbers of subjects.

had above average placental weight. Division of the data by placental weight revealed strong and opposing trends. At placental weights of 1.25 lb or less (≤591 g) a low ponderal index was associated with high adult blood pressure. At placental weights of more than 1.25 lb (>591 g), a high ponderal index was associated with high adult blood pressure.

The mean ponderal index of the babies in Sheffield was higher than that in Preston: fewer of the babies were thin.[18] Table 4.3 shows the strong association between birth length, abdominal circumference, and blood pressure in men and women born at term. Babies who were short and had a small abdominal circumference at birth had the highest blood pressures as adults.

In contrast to the associations between birth size and lipids (Chapter 5), glucose tolerance (Chapter 6) and coronary heart disease (Chapter 3) those between birthweight and blood pressure are generally as strong as those between thinness, stunting and blood pressure. Associations with thinness and stunting have been found in some studies[26] but not in others.[27] In a longitudinal study of young people in Adelaide associations between blood pressure and thinness and stunting were not apparent at age 8 years but emerged at age 20 (Moore, personal communication).

Table 4.3 Mean systolic blood pressure in men and women aged 50 years, born after 38 completed weeks of gestation, according to length and abdominal circumference at birth

Variable	Mean systolic pressure, mmHg*	p value for trend
Length, inches (cm)		
<20 (51)	154 (69)	
–20 (51)	153 (86)	
>20 (51)	143 (65)	0.0001
Abdominal circumference, inches (cm)		
<11.5 (29)	160 (45)	
–12.25 (31)	148 (52)	
–13 (33)	150 (74)	
>13 (33)	146 (47)	0.002

* Adjusted for sex, current body mass and alcohol intake.
Figures in parentheses are numbers of subjects.

The pattern of cardiovascular disease in China differs from that in Europe. Rates of stroke are higher, and more of the strokes are haemorrhagic rather than thrombotic.[28] Despite a high prevalence of hypertension and cigarette smoking among men, rates of coronary heart disease are low.[29, 30]

Figure 4.3 shows the Peking Union Medical College Hospital, a government hospital once owned by the Rockefeller Foundation, who purchased it from the London Missionary Society. The hospital kept exceptionally detailed obstetric records. Table 4.4 shows the blood pressures of a group of men and women aged 45 years who were born in the hospital during 1948–51, momentous years in Chinese history. Consistent with other studies systolic and diastolic pressures were higher in men than women and rose with increasing body mass index. They were inversely related to birthweight and ponderal index but were not related to length. It seems that in China it is the

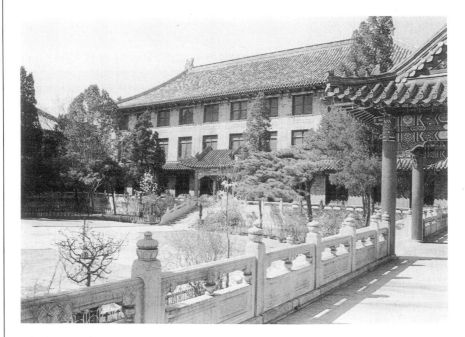

Fig. 4.3 The Peking Union Medical College Hospital.

Table 4.4 Blood pressure in Chinese men and women aged 45 years, according to ponderal index at birth

	Ponderal index at birth, kg/m³					
	≤24	–26	–28	>28	All	p value for trend
Systolic pressure*, mmHg	126	125	124	122	124	0.02
Diastolic pressure*, mmHg	76	76	75	73	75	0.001
Number of people	109	199	208	110	626	

* Adjusted for sex and body mass index.

thin rather than the stunted baby who has raised blood pressure. Blood pressure was also raised in people who had low placental weight. We know an unusual amount about the placentas of these men and women because, remarkably, there are detailed ink drawings of each placenta in the birth records.

FETAL GROWTH AND CHILDHOOD BLOOD PRESSURE

Figure 4.2 shows that the associations between birthweight and blood pressure which are consistently found in adults are also apparent in children before puberty. The children represented in Figure 4.2 come from Britain,[31] France,[32] Italy,[16] Japan,[33] India,[34] and Jamaica.[35] Current body size is the most powerful predictor of blood pressure in childhood, heavier children having higher blood pressure, and the data shown in Figure 4.2 are adjusted for this. Children's weight indicates biological maturity: at any age a heavier, taller child is likely to be more biologically mature than a lighter, shorter child. Although blood pressure variation in childhood is dominated by differences in the rate of development, it is not known whether these differences establish patterns of blood pressure in adult life.

In studies of adolescents the association between low birthweight and raised blood pressure is less consistently found.[13, 16, 36,37] It was, however, apparent in a recent large study of 150,000 military conscripts in Sweden.[38] This inconsistency may be related to the spurt in growth during adolescence and the accompanying perturbation of tracking of both blood pressure and growth.[39] Studies of neonates have shown that blood pressure is positively related to birthweight during the first 4 days of life.[13, 40] A study in Holland has shown that among small babies there is a relatively large increase in blood pressure during early infancy.[40] This accelerated rise in blood pressure may reset blood pressure onto a higher track. The same study found a different pattern of blood pressure development in babies with high birthweight. Their blood pressure was high at birth and remained high so that at the age of 4 years the association between birthweight and blood pressure was U-shaped. We know little about the processes which underlie this. U-shaped associations with birth size have also been reported with coronary heart disease[41] and non-insulin-dependent diabetes.[42]

PLACENTAL WEIGHT AND BLOOD PRESSURE

Table 4.5 shows the systolic pressure of a group of men and women who were born, at term, in Sharoe Green Hospital in Preston, 50 years ago.[21, 24] The subjects are grouped according to their birthweight and placental weight. Consistent with findings in other studies systolic pressure falls between subjects with low and high birthweight. In addition, however, there is a hitherto unsuspected increase in blood pressure with increasing placental weight. Subjects with a mean systolic pressure of 150 mmHg or more, a level sometimes used to define hypertension in clinical practice, comprise a group who as babies were relatively small in relation to the size of their placentas. There are similar trends with diastolic pressure. The differences in systolic pressure among all subjects, shown in the right-hand column of Table 4.5, are consistent with the

Table 4.5 Mean systolic blood pressure (mmHg) of men and women aged 50, born after 38 completed weeks of gestation, according to placental weight and birthweight

Birthweight, lb (kg)	Placental weight, lb (g)				
	≤1.0 (454)	−1.25 (568)	−1.5 (681)	>1.5 (681)	All
−6.5 (2.9)	149 (24)	152 (46)	151 (18)	167 (6)	152 (94)
−7.5 (3.4)	139 (16)	148 (63)	146 (35)	159 (23)	148 (137)
>7.5 (3.4)	131 (3)	143 (23)	148 (30)	153 (40)	149 (96)
All	144 (43)	148 (132)	148 (83)	156 (69)	149* (327)

Figures in parentheses are numbers of subjects.

difference in pressure associated with a 1-kg difference in birthweight found in other surveys of adults (see Fig. 4.2). The fall in systolic pressure of 10 mmHg, across the range of birthweight, is however statistically opposed by the rise of 12 mmHg associated with increasing placental weight. These two large and independent trends are concealed when all pressures at a given birthweight are combined as in the right-hand column.

A rise in blood pressure with increasing placental weight was also found in 4-year-old children in Salisbury, UK,[26] and among 8-year-old children in Adelaide, Australia.[43] Table 4.6 shows the findings in Adelaide. In studies of children and adults the association between placental enlargement and raised blood pressure has, however, been inconsistent.[44] Animal studies offer a possible explanation of this. In sheep the placenta enlarges in response to moderate undernutrition in mid-pregnancy.[45, 46] This is thought to be an adaptive response to extract more nutrients from the mother. It is not, however, a consistent response but occurs only in ewes that were well nourished before pregnancy. In a study of men and women born in Aberdeen, Scotland, after the Second World War, at a time when food was still rationed, raised blood pressure was associated with small placental size.[17] In 3000 children in the UK blood pressure was inversely related to placental weight among the girls but was positively related to the placental weight to birthweight ratio in boys.[27]

Table 4.6 Mean systolic pressure (mmHg) among children aged 8 years, in Adelaide, Australia, according to birthweight and placental weight

Birthweight kg (lb)	Placental weight, g (lb)			
	≤500 (1.1)	−600 (1.3)	>600 (1.3)	All
≤3.2 (7.0)	101.4 (162)	102.3 (71)	103.0 (23)	102.2
−3.6 (7.9)	100.8 (75)	101.7 (107)	102.4 (63)	101.6
>3.6 (7.9)	99.7 (20)	100.5 (78)	101.3 (175)	100.5
All	100.6	101.5	102.2	

Figures in parentheses are numbers of children.

In some studies the blood pressures of the mothers during and after pregnancy have been recorded.[18, 26, 47] They correlate with the offspring's blood pressure. Correspondingly, in Japan children's blood pressure was higher in mothers who had had pretibial oedema, a marker of raised blood pressure, during pregnancy.[33] However, the associations between body size and proportions at birth and later blood pressure are independent of the mothers' blood pressures. In the Salisbury study the blood pressures of the fathers were also measured and found to be related to those of the children.[26] The relationship was, however, weaker than that with the mothers' systolic pressures. This has been found before and has been ascribed to X-linked genes. Another possibility is that raised blood pressure in a mother reflects her own adverse fetal experience, which independently restricts the delivery of nutrients to the fetus (Chapter 8).

Recent observations show that if the mother's blood pressure is measured throughout a 24-hour period, rather than by isolated readings at antenatal clinics, there is a continuous inverse association between birthweight and maternal blood pressure.[48] It could be argued therefore that the association between low birthweight and raised blood pressure reflects an association, possibly genetic, between a mother's ambulatory blood pressure and the blood pressure of her offspring. The demonstration that undernutrition during gestation programs blood pressure in animals (p. 22) argues against this interpretation; an alternative explanation is that raised blood pressure during pregnancy reflects failure of maternal cardiovascular adaptations to pregnancy, which include peripheral vasodilation, with consequent fetal undernutrition, low birthweight and raised blood pressure in the offspring.

Several lines of evidence support the thesis that it is poor delivery of nutrients and oxygen which programs raised blood pressure in humans. Maternal height and parity, which influence fetal growth, have not been found to be related to the offspring's blood pressure other than in small preterm babies. In Jamaica, children whose mothers had thin triceps skinfolds in early pregnancy and low weight gain during pregnancy[49] had raised blood pressure. There were similar findings in a group of children in Birmingham.[50] In the Gambia low pregnancy weight gain was associated with higher blood pressure in childhood.[51] In Aberdeen, Scotland, the blood pressures of middle-aged men and women were found to be related to their mother's intakes of carbohydrate and protein during pregnancy.[17] In the Dutch study of men and women exposed to famine in utero (p. 100) those exposed in late gestation had raised blood pressure, though this was not statistically significant (Roseboom, unpublished). Among people exposed in utero to the famine in Leningrad the effect of obesity on blood pressure was enhanced.[52] A randomised controlled trial of calcium supplementation in pregnancy found that the children of mothers who received the supplement had lower blood pressures than the placebo group.[53] These findings are discussed further in Chapter 11.

Information on maternal smoking has been collected in studies of children.[26, 54] Children's blood pressures were not related to whether their mothers smoked. Lucas & Morley have reported on the blood pressures of 8-year-old children all of whom were born before term and weighed under 1850 g (4.1 lb), and who were part of a trial of early feeding. Their blood pressures were not related to neonatal nutrient intakes,[55] but they were related to whether the mother smoked. Among babies who were born at or after 33 weeks of gestation those whose mothers smoked had raised blood pressure.[56] These findings may indicate that small, preterm babies are especially vulnerable to deleterious effects of maternal smoking. It is, however, difficult to generalise from these babies to the population as a whole. It is also difficult to interpret the lack of an association between their neonatal feeding and blood pressures. The programming effects of nutrition in the neonatal period may be quite different from the effects on babies still in utero. Findings described in this book suggest that the placenta plays a major role in programming, and brain-sparing cardiovascular adaptations that occur in utero are no longer possible after birth when the foramen ovale has closed.

AMPLIFICATION

Comparison of the results for adults and children in Figure 4.2 shows that the differences in blood pressure associated with birthweight in children are small compared with those between adults. Whereas in childhood a 1-kg increase in birthweight is equivalent to a fall in systolic pressure of 1–2 mmHg, in older adults the difference is around 5 mmHg. The regression coefficients in adults remain larger than those in children, even after dividing them by the standard deviation to take account of the increase in standard deviation with age.

An interpretation of these findings is that differences in blood pressure are established in utero but progressively amplified throughout life. Direct evidence of amplification comes from studies by Whincup and colleagues, who showed that blood pressure rose more rapidly with age in children who had low birthweight.[44] The existence of initiating and amplification mechanisms in the aetiology of essential hypertension was first postulated by Folkow.[57] In patients with secondary hypertension from phaeochromocytoma, Conn's syndrome, or renal artery stenosis, hypertension may persist even after the initiating cause, that is the tumour or stenosis, has been removed.[39, 58]

MECHANISMS

There are a number of possible mechanisms by which restricted intrauterine growth could either initiate or amplify raised blood pressure.

Childhood growth

Studies in the USA, the UK and Holland have shown that blood pressure in childhood predicts the likelihood of developing hypertension in adult life. These predictions are strongest after adolescence. In children the rise of blood pressure with age is closely related to growth and is accelerated by the adolescent growth spurt. These observations have led Lever & Harrap to propose that essential hypertension is a disorder of growth.[39] The hypothesis that hypertension is a disorder of accelerated childhood growth can be reconciled with the association with low birthweight by postulating that postnatal catch-up growth plays an important role in amplifying changes established in utero.

Renin–angiotensin system

There is evidence that the fetal renin–angiotensin system is activated in intrauterine growth retardation.[59] However, in a follow-up study of men and women born in Sheffield, those who had been small at birth had lower plasma concentrations of inactive and active renin.[60] Causes of raised blood pressure that are not mediated by increased rates of renin release tend to result in low concentrations of renin and therefore, at first sight, these findings suggest that the association between impaired fetal growth and raised blood pressure must involve mechanisms other than the renin–angiotensin system. However, low concentrations of renin in adult life do not exclude the possibility that the renin–angiotensin system has exerted an earlier but lasting influence.

Renal structure

An alternative explanation for the low plasma renin concentrations of people who were small at birth is that it reflects a relative deficit of nephrons. Brenner and colleagues have suggested that retarded fetal growth leads to reduced numbers of nephrons which in turn leads to increased pressure in the glomer- ular capillaries and the development of glomerular sclerosis.[61, 62] This sclerosis leads to further loss of nephrons and a self-perpetuating cycle of hypertension and progressive glomerular injury. The number of nephrons in the normal pop- ulation varies widely, from 300 000 to 1 100 000 or more.[61] Animal and human studies have shown that low rates of intrauterine growth are associated with reduced numbers of nephrons (p. 25).[63] Studies using fetal ultrasound have shown that babies that are small for gestational age have restricted renal growth during the critical period at 26–34 weeks of gestation. This restricted the anteroposterior size of the kidney but does not diminish kidney length.[64] It has been suggested that during normal childhood development kidney growth lags behind the increases in body weight, and blood pressure rises in order to main- tain renal homeostasis.[65]

Endocrine mechanisms

Chapter 2 described the animal studies which led to the hypothesis that fetal undernutrition leads to lifelong changes in the fetal hypothalamic–pitu- itary–adrenal axis, which in turn resets homeostatic mechanisms controlling blood pressure (p. 29). These findings could also explain the association between raised blood pressure and a high ratio of placental weight to birth- weight. A recent study of 9-year-old children in Salisbury showed that those who had been small at birth had increased urinary adrenal androgen and glucocorticoid metabolite excretion.[66] Further evidence that the hypothalamic– pituitary–adrenal axis is programmed in humans comes from a study of 370 men in Hertfordshire.[67] Those who had had low birthweight had higher fasting cortisol concentrations (Table 4.7) which in turn were associated with raised blood pressure.

Table 4.7 Mean 9.00 a.m. fasting cortisol concentration according to birthweight in 370 men aged 65 years born in Hertfordshire

Birthweight, lb (kg)	No. of men	9.00 a.m. fasting plasma cortisol, nmol/l	'Free' cortisol index
≤5.5 (2.5)	20	408	11.5
–6.5 (2.9)	47	354	9.7
–7.5 (3.4)	104	347	9.6
–8.5 (3.9)	117	340	9.3
–9.5 (4.3)	54	337	9.4
>9.5 (4.3)	28	309	9.1
All	370	344	9.5
(Standard deviation)		(112)	(3.2)
p value for trend		0.007	0.02
p value for trend*		0.02	0.04

* Adjusted for age and body mass index.

The growth hormone insulin-like growth factor 1 (IGF-1) axis may also be programmed in utero. Children in Salisbury, England, and Pune, India, who had low birthweight were found to have raised plasma IGF-1 concentrations.[34] The highest concentrations were in children who had the lowest birthweights but attained the largest body size in childhood. Raised IGF-1 concentrations may therefore be linked to catch-up growth. IGF-1 is known to be important for the growth of blood vessels,[68] and raised concentrations could be one of the processes underlying the suggested association between catch-up growth and raised blood pressure in later life (p. 66).

Vascular structure

The elastic recoil of the aorta is important in maintaining blood flow in the peripheral circulation and in the coronary arteries during diastole. Reduced elasticity (compliance) in the aorta is a marker of cardiovascular disease.[69] It is associated with hypertension, and also with left ventricular hypertrophy because the work of the left ventricle is increased.[70, 71] In Sheffield 50-year-old men and women who were small at birth had reduced compliance in the large arteries of the trunk and legs.[18] Martyn & Greenwald have proposed that impaired synthesis of the scleroprotein elastin is one of the mechanisms underlying the association between low birthweight and raised blood pressure.[72] The elasticity of larger arteries largely depends on the scleroprotein elastin, which is laid down in utero and during infancy and thereafter turns over slowly.[73] Its half-life in humans is approximately 40 years.[74] Reduced elastin deposition leads to less compliant, that is 'stiffer', arteries which will lead to raised blood pressure.[72] The loss of elastin with ageing will amplify the increase in blood pressure. The elasticity of arteries is related to the blood flow in them during intrauterine life. In babies born with a single umbilical artery, the iliac artery which gave rise to it is elastic whereas the other iliac artery, in which blood flow was lower, is thin-walled and muscular.[75] In the growth-retarded fetus there are changes in blood flow in several vascular beds, including the descending aorta and cerebral vasculature.[76] These are 'brain-sparing' adaptations which lead to preferential perfusion of the brain at the expense of the trunk.[77] If sustained they may lead to reduced growth of the abdominal viscera and stunting at birth. Reduced blood flow in the large arteries of the trunk and legs may be associated with reduced elastin deposition, less compliant arteries, and consequent hypertension.

Diversion of oxygenated blood away from the trunk to sustain the growth of the brain also increases peripheral resistance and the load on the heart.[76, 78] Echocardiography has shown that growth-retarded fetuses have hypertrophy of both ventricles.[79, 80] Cardiac myocytes become terminally differentiated before birth and their rate of maturation is influenced by the load on the heart. Early pressure loading leads to fewer, but larger, myocytes. Left ventricular enlargement is known to be a strong predictor of morbidity and death from coronary heart disease independently of its association with raised systolic blood pressure and increased body mass.[81] Among 67-year-old men in Hertfordshire, those who had had low weight at 1 year had concentric enlargement of the left ventricle.[82] This may reflect the long-term effects of prenatal blood diversion to the brain in a baby that is short at birth (Fig. 3.10) and whose growth does not catch up in infancy. An association between low weight around the age of 1 year and later concentric left ventricular hypertrophy has been confirmed in a sample of children and adults in Lorraine, France.[32]

Recent studies suggest that low birthweight is associated with persisting alterations in vascular structure and function in addition to its associations with compliance. Among men in Hertfordshire those who had had low birthweight had narrow bifurcation angles in their retinal blood vessels.[83] People with hypertension have similar changes in retinal vascular geometry. In a study of children in the UK those who had low birthweight had reduced flow-mediated dilatation in the brachial artery after the artery had been occluded and released. Flow-mediated dilatation depends on the endothelium. These findings suggest, therefore, a link between low birthweight and endothelial dysfunction.[84] Since endothelial dysfunction is an early event in atherogenesis this may be a mechanism underlying the strong association between low birthweight and carotid atheroma in later life (Martyn, unpublished).

Nervous system

People with high blood pressure tend to have a high resting pulse rate.[85] This is associated with high cardiac output, hyperdynamic circulation and features of increased sympathetic nervous system activity.[86] Among men and women in Preston those who had low birthweight had a higher resting pulse rate.[87] This is consistent with the hypothesis that increased sympathetic nervous activity is established through retarded growth in utero and leads to raised blood pressure in later life.

BLOOD PRESSURE AND FINGERPRINTS

Fingerprint patterns and the shape of the palm provide additional evidence that raised blood pressure originates in utero.[88] The patterns formed by the dermal ridges on the fingers reflect growth and development during early gestation and are established by the 19th week. Babies who are thin at birth (Fig. 3.9) tend to have 'whorls', patterns of ridges thought to result from swollen finger pads in early gestation. Studies in India and England have shown that people with a whorl on one or more fingers have raised blood pressure in adult life. Similarly, babies who are short at birth in relation to their head size tend to have narrow palms, and adults with hands that are narrow in relation to their length have raised blood pressure.

Interestingly the prognostic significance of fingerprint patterns differs in the right and left hands.[88] This may be explained by the different arterial supply to the two arms.[89] The right subclavian artery arises from the brachiocephalic artery, whose other branch is the right common carotid, whereas the left arises directly from the aorta. The right arm thus receives its blood supply from the same source as the brain, where there is increased blood flow in response to hypoxia, whereas the left arm vessels may constrict in response to hypoxia.

ADULT LIFESTYLE AND BLOOD PRESSURE

Although the customary explanation for the differences in people's blood pressure is that they depend on the environment during adult life, the findings described in this chapter raise the possibility that the intrauterine environment has a dominant effect. Birth measurements are associated with adult blood pressure, independently of current body weight or alcohol consumption. Research into the adult environment and hypertension has focused on salt.[90, 91] A cross-cultural study in 52 centres concluded that 'lowering the daily intake of sodium from 170 mmol to 70 mmol corresponds to a 2 mmHg reduction in systolic pressure'.[91] This is a small effect compared with those associated with fetal growth (Table 4.5, for example). Adult body mass, however, is strongly correlated with blood pressure, and it remains to be seen whether this association reflects diet and other aspects of adult lifestyle which influence weight, or settings of hormonal output and metabolism which are programmed in utero.

Summary

Studies in many countries have shown that babies who are small for dates have raised systolic pressure in childhood and during adult life. These associations are independent of the subject's current body mass and alcohol consumption. Raised blood pressure is not only associated with low birthweight but with thinness and stunting at birth and with variations in the ratio of birthweight to placental weight. This suggests that it may be programmed at different stages of gestation, possibly through different mechanisms. The mechanisms may include persisting changes in vascular and renal structure, or in hormonal systems that control blood pressure. The hypothesis advanced is that blood pressure is programmed by lack of nutrition. This is supported by animal studies and by the associations between maternal thinness, diet in pregnancy and raised blood pressure in humans.

References

1 Evans JG. The epidemiology of stroke. *Age and Ageing* 1979; **8 (Suppl)**: 50–56.
2 Hoffman A. Blood pressure in childhood: an epidemiological approach to the aetiology of hypertension. *J Hypertens* 1984; **2**: 232–238.

3 MacMahon S, Peto R, Cutler J, Collins R, Sorlie P, Neaton J, et al. Blood pressure, stroke and coronary heart disease. Part 1, Prolonged differences in blood pressure: prospective observational studies corrected for the regression dilution bias. *Lancet* 1990; **335**: 765–774.

4 de Swiet M, Fayers P, Shinebourne EA. Blood pressure survey in a population of newborn infants. *Br Med J* 1976; **2**: 9–11.

5 Beaglehole R, Salmond CE, Eyles EF. A longitudinal study of blood pressure in Polynesian children. *Am J Epidemiol* 1977; **105**: 87–89.

6 Clarke WR, Schrott HG, Leaverton PE, Connor WE, Lauer RM. Tracking of blood lipids and blood pressures in school age children: the Muscatine study. *Circulation* 1978; **58**: 626–634.

7 Voors AW, Webber LS, Berenson GS. Time course studies of blood pressure in children – the Bogalusa heart study. *Am J Epidemiol* 1979; **109**: 320–334.

8 Labarthe DR, Eissa M, Varas C. Childhood precursors of high blood pressure and elevated cholesterol. *Annu Rev Public Health* 1991; **12**: 519–541.

9 Wadsworth MEJ, Cripps HA, Midwinter RE, Colley JRT. Blood pressure in a national birth cohort at the age of 36 related to social and familial factors, smoking, and body mass. *Br Med J* 1985; **291**: 1534–1538.

10 Barker DJP, Osmond C, Golding J, Kuh D, Wadsworth MEJ. Growth in utero, blood pressure in childhood and adult life, and mortality from cardiovascular disease. *Br Med J* 1989; **298**: 564–567.

11 Gennser G, Rymark P, Isberg PE. Low birth weight and risk of high blood pressure in adulthood. *Br Med J* 1988; **296**: 1498–1500.

12 Law CM, de Swiet M, Osmond C, Fayers PM, Barker DJP, Cruddas AM, et al. Initiation of hypertension in utero and its amplification throughout life. *Br Med J* 1993; **306**: 24–27.

13 Law CM, Shiell AW. Is blood pressure inversely related to birth weight? The strength of evidence from a systematic review of the literature. *J Hypertens* 1996; **14**: 935–941.

14 Koupilova I, Leon DA, Vagero D. Can confounding by sociodemographic and behavioural factors explain the association between size at birth and blood pressure at age 50 in Sweden? *J Epidemiol Community Health* 1997; **51**: 14–18.

15 Rose G. Sick individuals and sick populations. *Int J Epidemiol* 1985; **14**: 32–38.

16 Vancheri F, Alletto M, Burgio A, Fulco G, Paradiso R, Piangiamore M. Inverse relation between fetal growth and blood pressure in children and adults. *G Ital Cardiol* 1995; **25**: 833–841.

17 Campbell DM, Hall MH, Barker DJP, Cross J, Shiell AW, Godfrey KM. Diet in pregnancy and the offspring's blood pressure 40 years later. *Br J Obstet Gynaecol* 1996; **103**: 273–280.

18 Martyn CN, Barker DJP, Jespersen S, Greenwald S, Osmond C, Berry C. Growth in utero, adult blood pressure, and arterial compliance. *Br Heart J* 1995; **73**: 116–121.

19 Leon DA, Koupilova I, Lithell HO, Berglund L, Mohsen R, Vagero D, et al. Failure to realise growth potential in utero and adult obesity in relation to blood pressure in 50 year old Swedish men. *Br Med J* 1996; **312**: 401–406.

20 Curhan GC, Chertow GM, Willett WC, Spiegelman D, Colditz GA, Manson JE, et al. Birth weight and adult hypertension and obesity in women. *Circulation* 1996; **94**: 1310–1315.

21 Barker DJP, Bull AR, Osmond C, Simmonds SJ. Fetal and placental size and risk of hypertension in adult life. *Br Med J* 1990; **301**: 259–262.

22 Petry CJ, Ozanne SE, Wang CL, Hales CN. Early protein restriction and obesity independently induce hypertension in 1-year-old rats. *Clin Sci* 1997; **93**: 147–152.

23 Ounsted MK, Cockburn JM, Moar VA, Redman CWG. Factors associated with the blood pressures of children born to women who were hypertensive during pregnancy. *Arch Dis Child* 1985; **60**: 631–635.

24 Barker DJP, Godfrey KM, Osmond C, Bull A. The relation of fetal length, ponderal index and head circumference to blood pressure and the risk of hypertension in adult life. *Paediatr Perinat Epidemiol* 1992; **6**: 35–44.

25 Barker DJP, Gluckman PD, Godfrey KM, Harding JE, Owens JA, Robinson JS. Fetal nutrition and cardiovascular disease in adult life. *Lancet* 1993; **341**: 938–941.

26 Law CM, Barker DJP, Bull AR, Osmond C. Maternal and fetal influences on blood pressure. *Arch Dis Child* 1991; **66**: 1291–1295.

27 Taylor SJC, Whincup PH, Cook DG, Papacosta O, Walker M. Size at birth and blood pressure; cross sectional study in 8–11 year old children. *Br Med J* 1997; **314**: 475–480.

28 WHO. *World Health Statistics Annual 1993*. Geneva: WHO, 1994.

29 Chen Z, Peto R, Collins R, MacMahon S, Lu J, Li W. Serum cholesterol concentrations and coronary heart disease in populations with low cholesterol concentrations. *Br Med J* 1991; **303**: 276–282.

30 Tao S, Huang Z, Wu X, Zhou B, Xiao Z, Hao J, et al. Coronary heart disease and its risk factors in the People's Republic of China. *Int J Epidemiol* 1989; **18 (Suppl 1)**: s8159–s8163.

31 Whincup PH, Cook DG, Papacosta O. Do maternal and intrauterine factors influence blood pressure in childhood? *Arch Dis Child* 1992; **67**: 1423–1429.

32 Zureik M, Bonithon-Kopp C, Lecomte E, Siest G, Ducimetiere P. Weights at birth and in early infancy, systolic pressure, and left ventricular structure in subjects aged 8 to 24 years. *Hypertension* 1996; **27(Part 1)**: 339–345.

33 Hashimoto N, Kawasaki T, Kikuchi T, Takahashi H, Uchiyama M. The relationship between the intrauterine environment and blood pressure in 3-year-old Japanese children. *Acta Paediatr* 1996; **85**: 132–138.

34 Fall CHD, Pandit AN, Law CM, Yajnik CS, Clark PM, Breier B, et al. Size at birth and plasma insulin-like growth factor-1 concentrations. *Arch Dis Child* 1995; **73**: 287–293.

35 Forrester TE, Wilks RJ, Bennett FI, Simeon D, Osmond C, Allen M, et al. Fetal growth and cardiovascular risk factors in Jamaican schoolchildren. *Br Med J* 1996; **312**: 156–160.

36 Kolacek S, Kapetanovic T, Luzar V. Early determinants of cardiovascular risk factors in adults: B blood pressure. *Acta Paediatr* 1993; **82**: 377–382.

37 Seidman DS, Laor A, Gale R, Stevenson DK, Mashiach S, Danon YL. Birth weight, current body weight, and blood pressure in late adolescence. *Br Med J* 1991; **302**: 1235–1237.

38 Nilsson PM, Ostergren PO, Nyberg P, Soderstrom M, Allebeck P. Low birth weight is associated with elevated systolic blood pressure in adolescence: a prospective study of a birth cohort of 149 378 Swedish boys. *J Hypertens* 1997; **15**: 1627-1631.

39 Lever AF, Harrap SB. Essential hypertension: a disorder of growth with origins in childhood? *J Hypertens* 1992; **10**: 101–120.

40 Launer LJ, Hofman A, Grobbee DE. Relation between birth weight and blood pressure: longitudinal study of infants and children. *Br Med J* 1993; **307**: 1451–1454.

41 Barker DJP, Martyn CN, Osmond C, Wield GA. Abnormal liver growth in utero and death from coronary heart disease. *Br Med J* 1995; **310**: 703–704.

42 McCance DR, Pettitt DJ, Hanson RL, Jacobsson LTH, Knowler WC, Bennett PH. Birth weight and non-insulin dependent diabetes: thrifty genotype, thrifty phenotype, or surviving small baby genotype? *Br Med J* 1994; **308**: 942–945.

43 Moore VM, Miller AG, Boulton TJC, Cockington RA, Hamilton Craig I, Magarey AM, et al. Placental weight, birth measurements, and blood pressure at age 8 years. *Arch Dis Child* 1996; **74**: 538–541.

44 Whincup P, Cook D, Papacosta O, Walker M. Birth weight and blood pressure: cross sectional and longitudinal relations in childhood. *Br Med J* 1995; **311**: 773–776.

45 McCrabb GJ, Egan AR, Hosking BJ. Maternal undernutrition during mid-pregnancy in sheep; variable effects on placental growth. *J Agric Sci* 1992; **118**: 127–132.

46 McCrabb GJ, Egan AR, Hosking BJ. Maternal undernutrition during mid-pregnancy in sheep. Placental size and its relationship to calcium transfer during late pregnancy. *Br J Nutr* 1991; **65**: 157–168.

47 Whincup PH, Cook DG, Shaper AG. Early influences on blood pressure: a study of children aged 5–7 years. *Br Med J* 1989; **299**: 587–591.

48 Churchill D, Perry IJ, Beevers DG. Ambulatory blood pressure in pregnancy and fetal growth. *Lancet* 1997; **349**: 7–10.

49 Godfrey KM, Forrester T, Barker DJP, Jackson AA, Landman JP, Hall JStE, et al. The relation of maternal nutritional status during pregnancy to blood pressure in childhood. *Br J Obstet Gynaecol* 1994; **101**: 398–403.

50 Clark PM, Atton C, Law CM, Shiell A, Godfrey K, Barker DJP. Weight gain in pregnancy, triceps skinfold thickness and blood pressure in the offspring. *Obstet Gynaecol* 1998; (in press).

51 Margetts BM, Rowland MGM, Foord FA, Cruddas AM, Cole TJ, Barker DJP. The relation of maternal weight to the blood pressures of Gambian children. *Int J Epidemiol* 1991; **20 (4)**: 938–943.

52 Stanner SA, Bulmer K, Andres C, Lantseva OE, Botodina V, Potean VV, et al. Does malnutrition in utero determine diabetes and coronary heart disease in adulthood?

Results from the Leningrad siege study, a cross sectional study. *Br Med J* 1997; **315**: 1342–1349.

53 Belizan JM, Villar J, Bergel E, del Pino A, Di Fulvio S, Galliano SV, et al. Long term effect of calcium supplementation during pregnancy on the blood pressure of offspring: follow up of a randomised controlled trial. *Br Med J* 1997; **315**: 281–285.

54 Whincup P, Cook D, Papacosta O, Walker M, Perry I. Maternal factors and development of cardiovascular risk: evidence from a study of blood pressure in children. *J Hum Hypertens* 1994; **8**: 337–343.

55 Lucas A, Morley R. Does early nutrition in infants born before term programme later blood pressure? *Br Med J* 1994; **309**: 304–308.

56 Morley R, Leeson Payne C, Lister G, Lucas A, Maternal smoking and blood pressure in 7.5 to 8 year old offspring. *Arch Dis Child* 1995; **72**: 120-124.

57 Folkow B. Cardiovascular structural adaptation; its role in the initiation and maintenance of primary hypertension. *Clin Sci & Molecular Med* 1978; **55 (Suppl)**: 3–22.

58 Ferriss JB, Brown JJ, Fraser R, Haywood E, Davies DL, Kay AW, et al. Results of adrenal surgery in patients with hypertension, aldosterone excess, and low plasma renin concentration. *Br Med J* 1975; **1**: 135–138.

59 Kingdom JCP, McQueen J, Connell JMC, Whittle MJ. Fetal angiotensin II levels and vascular (Type 1) angiotensin receptors in pregnancies complicated by intrauterine growth retardation. *Br J Obstet Gynaecol* 1993; **100**: 476–482.

60 Martyn CN, Lever AF, Morton JJ. Plasma concentrations of inactive renin in adult life are related to indicators of foetal growth. *J Hypertens* 1996; **14**: 881–886.

61 Mackenzie HS, Brenner BM. Fewer nephrons at birth: a missing link in the etiology of essential hypertension? *Am J Kidney Dis* 1995; **26**: 91–98.

62 Brenner BM, Chertow GM. Congenital oligonephropathy: an inborn cause of adult hypertension and progressive renal injury? *Curr Opin Nephrol Hypertens* 1993; **2**: 691–695.

63 Merlet-Benichou C, Leroy B, Gilbert T, Lelievre-Pegorier M. Retard de croissance intra-utérin et déficit en néphrons (Intrauterine growth retardation and inborn nephron deficit). *Médecine/Sciences* 1993; **9**: 777–780.

64 Konje JC, Bell SC, Morton JJ, de Chazal R, Taylor DJ. Human fetal kidney morphometry during gestation and the relationship between weight, kidney morphometry and plasma active renin concentration at birth. *Clin Sci* 1996; **91**: 169–175.

65 Weder AB, Schork NJ. Adaptation, allometry, and hypertension. *Hypertension* 1994; **24**: 145–156.

66 Clark PM, Hindmarsh PC, Shiell AW, Law CM, Honour JW, Barker DJP. Size at birth and adrenocortical function in childhood. *Clin Endocrinol* 1996; **45**: 721–726.

67 Phillips DIW, Barker DJP, Fall CHD, Seckl JR, Whorwood CB, Wood PJ, et al. Elevated plasma cortisol concentrations: a link between low birthweight and the insulin resistance syndrome? *J Clin Endocrinol Metab* 1998; (in press)

68 Ferns GAA, Motani AS, Anggard EE. The insulin-like growth factors: their putative role in atherogenesis. *Artery* 1991; **18**: 197–225.

69 Lehmann ED. Pulse wave velocity as a marker of vascular disease. *Lancet* 1996; **348**: 744

70 Safar ME, Levy BI, Laurent S, London GM. Hypertension and the arterial system: clinical and therapeutic aspects. *Hypertension* 1990; **8 (Suppl 7)**: S113–S119.

71 Folkow B. Structure and function of the arteries in hypertension. *Am Heart J* 1987; **114**: 938–948.

72 Martyn CN, Greenwald SE. Impaired synthesis of elastin in walls of aorta and large conduit arteries during early development as an intiating event in pathogenesis of systemic hypertension. *Lancet* 1997; **350**: 953–955.

73 Rucker RB, Tinker D. Structure and metabolism of arterial elastin. *Int Rev Exp Pathol* 1977; **17**: 1–47.

74 Rucker RB, Dubick MA. Elastin metabolism and chemistry: potential roles in lung development and structure. *Environ Health Perspect* 1984; **55**: 179–191.

75 Berry CL, Gosling RG, Laogun AA, Bryan E. Anomalous iliac compliance in children with a single umbilical artery. *Br Heart J* 1976; **38**: 510–515.

76 Al-Ghazali W, Chita SK, Chapman MG, Allan LD. Evidence of redistribution of cardiac output in asymmetrical growth retardation. *Br J Obstet Gynaecol* 1989; **96**: 697–704.

77 Dicke JM. Poor obstetrical outcome. In: Pauerstein CJ, ed. *Clinical Obstetrics*. New York: John Wiley, 1987; 421–439.

78 Rizzo G, Arduini D. Fetal cardiac function in intrauterine growth retardation. *Am J Obstet Gynecol* 1991; **165**: 876–882.

79 Veille JC, Hanson R, Sivakoff M, Hoen H, Ben-Ami M. Fetal cardiac size in normal, intrauterine growth retarded, and diabetic pregnancies. *Am J Perinatol* 1993; **10**: 275–279.

80 Murotsuki J, Challis JRG, Han VKM, Fraher LJ, Gagnon R. Chronic fetal placental embolization and hypoxemia cause hypertension and myocardial hypertrophy in fetal sheep. *Am J Physiol* 1997; **272**: R201–R207.

81 Levy D, Garrison RJ, Savage DD, Kannel WB, Castelli WP. Prognostic implications of echocardiographically determined left ventricular mass in the Framingham Heart Study. *N Engl J Med* 1990; **322**: 1561–1566.

82 Vijayakumar M, Fall CHD, Osmond C, Barker DJP. Birth weight, weight at one year, and left ventricular mass in adult life. *Br Heart J* 1995; **73**: 363–367.

83 Chapman N, Mohamudally A, Stanton A, Aihie Sayer A, Cooper C, Barker DJP, et al. Low birth weight is associated with alterations of retinal vascular network geometry in an elderly male cohort. *J Hypertens* 1997; **15**: 1449–53.

84 Leeson CPM, Whincup PH, Cook DG, Donald AE, Papacosta O, Lucas A, et al. Flow-mediated dilation in 9- to 11-year old children. The influence of intrauterine and childhood factors. *Circulation* 1997; **96**: 2233–2238.

85 Julius S, Krause L, Schork NJ, Mejia AD, Jones KA, van de Ven C, Johnson EH et al. Hyperkinetic borderline hypertension in Tecumseh, Michigan. *J Hypertens* 1991; **9**: 77–84.

86 Esler M, Julius S, Zweifler A. Mild high-renin essential hypertension: Neurogenic human hypertension? *N Engl J Med* 1977; **296**: 405–411.

87 Phillips DIW, Barker DJP. Association between low birthweight and high resting pulse in adult life: is the sympathetic nervous system involved in programming the insulin resistance syndrome? *Diabet Med* 1997; **14**: 673–677.

88 Godfrey KM, Barker DJP, Peace J, Cloke J, Osmond C. Relation of fingerprints and shape of the palm to fetal growth and adult blood pressure. *Br Med J* 1993; **307**: 405–409.

89 Sepulveda W, Bower S, Nicolaidis P, de Swiet M, Fisk NM. Discordant blood flow velocity waveforms in left and right brachial arteries in growth-retarded fetuses. *Obstet Gynaecol* 1995; **86**: 734–738.

90 Diet and hypertension [Editorial]. *Lancet* 1984; **ii**: 671–673.

91 Intersalt Cooperative Research Group. Intersalt: an international study of electrolyte excretion and blood pressure. Results for 24 hour urinary sodium and potassium excretion. *Br Med J* 1988; **297**: 319–328.

5

Cholesterol and blood clotting

SERUM CHOLESTEROL

The reasons why serum cholesterol concentrations differ between populations and among people within populations are not understood. They are important because cholesterol may be directly involved in the pathogenesis of atheroma and is strongly associated with the risk of coronary heart disease.[1,2] Cholesterol and triglycerides are the lipids of central importance in the development of atheroma. They are transported in the blood as lipoprotein complexes, which are classified into low density lipoproteins (LDLs) and high density lipoproteins (HDLs). Around 65% of the serum total cholesterol is carried in the LDL fraction and 25% in the HDL fraction. Raised LDL concentrations are associated with an increased risk of coronary heart disease, whereas raised HDL concentrations seem to be protective.

Chapter 2 gave an account of animal experiments in which lipid metabolism was permanently changed by interference with diet, and other manipulations during gestation and shortly after birth. Speculation that the high cholesterol and saturated fat content of human milk influence lipid metabolism throughout life has not been supported by animal experiments or follow-up studies of children. The concentration of cholesterol in infant food seems to have only a transient effect on serum cholesterol concentrations. Animal studies unequivocally demonstrate, however, that interference with cholesterol metabolism during development affects lipid metabolism permanently, and that undernutrition in utero has persisting effects on the structure and function of the liver, which regulates cholesterol. This chapter describes early evidence that similar phenomena occur in humans. Follow-up studies have shown that children maintain their rank order by serum cholesterol concentrations from the age of 6 months.[3,4] Put another way cholesterol `tracks' from childhood into adult life.[5]

We do not yet know the relative contributions of pre- and early postnatal experience which establish an individual in his or her track.

FETAL GROWTH AND ADULT SERUM CHOLESTEROL CONCENTRATIONS

The unusually detailed birth measurements recorded at the Jessop Hospital for Women in Sheffield included not only birthweight, length and head circumference but abdominal and chest circumferences (Fig. 3.8). Out of 1039 singleton infants born in the hospital during 1939–40, there were 219 who still lived in Sheffield and took part in a study which included measurement of fasting serum lipid concentrations.[6]

LDL cholesterol

Serum concentrations of total cholesterol, LDL cholesterol and apolipoprotein B, which is the structural apolipoprotein linked to LDL cholesterol, tended to be higher in men and women with lower birthweight, although these were weak associations. The striking associations were with a specific pattern of disproportionate growth, leading to a small abdominal circumference at birth. Table 5.1 shows that the serum concentrations fell between men and women whose abdominal circumference was 11.5 inches (29 cm) or less at birth and those whose abdominal circumference was more than 13 inches (33 cm). The statistical significance of these trends was increased by adjustment for length of gestation. Figure 5.1 shows the trends in LDL cholesterol with abdominal circumference. In a simultaneous analysis with abdominal circumference, no other birth measurement was related to lipid concentration.

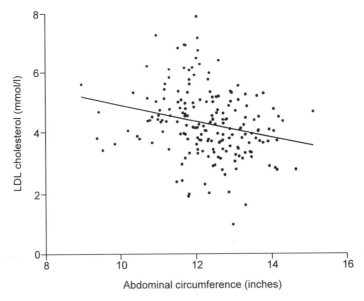

Fig. 5.1 Low density lipoprotein cholesterol concentrations plotted against abdominal circumference at birth, adjusted for duration of gestation, in men and women aged 50–53 years.

Table 5.1   Mean serum lipid concentrations according to abdominal circumference at birth in men and women aged 50–53 years

Abdominal circumference, inches (cm)	No. of people		Total cholesterol, mmol/l			LDL cholesterol, mmol/l			Apolipoprotein B, g/l		
	Men	Women	Men	Women	All	Men	Women	All	Men	Women	All
≤11.5 (29)	28	25	6.5	6.8	6.7	4.5	4.6	4.5	0.96	0.99	0.97
−12.0 (30)	22	21	6.8	6.9	6.9	4.8	4.4	4.6	0.95	0.97	0.96
−12.5 (32)	13	18	6.7	6.8	6.8	4.6	4.2	4.4	0.99	0.97	0.98
−13.0 (33)	21	24	6.0	6.5	6.2	3.8	4.2	4.0	0.90	0.93	0.91
>13.0 (33)	26	19	6.0	6.4	6.1	3.9	4.1	4.0	0.87	0.88	0.87
All	110	107	6.4	6.7	6.5	4.3	4.3	4.3	0.93	0.95	0.94
p value adjusted for gestational age by regression			0.009	0.16	0.003	0.003	0.12	0.0007	0.01	0.07	0.002*

LDL, low density lipoprotein.
* Adjusted for body mass index.

Table 5.2 Mean serum low density lipoprotein concentrations according to current body mass index in men and women aged 50–53 years

Current body mass index, kg/m²	Men	Women
≤23	4.0 (14)	4.1 (17)
–25	4.5 (19)	4.4 (32)
–27	4.5 (30)	4.0 (20)
–30	4.1 (30)	4.8 (15)
>30	4.1 (17)	4.3 (23)
All	4.3 (110)	4.3 (107)

Figures in parentheses are numbers of subjects.

In Table 5.2 the men and women are divided into five groups according to current body mass index. The weak, statistically non-significant trends in serum LDL cholesterol concentrations with current body mass contrast with the strong trends with abdominal circumference (Table 5.1). This is particularly remarkable because abdominal circumference was one of a series of routine measurements at birth and is liable to considerable error. The differences in serum cholesterol concentrations associated with the range of abdominal circumference at birth are clinically significant. Lowering serum cholesterol concentrations from 6.5 to 6.0 mmol/l has been estimated to reduce risk of coronary heart disease by 30%.[7] The differences associated with abdominal circumference are at least as great as this.

Cigarette smoking and alcohol consumption were associated with higher serum concentrations of total and LDL cholesterol and apolipoprotein B, but adjusting for these aspects of adult lifestyle strengthened the association between serum lipid concentrations and abdominal circumference at birth. Serum lipid concentrations did not differ by social class, either currently or at birth, and the association with abdominal circumference occurred within each social class group.

In Hertfordshire serum total cholesterol and LDL cholesterol concentrations were not related to birthweight, in either men or women, though there were associations with infant feeding that will be described later.[8, 9] A study in Jamaica examined the association between body proportions at birth and serum cholesterol concentrations in 485 prepubertal children.[10] Fatter children and those from more affluent families had higher cholesterol concentrations. Again cholesterol concentrations were not related to birthweight but they were inversely related to birth length, being higher in children who were short at birth. The abdominal circumferences at birth of these children were not recorded.

HDL cholesterol and triglycerides

In the study in Sheffield serum concentrations of HDL cholesterol and triglycerides were unrelated to abdominal circumference or other measures of size at birth. In Hertfordshire, however, HDL and triglyceride concentrations were associated with birthweight.[9] In women serum HDL concentrations rose from 1.32 mmol/l in those who weighed 5.5 lb (2.5 kg) or less to 1.57 mmol/l in those who weighed more than 9.5 lb (4.3 kg). As might be expected, triglyceride concentrations showed an opposite trend falling from 1.6 to 1.2 mmol/l. Trends in men were similar, though weaker.

LIVER GROWTH IN UTERO AND CORONARY HEART DISEASE

As was described in Chapter 2 undernutrition in early intrauterine life tends to produce small but normally proportioned animals, whereas undernutrition later in development leads to selective organ damage and disproportionate growth in animals whose birthweight may be normal.[11] The associations between birth size and LDL cholesterol can be understood in the light of this. During periods of undernutrition those tissues that are more mature have a greater priority of growth, and may continue to grow at the expense of other tissues. The timing of undernutrition therefore determines which tissues and systems are selectively damaged, and hence the pattern of disproportion in organ size at birth. Chapter 4 (p. 74) described how the human fetus may respond to nutrient deprivation in late gestation by sustaining the brain at the expense of trunk growth.[12] The liver, which is growing rapidly at this time, may be particularly compromised and its weight at birth is found to be low when compared with either the weight of the brain or with total body weight.[13] During ultrasonography of the fetus, the ratio of head circumference to abdominal circumference is used as a measure of the ratio of brain to liver size in disproportionate growth of this kind.[14] The association of serum total and LDL cholesterol concentrations with low abdominal circumference, but not independently with low head circumference, suggests that raised concentrations of these lipids in adult life are related to growth failure in late gestation.[6] The findings among children in Jamaica are consistent with this.[10] In the Sheffield study, chest circumference at birth did not predict serum lipid concentrations independently of abdominal circumference, which points to a specific association with growth failure of abdominal viscera, including the liver, rather than failure of growth of the trunk as a whole.

One possible explanation of these findings is that impaired growth of the liver in late gestation leads to permanent changes in LDL cholesterol metabolism. The liver is thought to be the major site for synthesis of LDL cholesterol in late gestation, and the human fetus requires large quantities at this time to sustain its metabolic activities, which include high rates of secretion of steroid hormones by the adrenal glands.[15] Just before birth, rates of cholesterol synthesis in the liver, as judged by the activity of the rate-limiting enzyme in cholesterol synthesis, are more than twice those in the adult.[16] The processes by which impaired liver growth in late gestation could lead, paradoxically, to persistently raised serum concentrations of LDL are unknown. A study of LDL metabolism in samples of middle-aged men in five countries has, however, led to the suggestion that differences in serum concentrations depend on different activity of LDL receptors in the liver.[17] Persistent reduction of LDL receptor activity, associated with failure of fetal liver growth, is one possible explanation for persisting elevation of serum cholesterol concentrations. Animal studies, described in Chapter 2 (p. 25)

Table 5.3 Standardised mortality ratios for coronary heart disease according to abdominal circumference at birth in 1819 men

Abdominal circumference, inches (cm)	Average birthweight or less (≤7.5 lb, 3.4 kg)	Above average birthweight (>7.5 lb, 3.4 kg)	All
≤11.5 (29)	123 (39)	48 (2)	114 (41)
–12.0 (30)	113 (36)	58 (11)	93 (47)
–12.5 (32)	79 (12)	102 (14)	90 (26)
–13.0 (33)	68 (7)	110 (26)	97 (33)
>13.0 (33)	101 (3)	125 (24)	122 (27)
All	106 (97)	97 (77)	101 (174)

Figures in parentheses are numbers of deaths.

suggest that alterations in the relative numbers of hepatocytes in the periportal and perivenous areas may be important.

The association between abdominal circumference at birth and death from coronary heart disease is shown in Table 5.3.[18] It is U-shaped; but further examination shows that this is the result of opposing trends at birthweights below and above the average. Among men whose birthweights were below average, those who had a small abdominal circumference at birth had raised death rates from coronary heart disease. This is consistent with the associations between small abdominal circumference and raised serum LDL cholesterol (Table 5.1) and raised plasma fibrinogen concentration (described later in this chapter). Among men with above average birthweight, those who had a large abdominal circumference at birth had raised death rates from coronary heart disease (Table 5.3). The babies of women who develop impaired glucose tolerance in pregnancy become macrosomic. During their accelerated growth in late gestation the fetus' abdomen enlarges rapidly.[19] The processes underlying this are not known, though deposition of glycogen in the liver has been suggested. It seems that both reduced and accelerated liver growth in late gestation are early determinants of coronary heart disease.

INFANT FEEDING AND ADULT SERUM CHOLESTEROL CONCENTRATIONS

During analyses of death from cardiovascular disease in Hertfordshire, which were described in Chapter 3, death rates were found to differ according to the method of infant feeding.[8, 20] When the health visitors in Hertfordshire visited the babies during infancy they recorded how each baby was being fed. In the period up to 1930, 66% of the babies were recorded as breast fed, 27% as breast and bottle fed, and 7% as exclusively bottle fed. When the infants were 1 year old a record was made of whether or not they were weaned. The term 'weaned' can imply that either breast feeding has stopped or solid food has been introduced. The evidence from the Hertfordshire Chief Health Visitor's annual reports, together with anecdotal evidence from health visitors who worked in Hertfordshire around this period, suggest that 'weaned' usually meant cessation of breast feeding. In her annual reports, Miss Burnside, the Chief Health Visitor for Hertfordshire, quoted percentages of breast fed babies weaned at 12 months, but gave no comparable information for bottle fed babies, presumably because the word did not usually apply to these babies.[21] In England, at the beginning of the century breast feeding was continued for longer than is now usual, but was commonly stopped at around 9 months and usually before 1 year.[22, 23] Around 20% of the babies in Hertfordshire were, however, breast fed beyond a year, and these babies tended to be from poorer families. Anecdotal evidence from Hertfordshire suggests that women in lower socioeconomic groups prolonged breast feeding beyond 1 year as a form of contraception.

It was surprising to find that death rates from cardiovascular disease were higher in two groups of people: those who had been breast fed beyond 1 year and those who had been exclusively bottle fed. Table 5.4 shows that raised death rates were found only in men who had been breast fed beyond 1 year, and not in women, whereas both men and women who had been exclusively bottle fed had raised rates, although this was not statistically significant. There were no important differences in mortality from non-cardiovascular causes in relation to the method of infant feeding.

Fall and colleagues measured the serum lipids in a sample of men who still lived in Hertfordshire.[8] Table 5.5 shows that men who had been breast fed

Table 5.4 Standardised mortality ratios (SMR) from cardiovascular disease at ages below 65 years according to method of infant feeding

Infant Feeding	Men			Women		
	SMR	(95% CI)	No. of deaths	SMR	(95% CI)	No. of deaths
Breast and bottle fed	73	(63–82)	213	65	(47–89)	40
Breast fed, weaned before 1 year	72	(64–79)	377	65	(51–82)	73
Breast fed, beyond 1 year	93	(80–107)	181	63	(39–98)	20
Bottle fed only	81	(62–103)	64	108	(60–178)	15

CI, confidence interval.

Table 5.5 Mean serum lipid concentrations in men aged 59–70 years according to infant feeding

	Breast and bottle fed (1)	Breast fed, weaned before 1 year (2)	Breast fed beyond 1 year (3)	Bottle fed only (4)	All	SD
Cholesterol, mmol/l	6.4	6.4	6.9**	7.1**	6.5	1.2
LDL cholesterol, mmol/l	4.6	4.6	5.0**	5.1*	4.7	1.1
LDL:HDL ratio	3.8	3.8	4.2**	4.2	3.9	1.5
Apolipoprotein B, g/l	1.08	1.08	1.14	1.14	1.09	1.3
Number of men	116	253	91	25	485	

* $p < 0.05$, **$p < 0.01$; comparison with groups (1) and (2) combined.
SD, standard deviation.
LDL, low density lipoprotein; HDL, high density lipoprotein.

beyond 1 year, and those who had been exclusively bottle fed, had higher serum concentrations of total cholesterol and LDL cholesterol, and higher LDL:HDL cholesterol ratios than men in the other two feeding groups.

There were no differences between feeding groups for other cardiovascular risk factors, including body mass, blood pressure, plasma glucose, insulin, fibrinogen and factor VII concentrations. The percentages of men who were either current smokers or who were in social class IV or V were similar in all the feeding groups. In spite of the similarity in current social class, a higher percentage of men who had been breast fed beyond 1 year had been born into families of social class IV or V. Table 5.6 shows, however, that the raised concentrations of LDL cholesterol in these men were found in each social class. Findings for total cholesterol and apolipoprotein B were similar.

These findings suggest that in men born 70 years ago who were breast fed and weaned relatively late, a process was established which led to raised serum concentrations of LDL cholesterol and increased death rates from coronary heart disease in adult life. This process was not linked to other lipids or other cardiovascular risk factors. Interestingly serum LDL cholesterol concentrations in women in Hertfordshire are unrelated to the method of infant feeding.[9] The regulation of serum lipid concentrations involves several tissues, most importantly the liver and gut. Mechanisms by which late weaning of infants might program lipid metabolism in adults are a matter for speculation. Breast milk contains several hormones and growth factors which can influence lipid metabolism, including thyroid hormones and steroids.[24, 25] One possible explanation of the findings, which derives from observations on baboons, is that thyroid hormones present in breast milk may down regulate the suckling infant's thyroid function in later life, thereby influencing cholesterol metabolism.[26, 27]

Breast milk provides ideal nourishment for the young infant, but there is evidence that some babies who are exclusively breast fed after 6 months receive inadequate energy.[28] Human breast milk contains low iron concentrations, and exclusively breast fed babies commonly develop low iron stores in the second half of infancy.[29] Breast milk may also be deficient in vitamins, notably vitamin D, if the mother is poorly nourished.[30] In Hertfordshire infants who were breast fed beyond 1 year weighed less at 1 year of age than those who were weaned. This may be evidence of poor nutrition.

Table 5.6 Mean serum LDL cholesterol concentrations (mmol/l) in men aged 59–70 years according to infant feeding and social class at birth

Social class at birth	Breast and bottle fed	Breast fed, weaned before 1 year	Breast fed, beyond 1 year	Bottle fed only	All groups	SD
I, II, III (N)	4.8	4.6	5.1	4.9	4.7 (62)	1.0
III (M)	4.5	4.7	5.0	5.6	4.7 (157)	1.1
IV, V	4.6	4.6	5.0	5.0	4.7 (225)	1.2
All classes	4.6	4.6	5.0	5.2	4.7 (444)	1.1

N = non manual; M = manual.
Figures in parentheses are numbers of men.

The men and women who had been exclusively bottle fed, comprising only 7% of the sample, also had raised death rates from coronary heart disease and, at least in the men, higher serum LDL cholesterol concentrations. We do not know what was contained in the bottle feeds because this was not specified in the Hertfordshire records. Bottle foods available 70 years ago included patent preparations of dried cows' milk, unmodified cows' milk, diluted condensed milk, and patent foods made from wheatflour or arrowroot.[31] Modern formula milks differ from these foods: they are fortified with iron and vitamins; the fat content is mainly unsaturated, and the electrolyte content is similar to that of breast milk. It is therefore difficult to assess the relevance of these findings for bottle fed babies today. They may, be another demonstration of the adverse effects of cows' milk in infancy.[32] They do, however, add to the evidence that in humans, as in animals, nutrition during infancy may have a permanent influence on lipid metabolism and the risk of coronary heart disease. A recent study in Croatia has added further evidence: young men and women breast fed for less than 3 months after birth had higher serum cholesterol concentrations than those breast fed for longer.[33]

BLOOD CLOTTING

After the Second World War, research into coronary heart disease centred almost exclusively on atheroma and, because of its lipid content, the role of dietary fat and serum cholesterol concentrations. The role of blood clotting, though implied in the term 'coronary thrombosis', was until recently overlooked. In 1951 Morris[34] drew attention to the probable role of processes other than atheroma in the genesis of coronary heart disease. Analysing postmortem findings at the London Hospital from the early years of the century, he showed that the prevalence of advanced atheroma had remained unchanged over a period of time in which mortality from coronary heart disease had increased several-fold. Clearly processes other than atheroma were involved in this steep rise. Interest in the role of thrombosis re-emerged when it was shown that thrombosis in the coronary vessels often preceded myocardial infarction and sudden coronary death.[35, 36]

During the evolution of a thrombus, platelets adhere rapidly to damaged endothelium and to each other. Thereafter fibrin becomes incorporated into the clot, giving it stability and volume. The importance of plasma concentrations of fibrinogen, the precursor of fibrin, as a predictor of death was first shown by Meade and colleagues in the Northwick Park Heart Study.[37, 38] Men with high plasma concentrations of fibrinogen were shown to be at increased risk of myocardial infarction. Raised plasma levels of factor VII activity, part of the 'extrinsic' pathway of the coagulation cascade involved in the production of thrombin, were also found to be associated with increased risk. Raised concentrations of fibrinogen and factor VII predispose to thrombosis, and may contribute to the development and progression of atheroma.[39] Fibrinogen is also an important determinant of plasma viscosity. People living in an area of high coronary heart disease mortality in western Scotland have been shown to have higher plasma viscosity than those in an area of low mortality in southern

Germany.[40] A suggestion from this finding is that the flow properties of blood may be important in causing coronary thrombosis.

Other studies have confirmed strong relationships between fibrinogen and coronary heart disease and stroke.[41–44] The association of coronary heart disease with fibrinogen is at least as strong as that with cholesterol.[38] Fibrinogen is an acute phase protein and rises in response to several stimuli.[45] Plasma concentrations are increased by cigarette smoking and much of the relationship between smoking and coronary heart disease may be mediated through this effect.[39] Smoking is also partly responsible for the higher plasma fibrinogen concentrations of men with low socioeconomic status.[46] Factor VII activity is increased by eating fat, and dietary fat may therefore increase the risk of coronary heart disease through an immediate effect on thrombosis as well as a long- term effect on atheroma.[47, 48]

FETAL AND INFANT GROWTH AND ADULT HAEMOSTATIC FACTORS

Table 5.7 shows mean plasma fibrinogen and factor VII concentrations in a sample of men in Hertfordshire.[49] Concentrations of both factors fell between those who had low and those who had high weight at 1 year. Neither factor showed a significant trend with birthweight, although the highest concentrations of each were found in men with birthweights of 5.5 lb (2.5 kg) or less. The difference in plasma fibrinogen concentrations between men who weighed more than 26 lb (11.8 kg) and those who weighed 18 lb (8.2 kg) or less at 1 year is statistically equivalent to an increase in cardiovascular death rate of around 40%.[38]

When the men were grouped into current smokers, ex-smokers, and those who had never smoked, mean plasma fibrinogen concentrations were, as expected, highest in smokers; they were also higher in ex-smokers than in men who had never smoked (Table 5.8). Adjustments for smoking did not, however, change the correlation of mean plasma fibrinogen concentrations with weight at 1 year. Regression analysis showed that the concentration fell with increasing weight at 1 year in each smoking group. Table 5.8 provides an example of the adverse effects of adult lifestyle adding to those associated with failure of early growth. The highest plasma fibrinogen concentrations were in those men

Table 5.7 Mean plasma fibrinogen and factor VII concentrations in men aged 59–70 years according to weight at one year

Weight at 1 year, lb (kg)	No. of men	Fibrinogen, g/l	Factor VII (% of standard)
≤18 (8.2)	38	3.21	122
–20 (9.1)	93	3.10	111
–22 (10.0)	178	3.13	108
–24 (10.9)	173	2.97	106
–26 (11.8)	82	2.93	106
>26 (11.8)	33	2.93	103
p value for trend		<0.001	<0.005

Table 5.8 Mean plasma fibrinogen concentration (g/l) in men aged 59–70 years according to their weight at 1 year of age and smoking habits

Weight at 1 year, lb (kg)	Non-smokers	Ex-smokers	Current smokers
≤18 (8.2)	2.87 (6)	3.25 (19)	3.33 (12)
–20 (9.1)	3.25 (11)	2.94 (48)	3.28 (31)
–22 (10.0)	2.98 (31)	3.10 (96)	3.29 (50)
–24 (10.9)	2.81 (32)	2.95 (97)	3.14 (42)
–26 (11.8)	2.78 (16)	2.93 (46)	3.05 (18)
>26 (11.8)	2.62 (4)	3.00 (22)	2.87 (7)
All	2.90 (100)	3.01 (328)	3.20 (160)

Figures in parentheses are numbers of men.

who had the lowest weight at 1 year and who smoked. The lowest concentrations were in those men who had the highest weight at 1 year and who had never smoked.

An analysis of plasma fibrinogen concentrations in the Preston sample of men (p. 65), whose size at birth had been measured in detail, showed that those who were stunted at birth, having a low crown–heel length, had raised concentrations. This finding was subsequently confirmed in men in Sheffield, where men with low birthweight, short length, and reduced abdominal circumference at birth were found to have raised plasma fibrinogen concentrations. Table 5.9 shows the trend with abdominal circumference, which was strengthened after adjustment for the current waist:hip circumference ratio of the subjects. A high waist:hip ratio is independently associated with raised plasma fibrinogen concentrations.[49, 50] Plasma fibrinogen concentrations among women were not linked to measurements at birth in Hertfordshire, Preston or Sheffield. One possible explanation for this is that in women aged 50 years and more a relation with fetal growth is transiently obscured by the increase in fibrinogen concentrations that occur at the menopause. Little is known about the association between plasma fibrinogen and cardiovascular disease in women.[44] In the Framingham study[42] plasma fibrinogen was linked to coronary heart disease in younger women but not to stroke.

The associations between the two haemostatic factors and failure of early growth in men were independent of smoking, social class, alcohol consumption, and adult body mass. It therefore does not seem possible to sustain the argument that the associations merely reflect the effects of confounding

Table 5.9 Mean plasma fibrinogen concentrations (g/l) in men aged 50–53 years according to abdominal circumference at birth

Abdominal circumference inches (cm)	Unadjusted	Adjusted for smoking and waist:hip ratio	No. of men
≤11.5 (29)	2.60	2.66	25
–12.25 (31)	2.53	2.51	22
–13 (33)	2.49	2.47	35
>13 (33)	2.37	2.36	22
p value for trend	0.03	0.006	

variables linked to both early growth failure and adult lifestyle.[49] This conclusion is supported by findings in the Whitehall study of middle-aged civil servants in London. Those whose fathers had had low socioeconomic status and who themselves had worse education had raised plasma fibrinogen concentrations, which were not explained by the subjects' own life circumstances.[51] These results suggest that there is a critical period in early life when the metabolism of haemostatic factors is programmed. Plasma concentrations of fibrinogen and factor VII are known to reach values within the adult range by the age of 1 year.[52]

Relative failure of growth in infancy, which is a strong predictor of fibrinogen and factor VII concentrations (see Table 5.7), may result from either postnatal or prenatal influences; postnatal influences include feeding and illness. In Hertfordshire, where postnatal development was recorded, concentrations of the haemostatic factors did not vary in relation to differences in infant feeding and weaning, although these differences were related to adult cholesterol concentrations (see Table 5.5). They were also not related to illness during infancy, although illness was related to adult lung function (see Chapter 7). The findings in Preston and Sheffield (see Table 5.9) suggest that prenatal influences may underlie the reduction in infant growth which is associated with high concentrations of the factors. The babies who subsequently have raised concentrations tend to be short at birth with a reduced abdominal circumference. As already described, the human fetus may respond to nutrient deprivation in late gestation by sustaining the brain at the expense of trunk growth;[12] the liver may be particularly compromised. After birth the growth of these babies, who tend to be short at birth, does not 'catch up'.[53, 54] High adult concentrations of haemostatic factors could be associated with infant growth failure through a common origin in fetal undernutrition in late gestation. Table 5.10 shows that mean plasma fibrinogen concentrations among men in Preston rose progressively as the placental weight:birthweight ratio increased. As already described (p. 70) a high placental weight:birthweight ratio is thought to indicate fetal undernutrition.

Circulating fibrinogen and factor VII concentrations are largely regulated by the liver. High adult concentrations may be a persistent response to impaired liver development during a critical early phase. One possibility, discussed further in Chapter 8, is that an aspect of this impaired liver development could be its sensitivity to growth hormone and production of insulin-like growth factor 1. Consistent with this, both fibrinogen and factor VII concentrations are linked to adult height, being lower in taller men.[49, 51] It is interesting that when con-

Table 5.10 Mean plasma fibrinogen concentrations in men aged 46–54 years according to ratio of placental weight:birthweight

Placental weight:birthweight	Mean plasma fibrinogen, g/l	No. of men
≤0.162	2.87	28
−0.182	2.89	30
−0.200	2.92	27
−0.229	2.90	28
>0.229	3.15	29
All	2.94	142

centrations of either factor are simultaneously regressed with adult height and with weight at 1 year of age, the association with adult height is abolished whereas that with infant weight remains – further evidence of the importance of early life. An inverse relation between height and cardiovascular disease has been found in prospective studies of at least three populations: 1.8 million people in Norway who attended for mass radiography, 17 000 male civil servants in London, and 1700 men in Finland.[55–57]

Although raised concentrations of fibrinogen and factor VII may both reflect impaired liver development in utero the underlying mechanisms may be different. Fibrinogen and factor VII concentrations are only weakly associated and, although fibrinogen concentrations are strongly related to blood pressure, factor VII concentrations are not.[48, 49]

Summary

Animal studies show that interference with cholesterol metabolism during development permanently changes lipid metabolism. There is now evidence that similar phenomena occur in humans. Raised serum concentrations of total and LDL cholesterol are found in men and women who had reduced liver size at birth, as measured by abdominal circumference. This suggests that impaired liver growth in late gestation may bring about a permanent alteration of LDL cholesterol metabolism. Raised LDL cholesterol concentrations and an increased risk of coronary heart disease are also found in men who had been breast fed for more than a year. This may reflect prolonged exposure to maternal hormones in breast milk.

Raised plasma concentrations of two haemostatic factors – fibrinogen and factor VII – are associated with an increased risk of cardiovascular disease. Raised concentrations of these factors are found in men who, at birth, were short with reduced abdominal circumferences, and who failed to gain weight in infancy. Circulating fibrinogen and factor VII concentrations are largely regulated by the liver. Impaired liver development during late gestation may program higher plasma concentrations in later life.

References

1 Keys A. *Seven countries*. Cambridge, MA: Harvard University Press, 1980.

2 Lewis B. The lipoproteins: predictors, protectors and pathogens. *Br Med J* 1983; **287**: 1161–1164.

3 Labarthe DR, Eissa M, Varas C. Childhood precursors of high blood pressure and elevated cholesterol. *Annu Rev Public Health* 1991; **12**: 519–541.

4 Sporik R, Johnstone JH, Cogswell JJ. Longitudinal study of cholesterol values in 68 children from birth to 11 years of age. *Arch Dis Child* 1991; **66**: 134–137.

5 Boulton TJC. 'The notion of tracking'. In: Boulton J, Laron Z, Rey J, eds. *Long-term consequences of early feeding*. Philadelphia: Lippincott-Raven, 1996.

6 Barker DJP, Martyn CN, Osmond C, Hales CN, Fall CHD. Growth in utero and serum cholesterol concentrations in adult life. *Br Med J* 1993; **307**: 1524–1527.

7 Wald NJ. Cholesterol and coronary heart disease: to screen or not to screen. In: Marmot M, Elliott P, eds. *Coronary heart disease epidemiology*. Oxford: Oxford University Press, 1992; 358–368.

8 Fall CHD, Barker DJP, Osmond C, Winter PD, Clark PMS, Hales CN. Relation of infant feeding to adult serum cholesterol concentration and death from ischaemic heart disease. *Br Med J* 1992; **304**: 801–805.

9 Fall CHD, Osmond C, Barker DJP, Clark PMS, Hales CN, Stirling Y, et al. Fetal and infant growth and cardiovascular risk factors in women. *Br Med J* 1995; **310**: 428–432.

10 Forrester TE, Wilks RJ, Bennett FI, Simeon D, Osmond C, Allen M, et al. Fetal growth and cardiovascular risk factors in Jamaican schoolchildren. *Br Med J* 1996; **312**: 156–160.

11 McCance RA, Widdowson EM. The determinants of growth and form. *Proc R Soc Lond B* 1974; **185**: 1–17.

12 Pauerstein CJ. *Clinical obstetrics.* New York: John Wiley, 1987.

13 Gruenwald P. Pathology of the deprived fetus and its supply line. In: Elliott K, Knight J, eds. *Size at birth. Ciba Foundation Symposium No. 27.* Amsterdam: Elsevier, 1974; 3–19.

14 Campbell S, Thoms A. Ultrasound measurement of the fetal head to abdomen circumference ratio in the assessment of growth retardation. *Br J Obstet Gynaecol* 1977; **84**: 165–174.

15 Carr BR, Simpson ER. Cholesterol synthesis in human fetal tissues. *J Clin Endocrinol Metab* 1982; **55**: 447–452.

16 McNamara DJ, Quackenbush FW, Rodwell VW. Regulation of hepatic 3-hydroxy-3-methylglutaryl coenzyme A reductase. *J Biol Chem* 1972; **247**: 5805–5810.

17 International Collaborative Study Group. Metabolic epidemiology of plasma cholesterol: mechanisms of variation of plasma cholesterol within populations and between populations. *Lancet* 1986; **ii**: 991–996.

18 Barker DJP, Martyn CN, Osmond C, Wield GA. Abnormal liver growth in utero and death from coronary heart disease. *Br Med J* 1995; **310**: 703–704.

19 Bochner CJ, Medearis AL, Williams J, Castro L, Hobel CJ, Wade ME. Early third-trimester ultrasound screening in gestational diabetes to determine the risk of macrosomia and labor dystocia at term. *Am J Obstet Gynecol* 1987; **157**: 703–708.

20 Osmond C, Barker DJP, Winter PD, Fall CHD, Simmonds SJ. Early growth and death from cardiovascular disease in women. *Br Med J* 1993; **307**: 1519–1524.

21 Burnside EM. Annual report of the Lady Inspector of Midwives. In: *The County Medical Officer of Health's Annual Report.* Hertfordshire, 1915.

22 Breast feeding and weaning. In: *Series II: Baby. Ten minute talks to centre mothers prepared for the use of health visitors.* Women Public Health Officers' Association. London, 1942; 1–5.

23 Whitehead R, Paul A. Changes in infant feeding in Britain during the last century. In: *Infant feeding and cardiovascular disease: Medical Research Council Environmental Epidemiology Unit Scientific Report No 8.* Southampton: 1987; 1–10.

24 Koldovsky O, Thornburg W. Hormones in milk: a review. *J Pediatr Gastroenterol Nutr* 1987; **6**: 172–196.

25 Salter AM, Fisher SC, Brindley DN. Interactions of triiodothyronine, insulin and dexamethasone on the binding of human LDL to rat hepatocytes in monolayer culture. *Atherosclerosis* 1988; **71**: 77–80.

26 Lewis DS, McMahan CA, Mott GE. Breast feeding and formula feeding affect differently plasma thyroid hormone concentrations in infant baboons. *Biol Neonate* 1993; **63**: 327–335.

27 Phillips DIW, Barker DJP, Osmond C. Infant feeding, fetal growth and adult thyroid function. *Acta Endocrinol* 1993; **129**: 134–138.

28 Whitehead RG, Paul AA, Ahmed EA. Weaning practices in the U.K. and variations in anthropometric development. *Acta Paediatr Scand Suppl* 1986; **323**: 14–23.

29 Saarinen UM. Need for iron supplementation in infants on prolonged breast feeding. *J Pediatr* 1978; **93**: 177–180.

30 Belton NR. Rickets – not only the 'English Disease'. *Acta Paediatr Scand Suppl* 1986; **323**: 68–75.

31 Paterson D. The next best thing: correct artificial feeding. In: *A chance for every child, A report of lectures given at the 9th Winter school for health visitors and school nurses held at Bedford College for Women, University of London, December 30th 1929 to January 10th 1930.* London: Women Sanitary Inspectors' and Health Visitors' Association, 1930; 22–26.

32 Miller MJS, Witherly SA, Clark DA. Casein: a milk protein with diverse biological consequences. *Proc Soc Exp Biol Med* 1990; **195**: 143–159.

33 Kolacek S, Kapetanovic T, Zimolo A, Luzar V. Early determinants of cardiovascular risk factors in adults. A. Plasma lipids. *Acta Paediatr* 1993; **82**: 699–704.

34 Morris JN. Recent history of coronary disease. *Lancet* 1951; **i**: 1–7.

35 DeWood MA, Spores J, Notske R, Mouser LJ, Burroughs R, Golden MS et al. Prevalence of total coronary occlusion during the early hours of transmural myocardial infarction. *N Engl J Med* 1980; **303**: 897–902.

36 Davies MJ, Thomas A. Thrombosis and acute coronary artery lesions in sudden cardiac ischemic death. *N Engl J Med* 1984; **310**: 1137–1140.

37 Meade TW, North WRS, Chakrabarti R, Stirling Y, Haines AP, Thompson SG et al. Haemostatic function and cardiovascular death: early results of a prospective study. *Lancet* 1980; **i**: 1050–1054.

38 Meade TW, Mellows S, Btozovic M, Miller GJ, Chakrabarti RR, North WRS et al. Haemostatic function and ischaemic heart disease: principal results of the Northwick Park heart study. *Lancet* 1986; **2**: 533–537.

39 Meade TW. The epidemiology of haemostatic and other variables in coronary artery disease. In: Verstraete M, Vermylen J, Lijnen R, Arnout J, eds. *Thrombosis and haemostasis*. Leuven, Netherlands: Leuven University Press, 1987; 36–66.

40 Koenig W, Sund WKM, Lowe GDO, Lee AJ, Resch KL, Tunstall-Pedoe H, et al. Geographical variations in plasma viscosity and relation to coronary event rates. *Lancet* 1994; **344**: 711–714.

41 Wilhelmsen L, Svardsudd K, Korsan-Bengtsen K, Larsson B, Welin L, Tibblin G. Fibrinogen as a risk factor for stroke and myocardial infarction. *N Engl J Med* 1984; **311**: 501–505.

42 Kannel WB, Wolf PA, Castelli WP, D'Agostino RB. Fibrinogen and risk of cardiovascular disease. *J Am Med Assoc* 1987; **258**: 1183–1186.

43 Yarnell JWG, Baker IA, Sweetnam PM, Bainton D, O'Brien JR, Whitehead PJ et al. Fibrinogen, viscosity, and white blood cell count are major risk factors for ischemic heart disease. *Circulation* 1991; **83**: 836–844.

44 Ernst E, Resch KL. Fibrinogen as a cardiovascular risk factor: a meta-analysis and review of the literature. *Ann Intern Med* 1993; **118**: 956–963.

45 Brozovic M. Physiological mechanisms in coagulation and fibrinolysis. *Br Med Bull* 1977; **33**: 231–238.

46 Brunner EJ, Marmot MG, White IR, O'Brien JR, Etherington MD, Slavin BM et al. Gender and employment grade differences in blood cholesterol, apolipoproteins and haemostatic factors in the Whitehall 11 study. *Atherosclerosis* 1993; **102**: 195–207.

47 Miller GJ, Martin JC, Webster J, Wilkes H, Miller NE, Wilkinson WH et al. Association between dietary fat intake and plasma factor VII coagulant activity – a predictor of cardiovascular mortality. *Atherosclerosis* 1986; **60**: 269–277.

48 Miller GJ, Cruickshank JK, Ellis LJ, Thompson RL, Wilkes HC, Stirling Y et al. Fat consumption and factor VII coagulant activity in middle-aged men. An association between a dietary and thrombogenic coronary risk factor. *Atherosclerosis* 1989; **78**: 19–24.

49 Barker DJP, Meade TW, Fall CHD, Lee A, Osmond C, Phipps K, et al. Relation of fetal and infant growth to plasma fibrinogen and factor VII concentrations in adult life. *Br Med J* 1992; **304**: 148–152.

50 Eliasson M, Evrin PE, Lundblad D. Fibrinogen and fibrinolytic variables in relation to anthropometry, lipids and blood pressure. The northern Sweden Monica Study. *J Clin Epidemiol* 1994; **47**: 513–524.

51 Brunner E, Davey Smith G, Marmot M, Canner R, Beksinska M, O'Brien J. Childhood social circumstances and psychosocial and behavioural factors as determinants of plasma fibrinogen. *Lancet* 1996; **347**: 1008–1013.

52 Andrew M, Paes B, Johnston M. Development of the hemostatic system in the neonate and young infant. *Am J Pediatr Hematol Oncol* 1990; **12**: 95–104.

53 Holmes GE, Miller HC, Hassanein K, Lansky SB, Goggin JE. Postnatal somatic growth in infants with atypical fetal growth patterns. *Am J Dis Child* 1977; **131**: 1078–1083.

54 Villar J, Smeriglio V, Martorell R, Brown CH, Klein RE. Heterogeneous growth and mental development of intrauterine growth-retarded infants during the first 3 years of life. *Pediatrics* 1984; **74**: 783–791.

55 Marmot MG, Shipley MJ, Rose G. Inequalities in death – specific explanations of a general pattern? *Lancet* 1984; **i**: 1003–1006.

56 Waaler HT. Height, weight and mortality. The Norwegian experience. *Acta Med Scand (Suppl)* 1984; **679**: 1–56.

57 Notkola V. *Living conditions in childhood and coronary heart disease in adulthood*. Helsinki: Finnish Society of Sciences and Letters, 1985.

6

Non-insulin-dependent diabetes and obesity

Non-insulin-dependent diabetes increases the risk of coronary heart disease and is associated with hypertension.[1, 2] Insulin has a central role in fetal growth, and disorders of glucose and insulin metabolism are therefore an obvious possible link between early growth and cardiovascular disease.[3] Although obesity and a sedentary lifestyle are known to be important in the development of non-insulin-dependent diabetes, they seem to lead to the disease only in predisposed individuals. Family and twin studies have suggested that the predisposition is familial, but the nature of this predisposition is unknown. The disease tends to be transmitted through the maternal rather than paternal side of the family.[4] Chapter 2 described how low protein diets given to pregnant rats, and increased maternal plasma glucose concentrations, both cause major changes in the structure and function of the offspring's pancreatic beta cells (p. 28). In the human fetus growth retardation is associated with reduced numbers of beta cells and reduced insulin secretion, while gestational diabetes leads to hyperinsulinaemia.[5–7] This chapter describes studies of the relationship between fetal growth and diabetes which have led to a new explanation of the origins of the disease, the so-called 'thrifty phenotype' hypothesis.[8]

LOW BIRTHWEIGHT AND DIABETES

Table 6.1 shows the results of a study in which 370 men in Hertfordshire were given a standard oral glucose challenge.[9] Plasma glucose concentrations 2 hours after ingestion of glucose were used to identify men with diabetes (plasma glucose $\geq$ 11.1 mmol/l) or the precursor disorder, impaired glucose tolerance (plasma glucose 7.8–11.0 mmol/l). The percentage of men with either disorder fell progressively between those with the lowest and highest birthweights. The differences in prevalence were threefold and the differences in relative risk, taking account of current body mass, were sevenfold. Trends with weight at 1 year were similar to those with birthweight (Table 6.2). In each social class and at each level of body mass, there was the same relationship between low weight gain in utero and during infancy, and impaired glucose tolerance 60 years later.

Table 6.1 Percentages of men aged 64 years with impaired glucose tolerance (2-hour glucose 7.8–11.0 mmol/l) or diabetes (2-hour glucose ≥ 11.1 mmol/l) according to birthweight

Birthweight, lb (kg)	No. of men	Percentage of men with 2-hour glucose (mmol/l) of:			Odds ratio adjusted for body mass index (95% CI)
		7.8–11.0	≥11.1	≥7.8	
≤5.5 (2.5)	20	30	10	40	6.6 (1.5–28)
–6.5 (2.9)	47	21	13	34	4.8 (1.3–17)
–7.5 (3.4)	104	25	6	31	4.6 (1.4–16)
–8.5 (3.9)	117	15	7	22	2.6 (0.8–8.9)
–9.5 (4.3)	54	4	9	13	1.4 (0.3–5.6)
>9.5 (4.3)	28	14	0	14	1.0
All	370	18	7	25	p value for trend <0.001

CI, confidence interval.

Among women in Hertfordshire there were both similarities to the men and differences in the associations between early growth and glucose–insulin metabolism.[10] Similarly to men the prevalence of non-insulin-dependent diabetes and 2-hour plasma glucose and insulin concentrations fell with increasing birthweight. In contrast to men fasting glucose and insulin concentrations were higher in women who had low birthweight, whereas they were unrelated to birthweight in men. An interpretation of this is that in women low birthweight is more strongly associated with insulin resistance than it is in men. Women also differed from men in that weight at 1 year of age was not associated with impaired glucose tolerance or non-insulin-dependent diabetes, which is consistent with the lack of an association between low weight at 1 year and death rates from coronary heart disease in women[11] (Ch. 3).

Table 6.3 shows the plasma glucose concentrations at 2 hours with the men divided into approximate thirds according to weight at 1 year of age and adult body mass index. The values rise from 5.8 mmol/l, in men with the highest weights at 1 year of age and lowest body mass indices, to 7.7 mmol/l in men with the lowest weights at 1 year and highest body mass indices. Fetal and

Table 6.2 Percentages of men aged 64 years with impaired glucose tolerance or diabetes according to weight at 1 year.

Weight at 1 year, lb (kg)	No. of men	Percentage of men with 2-hour glucose (mmol/l) of:			Odds ratio adjusted for body mass index (95% CI)
		7.8–11.0	≥11.1	≥7.8	
≤18 (8.2)	23	26	17	43	8.2 (1.8–38)
–20 (9.1)	63	21	11	32	4.8 (1.2–19)
–22 (10.0)	107	22	7	30	4.2 (1.1–16)
–24 (10.9)	105	13	5	18	2.1 (0.5–7.9)
–26 (11.8)	48	13	6	19	2.1 (0.5–9.0)
>26 (11.8)	24	13	0	13	1.0 —
All	370	18	7	25	p value for trend < 0.001

CI, confidence interval

Table 6.3 Mean plasma glucose 2 hours after 75-g oral glucose load, according to weight at 1 year and adult body mass index, in men aged 64 years

Adult body mass index, kg/m²	Weight at 1 year in lb (kg)			
	≤21.5 (9.8)	–23.5 (10.7)	>23.5 (10.7)	All
≤25.4	6.6 (45)	6.1 (39)	5.8 (36)	6.2 (120)
–28	6.7 (47)	6.9 (44)	5.9 (36)	6.5 (127)
>28	7.7 (39)	7.4 (43)	6.6 (41)	7.2 (123)
All	7.0 (131)	6.8 (126)	6.1 (113)	6.6 (370)

Figures in parentheses are numbers of men.

infant growth therefore protect against the deleterious effect of higher body mass in adult life and, conversely, lower body mass protects against the deleterious effect of reduced early growth. Of the men whose birthweight and weight at 1 year of age were below the median, and whose body mass indices were above the median, 41% had impaired glucose tolerance or diabetes. Only 6% of men who were above the median for early weights and below the median for body mass index were affected.

In the Hertfordshire study the only recorded measurement of body size at birth was birthweight; the study was therefore repeated among the men and women in Preston.[12] Again the prevalence of non-insulin-dependent diabetes and impaired glucose tolerance fell with increasing birthweight, from 27% in those with birthweight of 5.5 lb (2.5 kg) or less to 6% in those with birthweight of 7.5 lb (3.4 kg) or more. After allowing for differences in current body mass, the relative risks fell from 6.4 to 1.0. The trends in plasma glucose and insulin concentrations were similar to those in Hertfordshire. They were little changed by adjustments for duration of gestation, and therefore reflected differences in fetal growth rates. In Preston both thin (Fig. 3.9) and short babies (Fig. 3.10) developed impaired glucose tolerance and diabetes, and the disorders were also associated with an increased placental weight:birthweight ratio, suggesting a link with fetal undernutrition (p. 70).

In Uppsala, Sweden, Lithell and colleagues confirmed the association between non-insulin-dependent diabetes and thinness at birth.[13] The prevalence of diabetes was three times higher (relative odds by logistic regression 4.4) among men in the lowest fifth of ponderal index at birth (Table 6.4). This was a stronger association than that with birthweight; the prevalence of diabetes being only twice as high among men in the lowest fifth of birthweight.

A number of other studies have confirmed the association between birthweight and non-insulin-dependent diabetes. In the Health Professionals Study, USA, the odds ratio for diabetes, after adjusting for current body mass, was 1.9 among men whose birthweights were less than 5.5 lb (2.5 kg) compared with those who weighed 7–8.5 lb (3.2–3.9 kg).[14] Among the Pima Indians, USA, the odds ratio for diabetes was 3.8 in men and women who had weighed less than 5.5 lb (2.5 kg) at birth.[15] Among pregnant women in Liverpool, England, plasma glucose concentrations at 2 hours in a standard glucose tolerance test fell between those who had had low and high birthweight.[16]

Table 6.4 Prevalence of non-insulin-dependent diabetes by ponderal index at birth among 60-year-old men in Uppsala, Sweden

Ponderal index at birth, kg/m³	No. of men	Prevalence of diabetes, %
<24.2	193	11.9
24.2–	193	5.2
25.9–	196	3.6
27.4–	188	4.3
≥29.4	201	3.5
All	971	5.7
p value for trend		0.001

HIGH BIRTHWEIGHT AND DIABETES

In the Hertfordshire and Preston studies 2-hour plasma glucose concentrations fell progressively up to the highest birthweights. As mothers with diabetes in pregnancy tend to have large babies one might expect some large babies to show evidence of impaired glucose metabolism. This effect may not be apparent in the two studies because the number of such babies may be small in relation to the number of babies who are heavy through good fetal nutrition and for other reasons. Among the Pima Indians in the USA, however, among whom diabetes in pregnancy is unusually common, young men and women with birthweights over 9.9 lb (4.5 kg) had an increased prevalence of non-insulin-dependent diabetes.[15] The association between birthweight and non-insulin-dependent diabetes was therefore U-shaped. The increased risk of diabetes among babies with high birthweights was associated with maternal diabetes in pregnancy. The previous chapter (Table 5.3) described another 'U-shaped' distribution, that of coronary heart disease with abdominal circumference at birth in Sheffield.[17] The association between coronary heart disease and large abdominal circumference at birth is thought to reflect the accelerated liver growth of babies whose mothers had impaired glucose tolerance in pregnancy.

High birthweight is also associated with insulin-dependent, childhood onset diabetes. In a large study of diabetic children in Sweden the relative risk rose progressively from 0.81 in those who were small for gestational age to 1.20 in those who were large.[18] This was unchanged if children whose mothers had diabetes in pregnancy were excluded. The mechanisms underlying this association are largely unknown.

FAMINE AND DIABETES

The brief but severe famine in western Holland during the Second World War has given a novel insight into the effects of mothers' diet in pregnancy on non-insulin-dependent diabetes.[19] The period of famine was clearly delineated, for it began abruptly in late November 1944 and ended with liberation by the Allied Forces in early May 1945. The official rations varied between 400 and 800 calories per day in the first months of 1945. The effects on fetal growth, which were modest, are described in Chapter 8. Van der Meulin and colleagues (Table 8.1) traced and examined a sample of 702 babies born in Amsterdam around the time of the famine.[19] Babies were considered to have been exposed to famine in utero if the average maternal daily food ration during any 13-week period of gestation was below 1000 calories. They were divided into those exposed in late gestation, whose mothers were pregnant when the famine began, those exposed in mid- or early gestation, and those who were conceived and born before or after the famine.

Figure 6.1 shows that men and women who were exposed to famine at any stage of gestation had higher plasma glucose concentrations 2 hours after a standard glucose load. They also had higher fasting proinsulin and 2-hour plasma insulin concentrations, which suggests that their poor glucose tolerance was mainly determined by insulin resistance. Glucose tolerance was most affected in people whose mothers were thin, who were exposed to famine in mid- or late gestation, and who became obese as adults.

Although, consistently with other studies, the people born in Amsterdam who had low birthweight had raised 2-hour plasma glucose concentrations, the effects of famine were largely independent of this. One explanation is that the fetus' initial adaptation to undernutrition is to alter its metabolism, including its glucose–insulin metabolism, and continue to grow. Only if this adaptation fails does it reduce its rate of growth. Whatever the explanation, the findings from the Dutch famine are important because they provide direct evidence that undernutrition in utero programs non-insulin-dependent diabetes, and they show that the mother's dietary intakes during pregnancy can program metabolism without altering size at birth.

A study of 169 men and women who were in utero during the siege of Leningrad in 1941–44 did not find any alterations in glucose–insulin

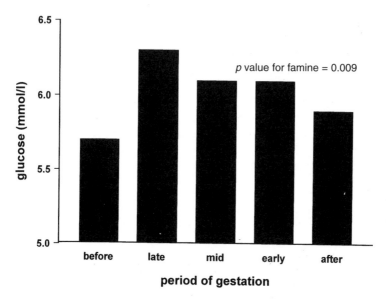

Fig. 6.1 Two-hour plasma glucose concentrations in 702 men and women exposed to famine in utero at different periods of gestation (see text).

metabolism. This study is, however, difficult to interpret because it lacks data on exposure – there being no information on the size of the babies at birth or the weight of their mothers.[20, 21]

INSULIN RESISTANCE

Both deficiency in insulin production and insulin resistance are thought to be important in the pathogenesis of non-insulin-dependent diabetes.[22] There is evidence that both may be determined in fetal life.

Men and women with low birthweight have a high prevalence of the 'insulin resistance syndrome', in which impaired glucose tolerance, hypertension and raised serum triglyceride concentrations occur in the same patient. The patients are insulin-resistant and have hyperinsulinaemia. Table 6.5 shows results for a sample of the men in the Hertfordshire study. The prevalence of the syndrome falls progressively from 30% in men who weighed 5.5 lb (2.5 kg) or less at birth to 6% in those who weighed 9.5 lb (4.3 kg) or more.[23] A study in Preston gave similar results, and showed a similar relationship in men and women.[23] The association with low birthweight was independent of the duration of gestation and therefore depended on low rates of fetal growth.

A recent study in San Antonio, Texas, confirmed the association in a different ethnic group. In 30-year-old Mexican-Americans and non-Hispanic white people, those with lower birthweight had a higher prevalence of the insulin resistance syndrome.[24] Among men and women in the lowest third of the birthweight distribution and the highest third of current body mass, 25% had the syndrome. By contrast none of the people in the highest third of birthweight and lowest third of current body mass had it. A study of young adults in the city of Haguenau, France showed that those who had had intrauterine growth retardation had raised plasma insulin concentrations when fasting and after a standard glucose challenge.[25] They did not show any of the other abnormalities that occur in the insulin resistance syndrome. An interpretation of this is that insulin resistance is a primary abnormality to which other changes are secondary.

These findings point to a link between impaired fetal growth and insulin resistance in later life. Phillips and colleagues[26] carried out insulin tolerance tests on 103 men and women in Preston. Table 6.6 shows the findings, with

Table 6.5 Prevalence of the insulin resistance syndrome in men aged 64 years according to birthweight

Birthweight, lb (kg)	No. of men	Percentage with insulin resistance syndrome	Odds ratio adjusted for body mass index (95% CI)
≤5.5 (2.5)	20	30	18 (2.6–118)
–6.5 (2.9)	54	19	8.4 (1.5–49)
–7.5 (3.4)	114	17	8.5 (1.5–46)
–8.5 (3.9)	123	12	4.9 (0.9–27)
–9.5 (4.3)	64	6	2.2 (0.3–14)
>9.5 (4.3)	32	6	1.0
All	407	14	p value for trend <0.001

CI, confidence interval

Table 6.6 Mean insulin resistance (half-life of blood glucose in minutes) in men and women aged 50 years according to ponderal index at birth and adult body mass

Ponderal index at birth, kg/m³	Body mass index, kg/m²				
	≤ 24.0	– 26.0	– 28.0	> 28.0	All
≤20.6	17.9 (8)	18.0 (8)	23.1 (4)	30.7 (6)	20.6 (26)
–22.3	15.8 (16)	17.3 (11)	17.8 (6)	27.1 (4)	17.3 (37)
–25.0	14.4 (8)	20.7 (4)	21.0 (3)	20.4 (8)	17.9 (23)
>25.0	14.1 (4)	16.1 (4)	17.8 (3)	18.5 (6)	16.6 (17)
All	15.6 (36)	17.7 (27)	19.5 (16)	22.6 (24)	18.0 (103)

Figures in parentheses are numbers of people.

insulin resistance expressed as the time taken for the plasma glucose concentration to fall to half its initial value after intravenous injection of insulin. The men and women are subdivided according to ponderal index at birth and current body mass index. At each body mass resistance was greater in people who had a low ponderal index at birth. Conversely at each ponderal index resistance was greater in those with high body mass, and the greatest mean resistance was therefore in those with low ponderal index at birth but high current body mass.

Insulin resistance and mother's body mass

The remarkable birth records kept at the Peking Union Medical College Hospital, in Beijing (Fig. 4.3) have extended our understanding of the fetal origins of insulin resistance, because they include information on the mother's height and weight. As in other studies, men and women born in the hospital who had low birthweight and were thin at birth had raised 2-hour plasma glucose and insulin concentrations (unpublished). Table 6.7 shows that the 2-hour plasma glucose and insulin concentrations, and triglyceride concentrations, were also raised in people whose mothers had a low body mass index in

Table 6.7 Plasma glucose, insulin, and triglyceride concentrations in Chinese men and women aged 45 years according to mother's body mass index (BMI) in late pregnancy

	Mother's body mass in late pregnancy, kg/m²					
	≤23.2 (146)	–24.6 (146)	–26.1 (147)	>26.1 (146)	All (585)	p for trend
Fasting glucose, mmol/l	5.29	5.40	5.41	5.37	5.37	NS
120-min glucose, mmol/l	6.92	6.55	6.64	6.26	6.59	0.004
Fasting insulin, pmol/l	43.0	45.6	41.9	41.0	42.8	NS
120-min insulin, pmol/l	259	252	256	207	243	0.005
Fasting triglyceride, mmol/l	1.30	1.32	1.29	1.15	1.26	0.09

Figures in parentheses are numbers of people. NS, not significant.
Adjusted for sex and body mass index.

Table 6.8 Plasma glucose, insulin, and triglyceride concentrations in Chinese men and women aged 45 years according to mother's body mass index (BMI) in early pregnancy

	Mother's body mass in early pregnancy, kg/m²					
	≤ 19.2 (56)	−20.5 (57)	−22.3 (57)	> 22.3 (56)	All (226)	p for trend
Fasting glucose, mmol/l	5.15	5.30	5.28	5.27	5.25	0.2
120-min glucose, mmol/l	7.37	6.95	7.07	5.59	6.72	0.03
Fasting insulin, pmol/l	48.7	50.1	40.7	39.8	44.6	0.05
120-min insulin, pmol/l	399	300	253	182	273	0.04
Fasting triglyceride, mmol/l	1.56	1.38	1.11	1.07	1.26	0.09

Figures in parentheses are numbers of people.
Adjusted for sex and body mass index.

late pregnancy. About half of the mothers also had their body mass index in early pregnancy recorded. Table 6.8 shows that the results were similar, other than the trend for fasting insulin which became statistically significant. These findings suggest that children of thin mothers become insulin-resistant.

Mechanisms

The processes that link thinness at birth with insulin resistance in adult life are not known. Babies born at term with a low ponderal index have a reduced mid-upper arm circumference, which implies that they have a low muscle bulk as well as less subcutaneous fat.[27] It is therefore possible that thinness at birth is associated with abnormalities in muscle structure and function which develop in mid-gestation and persist into adult life, interfering with insulin's ability to promote glucose uptake. Magnetic resonance spectroscopy studies show that people who were thin at birth have lower rates of glycolysis and glycolytic ATP (adenosine triphosphate) production during exercise.[28] In response to undernutrition a fetus may reduce its metabolic dependence on glucose and increase oxidation of other substrates, including amino acids and lactate (Fig. 8.2). This has led to the hypothesis that a glucose-sparing metabolism persists into adult life, and that insulin resistance arises as a consequence of similar processes, possibly because of reduced rates of glucose oxidation in insulin-sensitive peripheral tissues.

When the availability of nutrients to the fetus is restricted concentrations of anabolic hormones, including insulin and insulin-like growth factor 1 fall, while catabolic hormones, including glucocorticoids rise (Fig. 8.2). Persisting hormonal changes could underlie the development of insulin resistance. Experiments in rats (p. 29) show that hypothalamic–pituitary–adrenal responses are readily programmed in utero. Growth retarded human fetuses also have persisting changes in the growth hormone–IGF axis. Glucocorticoids and growth hormone are both powerful regulators of glucose metabolism. Bjorntorp has postulated that glucocorticoids, growth hormone and sex steroids may play a major role in the evolution of the metabolic syndrome.[29] Table 4.7 shows suggestive evidence that circulating concentrations of glucocorticoids are programmed in utero in humans. Among men in Hertfordshire plasma cortisol concentrations in fasting blood samples fell steeply between those with low and high birthweight. Higher plasma cortisol concentrations were associated with raised two-hour plasma glucose concentrations and insulin resistance.[30]

Recent advances in assay methodology make it possible to measure specifically plasma concentrations of the precursor of insulin, 32–33 split proinsulin.[30, 31] Higher concentrations are found in people who had low birthweight and low weight at 1 year.[9] The significance of raised plasma split proinsulin concentrations remains unclear but they are thought to indicate both insulin resistance and pancreatic beta cell dysfunction.

INSULIN DEFICIENCY

Infants who are small for dates have fewer beta cells.[6] There are conflicting reports on whether the beta-cell mass is reduced in patients with non-insulin-dependent diabetes.[31] In one study, however, in which diabetic patients were compared with people of the same weight, their beta-cell mass was found to be lower.[32] As a working hypothesis it seems reasonable to propose that nutritional and other factors determining fetal and infant growth influence the size and function of the adult pancreatic beta-cell complement. Whether and when non-insulin-dependent diabetes supervenes will be determined by the rate of attrition of beta cells with ageing, and by the development of insulin resistance, of which obesity is an important determinant.

Phillips and colleagues[33] measured insulin secretion following intravenous infusion of glucose in 103 men and women in Preston. The insulin response was not related to birthweight or other measurements at birth. This argues against a link between reduced fetal growth and insulin deficiency in adult life. Similarly a study of men in Stockholm found no association between birthweight and insulin responses to infused glucose.[34] Birth length and other measures of birth size were not available in that study. There was, however, an association between short stature and a low insulin response. It is possible that insulin resistance in adult life changes insulin secretion and obscures associations with fetal growth. Studies of younger people may resolve this: a study of men aged 21 years by Robinson and colleagues[35] showed that those with lower birthweight had reduced plasma insulin concentrations at 30 minutes. Another study of men of similar age showed that a low insulin response to glucose was associated with a high placental weight and a high ratio of placental weight to birthweight. This study also confirmed the association between low insulin secretion and short stature.[36] In contrast a study of young Pima Indians showed that those with low birthweight had evidence of insulin resistance but no defect in insulin secretion.[37]

Non-insulin-dependent diabetes in India

In Mysore, south India, men and women with non-insulin-dependent diabetes showed signs of both insulin resistance and insulin deficiency.[38] The high prevalence of central obesity, insulin resistance and non-insulin-dependent diabetes in people from south India living in Britain has been remarked on.[39, 40] The study of men and women born in the Holdsworth Memorial Hospital, Mysore,

(p. 58) showed this again. Those who had non-insulin-dependent diabetes also had a low insulin increment after a standard challenge, indicating that they were insulin-deficient as well as resistant. Whereas, however, insulin resistance was associated with low birthweight, non-insulin-dependent diabetes was associated with stunting at birth in relation to birthweight, that is a high ponderal index, and with maternal adiposity.

These findings led to a novel explanation for the epidemic of non-insulin-dependent diabetes in urban and migrant Indian populations (Fig. 6.2).[38] Widespread fetal undernutrition predisposes the Indian population to insulin resistance. On moving to cities people's levels of physical activity diminish. Young women, no longer required to do agricultural work, or walk long distances to fetch water and firewood, become fatter and therefore more insulin-resistant. They are therefore unable to maintain glucose homeostasis during pregnancy, even at relatively low levels of obesity, and become hyperglycaemic, though not necessarily diabetic. It is known that high plasma glucose concentrations within the normal range influence fetal growth and lead to macrosomia.[41] Figure 6.2 proposes that the fetuses become 'macrosomic', having a high ponderal index at birth, and impaired pancreatic beta-cell development which leads to insulin deficiency. Thus non-insulin-dependent diabetes in urban India reflects programmed insulin deficiency in the offspring of women rendered highly insulin-resistant by a combination of fetal undernutrition and urbanisation.

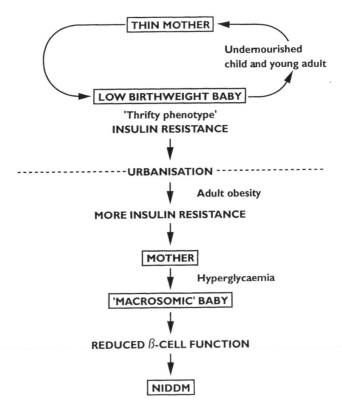

Fig. 6.2 A model to explain the epidemic of non-insulin-dependent diabetes (NIDDM) in urban India.

Findings in adults lead to the conclusion that fetal undernutrition gives rise to insulin resistance and also impairs the function of the endocrine pancreas. Surveys of young adults in Britain and the USA have shown similar relationships between reduced glucose tolerance and low birthweight as are seen in older adults.[24, 35–37] They raise the question as to whether these relationships could be demonstrated in children. This would be further evidence that the pathogenesis of non-insulin-dependent diabetes is set in train in fetal life, and would show that metabolism is already impaired within a few years of birth.

A total of 250 7-year-old children in Salisbury, England, who had taken part in a study of blood pressure at the age 4 years (p. 70), were still living in the district and were willing to take part in a study of glucose tolerance.[42] The test was not continued beyond 30 minutes after a standard oral glucose load. Children who had been the heaviest babies had the lowest plasma glucose concentrations at 30 minutes, although there was no trend from the lowest to the highest birthweight groups. Ponderal index at birth was more strongly related to 30-minute glucose. Table 6.9 shows that boys and girls who were thinnest at birth had the highest 30-minute glucose concentrations, and the highest blood pressures.[42]

Whincup and colleagues studied an older group of British children, aged 10–11 years, and found that those who had lower birthweight had raised plasma insulin concentrations, both fasting and after oral glucose.[43] This is consistent with the association between low birthweight and insulin resistance. Among these children, however, the plasma glucose concentrations of those who had low birthweight were unaltered, which implies that despite being insulin-resistant they were able to maintain glucose homeostasis. In contrast, Yajnik and colleagues found that 4-year-old Indian children who had low birthweight had raised plasma glucose and insulin concentrations (Table 6.10),

Table 6.9 Mean plasma glucose concentrations at 30 minutes and mean systolic pressures in 7-year-old children in England, by ponderal index at birth

Ponderal index, kg/m³	Mean plasma glucose concentration (mmol/l) at 30 minutes			Mean systolic pressure at 4 years, mmHg*
	Boys	Girls	All	
≤23.0	8.35 (24)	8.64 (22)	8.49 (46)	107 (46)
–25.0	8.18 (20)	8.16 (21)	8.17 (41)	107 (40)
–27.5	8.35 (29)	8.18 (29)	8.27 (58)	105 (57)
>27.5	7.61 (28)	8.27 (33)	7.97 (61)	103 (61)
All	8.11 (101)	8.30 (105)	8.21 (206)	105 (204)
SD	1.54	1.58	1.57	9
p value for trend			0.04	0.05

Figures in parentheses are numbers of children.
* After adjustment for weight at 4 years. SD, standard deviation.

Table 6.10 Mean 30-minute plasma glucose and insulin concentrations among 4-year-old children in India

Birthweight, kg (lb)	Number of children	Plasma glucose at 30 minutes, mmol/l	Plasma insulin at 30 minutes, pmol/l	Ratio of 30-minute insulin/glucose
≤2.4 (5.3)	36	8.1	321	4.4
–2.6 (5.7)	36	8.3	337	4.4
–2.8 (6.2)	44	7.8	309	4.3
–3.0 (6.6)	42	7.9	298	4.2
>3.0 (6.6)	43	7.5	289	4.2
All	201	7.9	310	4.3
p value for trend		0.01*	0.04†	0.08

* Allowing for the children's current weight.
† Allowing for the children's age, sex and current weight.

suggesting that at the levels of poor fetal growth and insulin resistance which prevail in India even young children are unable to maintain glucose homeostasis.[44] These findings in children provide further support for the hypothesis that non-insulin-dependent diabetes originates from impaired development in utero and that the seeds of diabetes in the next generation have already been sown and are apparent in today's children.

In the Salisbury study there were interesting differences in the associations of the two insulin precursors, proinsulin and 32–33 split proinsulin, with size at birth. Plasma concentrations of both precursors rose with increasing current weight, but split proinsulin concentrations, which were high in comparison with those found in adults, also rose with decreasing length at birth. One possibility is that this association reflects the effects of fetal undernutrition in late gestation, with consequent reduction in linear growth and failure of pancreatic development. Forrester and colleagues found an association between stunting at birth and reduced glucose tolerance among children in Jamaica, in whom the serum glycated haemoglobin levels rose progressively between those who were 52 cm (20.5 in) or more in length at birth and those who were 46 cm (18.1 in) or less.[45]

THE 'THRIFTY PHENOTYPE' HYPOTHESIS

The associations between body size at birth and impaired glucose tolerance in adults and children led Hales to propose what has been called the 'thrifty phenotype' hypothesis.[8] According to this hypothesis insulin resistance and deficiency are the outcome of the undernourished fetus and infant having to be nutritionally thrifty. For as long as an individual remains undernourished in postnatal life its glucose–insulin metabolism is adequate. A sudden move to over- or good nutrition, however, exposes the deficiencies in beta-cell function and tissue sensitivity, and non-insulin-dependent diabetes results. The 'thrifty phenotype' hypothesis is shown diagrammatically by Figure 6.3 which also outlines how the features of the insulin-resistance syndrome may originate in failure of early development. The hypothesis demands a reinterpretation of

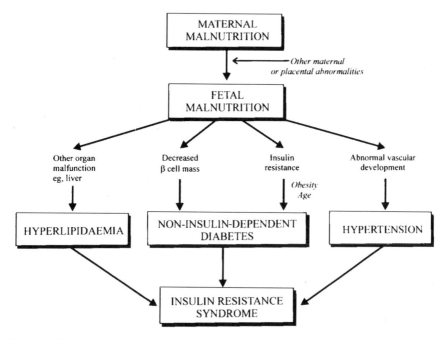

Fig. 6.3 The fetal origins of non-insulin-dependent diabetes and insulin resistance syndrome: the 'thrifty phenotype' hypothesis.

some data and explains other observations which at present are not easy to understand.

GEOGRAPHICAL VARIATIONS AND MIGRANT STUDIES

The prevalence of non-insulin-dependent diabetes varies in different countries and in different parts of the same country. Rates tend to be lower in places that have retained a traditional lifestyle, for example rural Africa, where the prevalence in adults is between 1 and 2%, or the highlands of Papua New Guinea, where there was a complete absence of diabetes in one survey.[46, 47] Prevalences in European and white North American populations are typically around 5% among adults.[48] Populations exposed to rapid westernisation have a higher prevalence than European populations. The highest known prevalences occur in North American and western Pacific societies where up to one-third of the adult population may be affected. The best studied of these are the Pima Indians and the Nauruan islanders.[49, 50]

The proposal that the disease is the outcome of reduced early growth is consistent with these geographical variations. If undernutrition during fetal life and infancy results in insensitivity to insulin and impaired function of the beta cells, later overnutrition may expose the impaired function and lead to diabetes. A rapid transition from subsistence to overnutrition could explain the high diabetes rate in the Nauruan islanders. These people suffered severe nutritional deficiency before and during the Second World War. After the war they suddenly became affluent as a result of phosphate mining, and diabetes became epidemic on the island, affecting 30% of the adult population.

A similarly sudden transition occurred when Ethiopian Jews were transported to Israel during one of the recent famines in Ethiopia. After only 4 years 9% of those under 30 years had developed non-insulin-dependent diabetes.[51]

GENETIC EFFECTS

Evidence for a genetic aetiology of non-insulin-dependent diabetes comes from twin studies and studies of family pedigrees. Three studies of twin pairs, two in the USA and one in the UK,[52–54] found a higher concordance rate in monozygotic twins when the age of onset in the proband was more than 40 years, that is, the diabetes was non-insulin-dependent. Although two of these studies are likely to have been affected by serious ascertainment bias, the most recent study was carried out using a population-based sample of twins identified from military records.[54] Twin pairs were examined twice, at a mean age of 47 years and then at 57 years. At the first examination, when the prevalence rate was 5.7%, there was no difference in concordance rates between monozygotic and dizygotic twins. However, 10 years later the disease prevalence rate was 13% and the concordance rate in monozygotic twins was 58.3%, compared with 17.4% in dizygotic twins.

One of the largest studies of the familial aggregation of non-insulin-dependent diabetes was based on 3117 patients in Canada.[55] The risk of the disease was increased between two- and fourfold in the siblings of these patients.[55] Findings in the Whitehall surveys of civil servants were similar.[56] In populations with a higher prevalence of glucose intolerance, familial clustering of the disease is even more marked. Thus in the Nauruan islanders, glucose intolerance develops in approximately 40% of the offspring of two diabetic parents, in 6% of offspring if one parent is diabetic, and in none of the children if the parents have normal glucose tolerance.[57] The observations of familial clustering of diabetes, a high concordance rate in monozygotic twins, and the high prevalence rate in communities that have abandoned their traditional lifestyle and adopted a western diet led Neel to suggest the 'thrifty genotype' hypothesis.[58] He proposed that genes existed which gave a survival advantage in harsh conditions when food was scarce. In times of plenty, however, the same genes were detrimental, leading to obesity and glucose intolerance. In the absence of any information about the particular genes involved this hypothesis remains wholly speculative. The evidence presented here raises a question about the interpretation of family and twin data as evidence for genetic inheritance. As maternal physique and nutrition have such a strong influence on fetal and infant growth (Ch. 8), the reason for the familial clustering of diabetes may be that family members share a similar intrauterine environment (p. 129). A stronger maternal than paternal influence on the development of diabetes is consistent with this.[59] Likewise, a genetic interpretation of high concordance rates in monozygous twins may not be justifiable because identical twins share a more similar intrauterine environment, usually having a common placenta, whereas non-identical twins have separate placentas.[60]

Fetal growth of twins

Because the fetal growth of twins is retarded it has been suggested that they should have an increased risk of coronary heart disease and non-insulin-dependent diabetes.[61] Twins are heterogeneous, however, and are a mixture of proportionately and disproportionately small babies.[62] A group of twins might have low or high rates of coronary heart disease depending on whether they had predominately been proportionately or disproportionately small babies. Studies of the long-term effects of retarded growth caused by twinning will, however, be of interest aside from this issue. In a recent study of twins in Denmark, those with non-insulin-dependent diabetes had lower mean birthweight than their unaffected twin pairs, whether identical or non-identical.[63]

OBESITY

Excess body weight may be initiated or 'entrained' during critical periods in early life.[64] Critical periods, during which changes tend to be irreversible, may be distinguished from high risk periods which occur throughout life and are associated with reversible increases in body weight. Pregnancy or times of emotional stress illustrate high risk periods. There is evidence for three critical periods for body weight, prenatal, childhood and adolescence. Early observations on prenatal effects come from studies of men born at the time of the Dutch famine of 1944–45. Those who were conceived during the famine became obese as adults.[65] It is, however, difficult to interpret this because many mothers, presumably the thinner ones, were infertile during the famine, and the second half of gestation of the babies conceived during the famine occurred when food had become abundant. People who had high birthweight or were heavy during infancy also have an increased risk of obesity in later life, but the effect is small.[9, 66, 67]

People who had low birthweight tend to accumulate fat on the trunk and abdomen, a pattern of adiposity found in the insulin-resistance syndrome and associated with an increased risk of coronary heart disease.[68] Men in Hertfordshire who had low birthweight and low weight at 1 year had high ratios of waist to hip circumference.[69] Among 30-year-old Mexican and non-Hispanic Americans low birthweight was not associated with abdominal fat deposition, as measured by a high waist to hip ratio, but rather was associated with fat storage on the trunk, reflected in a high ratio of subscapular to triceps skinfold thickness.[24] At younger ages, skinfolds may be better indicators of regional fat distribution than waist to hip size. Among English girls aged 14–16 years those who were smallest at birth but fattest as teenagers had the highest ratio of subscapular to triceps skinfold.[70] Among children aged 7–12 years in Philadelphia, USA, there was a similar association between low birthweight and truncal fat deposition with partial correlations between birthweight and the ratio of triceps to suscapular skinfolds of around 0.20, after allowing for body mass index.[71] Associations between central fat distribution and birthweight occur across the range of birthweight. They were not found in a comparison between 15-year-olds who had low birthweight and controls within the normal birthweight range.[72] This could reflect aspects of body composition specific to babies weighing less than 5.5 lb (2.5 kg), since the low birthweight adolescents were markedly thinner than the controls. The difference in study design makes it difficult to compare this study with the others. The processes which link reduced fetal growth with increased central fat deposition are unknown; but sustained adrenal overactivity initiated by early growth restraint is one possibility.[73]

Obese children tend to become obese adults. One study showed that 80% of children who were overweight at around 12 years of age were still obese at around 30 years.[74] Entrainment of body weight during childhood may depend on behavioural influences that determine patterns of food intake and activity.[75] The transition from childhood to puberty seems to be important in establishing individual patterns of body fat distribution. At puberty a more central pattern of subcutaneous fat distribution is established in both boys and girls.[76] These changes are linked to changes in sex steroids. The extent to which hormonal changes in puberty are programmed in fetal life is not known, but a number of studies, including one of a national cohort of British girls, shows that low birthweight is associated with an earlier menarche (p. 187).[77] Hormonal changes during the menopause may also lead to another critical period for body weight regulation, which becomes impaired with ageing and fetal growth may again contribute to this since women who had lower birthweight have an earlier menopause (p. 187).[78]

Summary

Men and women who had low birthweight have increased rates of non-insulin-dependent diabetes and impaired glucose tolerance. People who were thin at birth, having a low muscle bulk, tend to become insulin-resistant and develop the insulin resistance syndrome: diabetes, hypertension and abnormal blood lipids. The 'thrifty phenotype' hypothesis offers a new explanation of the epidemiology of non-insulin-dependent diabetes. The hypothesis proposes that poor nutrition in fetal and early infant life is detrimental to the mechanisms that maintain carbohydrate tolerance. It may affect the structure and function of the beta cells of the islets of Langerhans, and may change the tissues, primarily muscle, which respond to insulin and as a consequence lead to insulin resistance. Although these early changes determine susceptibility to non-insulin-dependent diabetes, additional factors such as obesity, ageing and physical inactivity must also play a part in determining the time of onset and severity of the disease.

References

1 Fuller JH, Shipley MJ, Rose G, Jarrett RJ, Keen H. Coronary-heart-disease risk and impaired glucose tolerance. *Lancet* 1980; i: 1373–1376.

2 Modan M, Halkin H, Almog S, Lusky A, Eshkol A, Shefi M, et al. Hyperinsulinaemia: A link between hypertension, obesity and glucose intolerance. *J Clin Invest* 1985; 75: 809–817.

3 Fowden AL. The role of insulin in prenatal growth. *J Dev Physiol* 1989; 12: 173–182.

4 Mitchell BD, Valdez R, Hazuda HP, Haffner SM, Monterrosa A, Stern MP. Differences in prevalence of diabetes and impaired glucose tolerance according to maternal or paternal history of diabetes. *Diabetes Care* 1993; 16: 1262–1267.

5 Aerts L, Holemans K, Van Assche FA. Maternal diabetes during pregnancy: consequences for the offspring. *Diabetes Metab Rev* 1990; 6: 147–167.

6 Van Assche FA, Aerts L. The fetal endocrine pancreas. *Contrib Gynecol Obstet* 1979; 5: 44–57.

7 Van Assche FA, de Prins F, Aerts L, Verjans M. The endocrine pancreas in small-for-dates infants. *Br J Obstet Gynaecol* 1977; 84: 751–753.

8 Hales CN, Barker DJP. Type 2 (non-insulin-dependent) diabetes mellitus: the thrifty phenotype hypothesis. *Diabetologia* 1992; **35**: 595–601.

9 Hales CN, Barker DJP, Clark PMS, Cox LJ, Fall C, Osmond C, et al. Fetal and infant growth and impaired glucose tolerance at age 64. *Br Med J* 1991; **303**: 1019–1022.

10 Fall CHD, Osmond C, Barker DJP, Clark PMS, Hales CN, Stirling Y, et al. Fetal and infant growth and cardiovascular risk factors in women. *Br Med J* 1995; **310**: 428–432.

11 Osmond C, Barker DJP, Winter PD, Fall CHD, Simmonds SJ. Early growth and death from cardiovascular disease in women. *Br Med J* 1993; **307**: 1519–1524.

12 Phipps K, Barker DJP, Hales CN, Fall CHD, Osmond C, Clark PMS. Fetal growth and impaired glucose tolerance in men and women. *Diabetologia* 1993; **36**: 225–228.

13 Lithell HO, McKeigue PM, Berglund L, Mohsen R, Lithell UB, Leon DA. Relation of size at birth to non-insulin dependent diabetes and insulin concentrations in men aged 50–60 years. *Br Med J* 1996; **312**: 406–410.

14 Curhan GC, Willett WC, Rimm EB, Stampfer MJ. Birth weight and adult hypertension and diabetes mellitus in US men. *Am J Hypertens* 1996; **9**: 11A (Abstract)

15 McCance DR, Pettitt DJ, Hanson RL, Jacobsson LTH, Knowler WC, Bennett PH. Birth weight and non-insulin dependent diabetes: thrifty genotype, thrifty phenotype, or surviving small baby genotype? *Br Med J* 1994; **308**: 942–945.

16 Olah KS. Low maternal birthweight – an association with impaired glucose tolerance in pregnancy. *J Obstet Gynaecol* 1996; **16**: 5–8.

17 Barker DJP, Martyn CN, Osmond C, Wield GA. Abnormal liver growth in utero and death from coronary heart disease. *Br Med J* 1995; **310**: 703–704.

18 Dahlquist G, Sandberg Bennich S, Kallen B. Intrauterine growth pattern and risk of childhood onset insulin dependent (type 1) diabetes: population based case-control study. *BMJ* 1996; **313**: 1174–1177.

19 Ravelli ACJ, van der Meulen JHP, Michels RPJ, Osmond C, Barker DJP, Hales CN, et al. Glucose tolerance in adults after prenatal exposure to the Dutch famine. *Lancet* 1998; **351**: 173–177.

20 Stanner SA, Bulmer K, Andres C, Lantseva OE, Borodina V, Poteen VV, et al. Does malnutrition in utero determine diabetes and coronary heart disease in adulthood? Results from the Leningrad siege study, a cross sectional study. *Br Med J* 1997; **315**: 1342–1348.

21 Rich-Edwards JW, Gillman MW. Commentary: a hypothesis challenged, *Br Med J* 1997; **315**: 1348–1349.

22 DeFronzo RA. The triumvirate: beta cell, muscle, liver. A collusion responsible for NIDDM. *Diabetes* 1988; **37**: 667–687.

23 Barker DJP, Hales CN, Fall CHD, Osmond C, Phipps K, Clark PMS. Type 2 (non-insulin-dependent) diabetes mellitus, hypertension and hyperlipidaemia (Syndrome X): Relation to reduced fetal growth. *Diabetologia* 1993; **36**: 62–67.

24 Valdez R, Athens MA, Thompson GH, Bradshaw BS, Stern MP. Birthweight and adult health outcomes in a biethnic population in the USA. *Diabetologia* 1994; **37**: 624–631.

25 Leger J, Levy-Marchal C, Bloch J, Pinet A, Chevenne D, Porquet D, et al. Reduced final height and indications for insulin resistance in 20 year olds born small for gestational age: regional cohort study. *Br Med J* 1997; **315**: 341–347.

26 Phillips DIW, Barker DJP, Hales CN, Hirst S, Osmond C. Thinness at birth and insulin resistance in adult life. *Diabetologia* 1994; **37**: 150–154.

27 Robinson SM, Wheeler T, Hayes MC, Barker DJP, Osmond C. Fetal heart rate and intrauterine growth. *Br J Obstet Gynaecol* 1991; **98**: 1223–1227.

28 Taylor DJ, Thompson CH, Kemp GJ, Barnes PRJ, Sanderson AL, Radda GK, et al. A relationship between impaired fetal growth and reduced muscle glycolysis revealed by ^{31}P magnetic resonance spectroscopy. *Diabetologia* 1995; **38**: 1205–1212.

29 Bjorntorp P. Insulin resistance: the consequence of a neuroendocrine disturbance? *Int J Obesity* 1995; **19 (Suppl 1)**: S6–S10.

30 Phillips DIW, Barker DJP, Fall CHD, Seckl JR, Whorwood CB, Wood PJ, et al. Elevated plasma cortisol concentrations: a link between low birthweight and the insulin resistance syndrome? *J Clin Endocrinol Metab* 1998; (in press).

31 Hellerström C, Swenne I, Andersson A. Islet cell replication and diabetes. In: Lefevre PJ, Pipeleers DG, eds. *The pathology of the endocrine pancreas in diabetes*. Heidelberg: Springer, 1988; 141–170.

32 Kloppel G, Lohr M, Habich K, Oberholzer M, Heitz PU. Islet pathology and the pathogenesis of type 1 and type 2 diabetes mellitus revisited. *Surv Synth Path Res* 1985; **4**: 110–125.

33 Phillips DIW, Hirst S, Clark PMS, Hales CN, Osmond C. Fetal growth and insulin secretion in adult life. *Diabetologia* 1994; **37**: 592–596.

34 Alvarsson M, Efendic S, Grill VE. Insulin responses to glucose in healthy males are associated with adult height but not with birth weight. *J Intern Med* 1994; **236**: 275–279.

35 Robinson S, Walton RJ, Clark PM, Barker DJP, Hales CN, Osmond C. The relation of fetal growth to plasma glucose in young men. *Diabetologia* 1992; **35**: 444–446.

36 Wills J, Watson JM, Hales CN, Phillips DIW. The relation of fetal growth to insulin secretion in young men. *Diabet Med* 1996; **13**: 773–774.

37 Leger J, Levy-Marchal C, Block J, Pinet A, Benali K, Porquet D, et al. Evidence for insulin resistance developing in young adults with intra-uterine growth retardation. *Diabetologia* 1997; **40**: A53 (Abstract)

38 Fall CHD, Stein CE, Kumaran K, Cox V, Osmond C, Barker DJP, et al. Size at birth, maternal weight, and non-insulin dependent diabetes in South India. *Diabet Med* 1998; (in press).

39 Mather HM, Keen H. The Southall diabetes survey: prevalence of known diabetes in Asians and Europeans. *Br Med J* 1985; **291**: 1081–1084.

40 McKeigue PM, Shah B, Marmot MG. Relation of central obesity and insulin resistance with high diabetes prevalence and cardiovascular risk in South Asians. *Lancet* 1991; **337**: 382–386.

41 Farmer G, Russell G, Hamilton-Nicol DR, Ogenbede HO, Ross IS, Pearson DWM, et al. The influence of maternal glucose metabolism on fetal growth, development and morbidity in 917 singleton pregnancies in nondiabetic women. *Diabetologia* 1988; **31**: 134–141.

42 Law CM, Gordon GS, Shiell AW, Barker DJP, Hales CN. Thinness at birth and glucose tolerance in seven year old children. *Diabet Med* 1995; **12**: 24–29.

43 Whincup PH, Cook DG, Adshead F, Taylor SJC, Walker M, Papacosta O, et al. Childhood size is more strongly related than size at birth to glucose and insulin levels in 10–11-year-old children. *Diabetologia* 1997; **40**: 319–326.

44 Yajnik CS, Fall CHD, Vaidya U, Pandit AN, Bavdekar A, Bhat DS, et al. Fetal growth and glucose and insulin metabolism in four-year-old Indian children. *Diabet Med* 1995; **12**: 330–336.

45 Forrester TE, Wilks RJ, Bennett FI, Simeon D, Osmond C, Allen M, et al. Fetal growth and cardiovascular risk factors in Jamaican schoolchildren. *Br Med J* 1996; **312**: 156–160.

46 McLarty DG, Swai BM, Kitange HM, Masukai G, Mtinangi BL, Kilima PM, et al. Prevalence of diabetes and impaired glucose tolerance in rural Tanzania. *Lancet* 1989; i: 871–875.

47 King H, Heywood P, Zimmet P, Alpeis M, Collins V, Collins A, et al. Glucose tolerance in a highland population in Papua New Guinea. *Diabetes Res* 1984; **1**: 45–51.

48 Butler WJ, Ostrander LD, Carman WJ, Lamphiear DE. Diabetes mellitus in Tecumseh, Michigan: prevalence, incidence, and associated conditions. *Am J Epidemiol* 1982; **116**: 971–980.

49 Knowle AWC, Bennett PH, Hamman RF, Miller M. Diabetes incidence and prevalence in Pima Indians: a 19-fold greater incidence than in Rochester, Minnesota. *Am J Epidemiol* 1978; **108**: 497–505.

50 Zimmet P, King H, Taylor R, Roper LR, Balkau B, Borges J, et al. The high prevalence of diabetes mellitus, impaired glucose tolerance and diabetic retinopathy in Nauru: the 1982 survey. *Diabetes Res* 1984; **1**: 13–18.

51 Cohen MP, Stern E, Rusecki Y, Zeidler A. High prevalence of diabetes in young adult Ethiopian immigrants to Israel. *Diabetes* 1988; **37**: 824–828.

52 Gottlieb MS, Root HF. Diabetes mellitus in twins. *Diabetes* 1968; **17**: 693–704.

53 Barnett AH, Eff C, Leslie RDG, Pyke DA. Diabetes in identical twins: a study of 200 pairs. *Diabetologia* 1981; **20**: 87–93.

54 Newman B, Selby JV, King MC, Slemenda C, Fabsitz R, Friedman GD. Concordance for type 2 (non-insulin-dependent) diabetes mellitus in male twins. *Diabetologia* 1987; **30**: 763–768.

55 Simpson NE. Diabetes in the families of diabetics. *Can Med Assoc J* 1968; **98**: 427–432.

56 Keen H, Jarrett RJ. Environmental factors and genetic interactions. In: Creutzfeldt W, Kobberling J, Neel JV, eds. *The genetics of diabetes mellitus*. Berlin: Springer-Verlag, 1976; 115–124.

57 Serjeantson SW, Zimmet P. Diabetes in the Pacific: evidence for a major gene. In: Baba S, Gould M, Zimmet P, eds. *Diabetes mellitus: recent knowledge on aetiology, complications and treatment*. Sydney: Academic Press, 1984; 23–30.

58 Neel JV. Diabetes mellitus: a 'thrifty' genotype rendered detrimental by 'progress'? *Am J Hum Genet* 1962; **14**: 353–362.

59 Alcolado JC, Alcolado R. Importance of maternal history of non-insulin dependent diabetic patients. *Br Med J* 1991; **302**: 1178–1180.

60 Phillips DIW. Twin studies in medical research: can they tell us whether diseases are genetically determined? *Lancet* 1993; **341**: 1008–1009.

61 Vagero D, Leon D. Ischemic heart disease and low birthweight: a test of the fetal-origins hypothesis from the Swedish twin registry. *Lancet* 1994; **343**: 260–263.

62 Leveno KJ, Santos-Ramos R, Duenhoelter JH, Reisch JS, Whalley PJ. Sonar cephalometry in twins: a table of biparietal diameters for normal twin fetuses and a comparison with singletons. *Am J Obstet Gynecol* 1979; **135**: 727–730.

63 Vaag A, Populsen P, Kyvik KO, Beck-Nielsen H. Etiology of NIDDM: Genetics versus pre- or post natal environments? Results from twin studies. *Clin Endocrinol Diabetes* 1996; **104**: 181–182. (Abstract)

64 Dietz WH. Early influences on body weight regulation. In: Bouchard C, Bray GA, eds. *Regulation of body weight*. Chichester: John Wiley, 1996.

65 Ravelli GP, Stein ZA, Susser MW. Obesity in young men after famine exposure in utero and early infancy. *New Engl J Med* 1976; **295**: 349–353.

66 Charney E, Chamblee Goodman H, McBride M, Lyon B, Pratt R. Childhood antecedents of adult obesity. Do chubby infants become obese adults? *New Engl J Med* 1976; **295**: 6–9.

67 Seidman DS, Laor A, Gale R, Stevenson DK, Danon YL. A longitudinal study of birth weight and being overweight in late adolescence. *AJDC* 1991; **145**: 782–785.

68 Larsson B, Svardsudd K, Welin L, Wilhelmsen L, Bjorntorp P, Tibblin G. Abdominal adipose tissue distribution, obesity, and risk of cardiovascular disease and death: 13 year follow up of participants in the study of men born in 1913. *Br Med J* 1984; **288**: 1401–1404.

69 Law CM, Barker DJP, Osmond C, Fall CHD, Simmonds SJ. Early growth and abdominal fatness in adult life. *J Epidemiol Community Health* 1992; **46**: 184–186.

70 Barker ME, Robinson S, Osmond C, Barker DJP. Birthweight and body fat distribution in adolescent girls. *Arch Dis Child* 1997; **77**: 381–383.

71 Malina RM, Katzmarzyk PT, Beunen G. Birthweight and its relationship to size attained and relative fat distribution at 7 to 12 years of age. *Obesity Research* 1996; **4**: 385–390.

72 Matthes JWA, Lewis PA, Davies DP, Bethel JA. Body size and subcutaneous fat patterning in adolescence. *Arch Dis Child* 1996; **75**: 521–523.

73 Bjorntorp P. The associations between obesity, adipose tissue distribution and disease. *Acta Med Scand Suppl* 1988; **723**: 121–134.

74 Abraham S, Nordseick M. Relationship of excess weight in children and adults. *Public Health Report* 1960; **75**: 263–273.

75 Barker DJP, Blundell JE, Dietz WH, Epstein LH, Jeffery RW, Remschmidt H, et al. What are the bio-behavioral determinants of body weight regulation? In: Bouchard C, Bray GA, eds. *Regulation of body weight. Biological and behavioral mechanisms*. Chichester: John Wiley, 1996; 158–177.

76 Malina RM, Bouchard C. Subcutaneous fat distribution during growth. In: Bouchard C, Juhiston FE, eds. *Fat distribution during growth and later health outcomes*. New York: AR Liss, 1988; 63–84.

77 Cooper C, Kuh D, Egger P, Wadsworth M, Barker DJP. Childhood growth and age at menarche. *Br J Obstet Gynaecol* 1996; **103**: 814–817.

78 Cresswell JL, Egger P, Fall CHD, Osmond C, Fraser RB, Barker DJP. Is the age of menopause determined in-utero? *Early Hum Dev* 1997; **49**: 143–148.

Fetal growth, childhood respiratory infection and chronic bronchitis

For many years there has been interest in the hypothesis that lower respiratory tract infection during infancy and early childhood causes chronic bronchitis in later life.[1-6] (In this chapter the term 'chronic bronchitis' is used instead of the more precise, but less familiar, 'chronic airflow obstruction'.) The broad similarity in the international geography and time trends of respiratory disease at different ages was an early pointer to this.[3] Migrant studies also suggested that determinants of chronic bronchitis act in early life. Among British-born men who migrated to the USA, the prevalence of chronic bronchitis was higher than among migrants from Norway.[7] The differences persisted after allowing for smoking habits and were unrelated to the men's age at migration. The prevalence was also higher among men born in urban rather than rural areas of Britain. It was later shown that people born in cities and large towns in Britain have an increased risk of death from chronic bronchitis irrespective of where they move to, either within or outside the country.[7, 8]

Until recently there was little direct evidence that respiratory infection in early life had long-term effects. Bronchiolitis, bronchitis and pneumonia in infancy were shown to be followed by persisting damage to the airways during childhood, with cough, wheeze, bronchial reactivity, and impaired ventilatory function;[9-12] and in the long-term follow up of a national sample of 3899 British children born in 1946, young adults who had had one or more lower respiratory infections before 2 years of age were found to have a higher prevalence of chronic cough.[13-15] Recently, however, a geographical study and two follow-up studies of men born 60 or more years ago have added to the evidence.

GEOGRAPHY

Death rates from chronic bronchitis vary widely between different places in England and Wales. Figure 7.1 shows rates among men in each of the 1366 local authority areas during 1968–78;[16] rates are highest in the cities and large towns, and lowest in the rural areas. The distributions are similar in men and women, although rates in women are much lower: 269 deaths per million per year

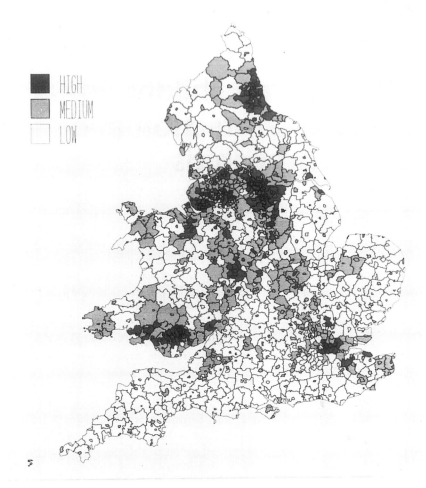

Fig. 7.1 Standardised mortality ratios for chronic bronchitis in England and Wales among men aged 35–74 years.

compared with 848 in men. Detailed studies of death certificates and the findings of prevalence surveys in Britain show that geographical differences in mortality certified as caused by chronic bronchitis and emphysema reflect differences in the prevalence of these diseases.[17] In Figures 7.2 and 7.3 the death rates among men and women are compared with infant deaths from bronchitis and pneumonia during 1921–25, the earliest period for which such data are available. In the same way as in the geographical studies of cardiovascular disease (see Ch. 1), the local authority areas are grouped into 212 areas, comprising county boroughs (large towns), London boroughs, all small towns within each county, and all rural areas within each county. The distribution of adult deaths from chronic bronchitis correlates remarkably strongly with past infant deaths from respiratory infection, the correlation coefficients being 0.84 in men (Fig. 7.2) and 0.80 in women (Fig. 7.3). The correlations are also specific. Past infant death rates from bronchitis and pneumonia correlate more closely with current adult death rates from chronic bronchitis than with any other cause of death, current or past, adult or infant.

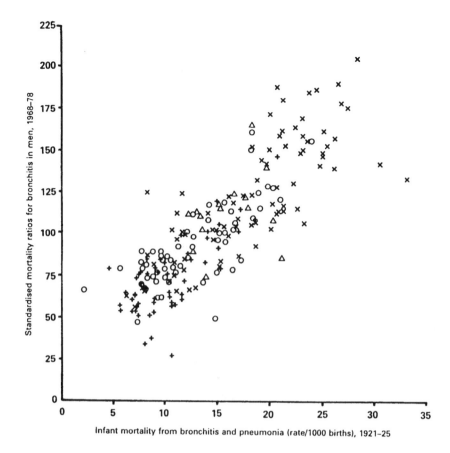

Fig. 7.2 Standardised mortality ratios for chronic bronchitis in men aged 35–74, and past infant mortality rates from bronchitis and pneumonia in England and Wales. Δ, London boroughs; X, county boroughs; O, urban districts; +, rural districts.

Most deaths from chronic bronchitis occurring at age 35–74 years during 1968–78 occurred among people born before 1921–25, the earliest years for which cause-specific infant mortality data were published. Total postneonatal death rates are, however, available from 1911 and may be used as a proxy for respiratory deaths in infants, because respiratory infection was the main cause of postneonatal mortality.[18] The correlation coefficients between postneonatal mortality and adult mortality from bronchitis during 1968–78, in both sexes, were the same ($r = 0.83$) for postneonatal rates throughout 1911–20 as for 1921–25.

It could be argued that the similar geographical distribution of infant deaths from respiratory infection and adult deaths from bronchitis simply reflects persistence over the years of geographical differences in environmental influences which determine respiratory disease at all ages. Air temperature is an example of such an influence.[19] Several determinants of respiratory disease, however, act only at certain ages.[20] The risk of infant respiratory infection is reduced by breast feeding, increased by overcrowding, and linked to the number and age of other siblings, their presence in the same room at night, respiratory infection among them, and parental smoking.[21-23] Domestic air pollution may also affect

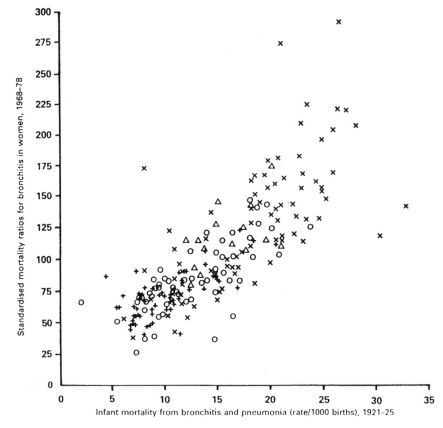

Fig. 7.3 Standardised mortality ratios for chronic bronchitis in women aged 35–74, and past infant mortality rates from bronchitis and pneumonia in England and Wales. Δ, London boroughs; X, county boroughs; O, urban districts; +, rural districts.

infant respiratory infection, though the balance of evidence suggests that the effect is small.[24]

Among adults cigarette smoking is the most important known determinant of chronic bronchitis.[25] Mortality from lung cancer in England and Wales does not, however, correlate with infant respiratory mortality.[17] This suggests that the geographical distribution of smoking differs from that of the determinants of respiratory infection in early childhood. By using current death rates from lung cancer as an indicator of cigarette smoking, the statistical dependence of the distribution of chronic bronchitis on infant respiratory infection and smoking can be explored. The results suggest that, in both men and women, smoking is subordinate to infant respiratory infection in determining the geographical distribution of chronic bronchitis within England and Wales.[17]

FOLLOW-UP STUDIES

Direct evidence of a link between lower respiratory tract infection in early childhood and chronic bronchitis has come from two follow-up studies in the counties of Hertfordshire and Derbyshire, England.[26, 27] In both places records of health visitors from the early years of the century have been preserved. Health visitors had visited each child born in the county periodically throughout infancy and early childhood, and noted the occurrence of illnesses. In Hertfordshire, the babies' birthweights and weights at 1 year of age were also recorded.

SIZE AT BIRTH AND DURING INFANCY

In an initial study of 5700 men born in Hertfordshire during 1911–30, death rates from chronic bronchitis fell from those with low to those with high birthweights and weights at 1 year of age.[26] Figure 7.4 shows more recent results for the full cohort of 10 141 men (unpublished data). Standardised mortality ratios among men with birthweights of 5.5 lb (2.5 kg) or less are twice those among men with birthweights of more than 9.5 lb (>4.3 kg). There is an even stronger trend with weight at 1 year of age. There are no similar trends in death rates for lung cancer. Rates of chronic bronchitis are lower in women, and there are too few deaths in the Hertfordshire cohort for useful study.

The lung function of a sample of 825 men was measured.[26] Their mean forced expiratory volume (FEV_1), which largely reflects airway size, rose between those with low and those with high birthweight (Table 7.1). The effect of birthweight on FEV_1, which was strongly statistically significant, was independent

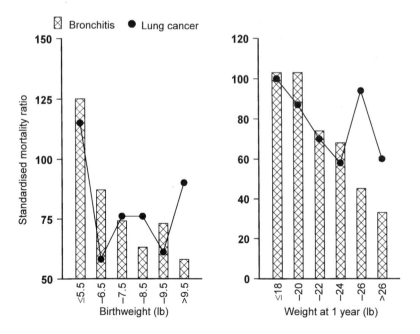

Fig. 7.4 Standardised mortality ratios for chronic bronchitis and lung cancer in 10 141 men according to birthweight and weight at 1 year.

Table 7.1 Mean forced expiratory volume in 1 second (FEV₁) (litres) adjusted for height and age among men aged 59–70 years according to birthweight and smoking habit

Birthweight, lb (kg)	Non-smokers	Ex-smokers	Current smokers	All
≤5.5 (2.5)	2.53 (4)	2.34 (16)	2.14 (13)	2.28 (33)
–6.5 (2.9)	2.48 (20)	2.46 (52)	2.29 (31)	2.41 (103)
–7.5 (3.4)	2.65 (37)	2.49 (154)	2.21 (67)	2.44 (258)
–8.5 (3.9)	2.77 (39)	2.53 (134)	2.35 (69)	2.52 (242)
–9.5 (4.3)	2.83 (19)	2.60 (75)	2.30 (38)	2.55 (132)
>9.5 (4.3)	2.79 (8)	2.60 (31)	2.43 (18)	2.57 (57)
All	2.69 (127)	2.52 (462)	2.29 (236)	2.48 (825)*
p value for trend				0.0007

* Standard deviation = 0.59.
Figures in parentheses are numbers of men.

of the effect of current height. FEV_1 was not related to weight at 1 year, independent of birthweight, which suggests that it is linked to growth in utero rather than growth during infancy. A link to fetal rather than early postnatal growth might be expected because growth of the airways is largely completed in utero (p. 24).[28] A study of children confirmed that low birthweight is associated with a lower FEV_1, independently of the duration of gestation.[29] Within a group of children who weighed less than 2000 g (4.4 lb) at birth, most of whom were preterm, low birthweight was also associated with low FEV_1.[30] Although only a small and statistically non-significant reduction in lung function was found in a group of adolescents who had low birthweight, these results cannot be compared with those of the studies which examined associations across the range of birthweight.[31] The findings suggest that retarded weight gain in utero is associated with a constraint on the growth of the airways which is never made up.

In a study of men and women in Mysore, South India, Stein and colleagues found that low birthweight was associated with a reduced FEV_1, after adjusting for height.[32] A small head circumference at birth was associated with a low ratio of FEV_1 to FVC which is consistent with impaired growth in early gestation leading to a reduced FEV_1 in adult life. Lung function in India is also influenced by tobacco smoking, which is common in men, and in women by domestic air pollution from cooking fuels.[33]

As would be expected, men who smoked had a lower FEV_1 than those who did not smoke. Table 7.1 shows that the trend of increasing FEV_1 with increasing birthweight occurred in men who had never smoked (non-smokers), in ex-smokers, and in current smokers. The trend also occurred at each level of social class. In contrast to FEV_1 the forced vital capacity (FVC) was not related to birthweight but was reduced in men with lower weights at 1 year of age. An interpretation of this is that aspects of lung physiology which determine FVC, as opposed to FEV_1, are programmed in infancy rather than intrauterine life. This interpretation is supported by a study of 7-year-old children whose FVC was not related to birthweight but whose FEV_1 was.[30]

In 1923 the health visitors in Hertfordshire began to visit children after infancy, continuing up to 5 years of age when the children went to school. Tables 7.2 and 7.3 show FEV_1 and FVC values for the 639 men born from 1923 onwards, 59 of whom were recorded as having had an attack of bronchitis or pneumonia during infancy. At each birthweight their mean FEV_1 and FVC values were lower than those of men not recorded as having had bronchitis or pneumonia. A total of 63 men were recorded as having had an attack of bronchitis or pneumonia between 1 and 5 years of age, but their mean FEV_1 and FVC values were similar to those of all the other men. Lower respiratory tract infection before the age of 1 year was associated with reduced lung function independently of smoking habit and social class.

Shaheen and colleagues provided further evidence of the long-term effects of respiratory infection in early life in a study of 70-year-old men in Derbyshire, England, which also made use of health visitors' records.[27] The FEV_1 of men who had had pneumonia before the age of 2 years was 0.65 litres less than that

Table 7.2 Mean forced expiratory volume in 1 second (FEV_1) (litres) adjusted for height and age among men aged 59–67 years according to birthweight and the occurrence of bronchitis or pneumonia in infancy

Birthweight, lb (kg)	Bronchitis or pneumonia in infancy	
	Absent	Present
≤5.5 (2.5)	2.39 (22)	1.81 (4)
–6.5 (2.9)	2.40 (70)	2.23 (10)
–7.5 (3.4)	2.47 (163)	2.38 (25)
–8.5 (3.9)	2.53 (179)	2.33 (12)
–9.5 (4.3)	2.54 (103)	2.36 (5)
>9.5 (4.3)	2.57 (43)	2.36 (3)
All	2.50 (580)	2.30 (59)

Figures in parentheses are numbers of men.

Table 7.3 Mean forced vital capacity (FVC) (litres) adjusted for height and age among men aged 59–67 years according to birthweight and the occurrence of bronchitis or pneumonia in infancy

Birthweight, lb (kg)	Bronchitis or pneumonia in infancy	
	Absent	Present
≤5.5 (2.5)	2.91 (22)	2.88 (4)
–6.5 (2.9)	3.02 (70)	2.81 (10)
–7.5 (3.4)	2.94 (163)	2.74 (25)
–8.5 (3.9)	3.03 (179)	2.76 (12)
–9.5 (4.3)	3.01 (103)	2.75 (5)
>9.5 (4.3)	3.11 (43)	2.57 (3)
All	3.00 (580)	2.76 (59)

Figures in parentheses are numbers of men.

of other men, a reduction in FEV_1 of approximately twice that associated with lifelong smoking. The finding was specific: other diseases occurring before the age of 2 years, including bronchitis, measles and whooping cough, had no effect on FEV_1.

The simplest explanation of these observations is that infection of the lower respiratory tract during a critical period in infancy has persisting deleterious effects. Taussig has proposed an alternative explanation, however, namely that occurrence of lower respiratory infection in infancy plays no part in the causation of chronic bronchitis but merely identifies people in whom airway growth is constrained in early life and who are therefore more likely to develop symptoms if infection occurs.[34] According to this explanation, symptomatic lower respiratory tract infection identifies people in whom impaired lung function has already been programmed in utero. Prospective studies of children whose lung function has been measured soon after birth may help to resolve this.[35]

GROWTH OF THE LUNG

Whatever the outcome of the above mentioned studies lung growth in utero seems to have a major effect on chronic bronchitis in adult life.[36] The high frequency of lung hypoplasia at postmortem examination of aborted fetuses or babies who died perinatally suggests that lung growth in utero is often impaired.[37] In humans, airway division down to the level of the terminal bronchioles is completed by week 16 of gestation.[28] This is followed by a period of rapid lung growth, so that between 17 and 20 weeks the lung cell population doubles. At 20 weeks the lungs are twice as large relative to the body weight as at term.[38] Alveoli can be detected as early as 30 weeks in the fetus.[39, 40] Early studies suggested that around 10% of the adult number of alveoli are present at birth,[41, 42] but more recent studies suggest that this is a considerable underestimate.[40, 43] Around 50% of the adult alveoli may be present at birth, although there is wide variation. After birth multiplication slows and is almost complete by 2 years of age, although during this period there is a rapid increase in alveolar size and complexity.[43] 95% of the adult alveolar surface area is formed postnatally.[40] In childhood the airway size may be inferred from measures of flow.[44, 45] Longitudinal studies suggest that airway growth 'tracks' through childhood and that the trajectory of growth is established before the age of 1 year.[46, 47]

Adverse influences may impair airway growth or enhance alveolar growth, depending on their nature and timing, and lead to airflow obstruction, as indicated by a reduction in FEV_1/FVC. Undernutrition in mid-late gestation is likely to impair airway growth, leading to a reduced FEV_1. Alveolar growth may, however, be stimulated by hypoxia leading to an increase in FVC. This is known to occur in animals and seems to occur in humans born at altitude.[48]

Since maternal smoking is associated with fetal growth retardation the higher rates of respiratory illness of infants whose mothers smoked may partly result from altered lung growth.[49-51] The effects of smoking on fetal lung development are, however, complex. Smoking accelerates lung maturation, possibly by enhancing the surge of cortisol production in late gestation, and infants of smoking mothers are at lower risk of neonatal respiratory distress syndrome.[52]

The pattern of early lung growth differs in boys and girls: in boys airway growth tends to lag behind parenchymal growth.[44] Boys have a larger lung volume than girls of a similar age and stature, but longer and narrower airways in relation to that volume.[43, 53] In the Hertfordshire study, the associations between birthweight and FEV_1 were weaker in women (unpublished data) and this could be explained by sex differences in early lung growth. In a similar way, the associations between lower respiratory tract infection in early childhood and FEV_1 were weaker in women in Hertfordshire and in Derbyshire.[27] This is consistent with the results of a study of children in whom pneumonia in early childhood was related to impaired lung function in boys but not in girls.[54] Boys are known to have more severe lower respiratory tract infection than girls in infancy, and they are more likely to be hospitalised with bronchiolitis.[55, 56] This has been attributed partly to the smaller airway size.[45]

CONCLUSIONS

In the past, discussion of the natural history of chronic bronchitis has tended to focus on the rate of decline of adult lung function.[57] The findings described here, however, suggest the disease is associated with impaired lung growth in early life. Influences which determine the rate of functional decline, of which smoking is the most important, add to the effects of impaired early growth.

Green and colleagues have suggested that the susceptibility to smoking damage may be linked to the pattern of lung growth and structure.[58] A moderate smoker who failed to attain maximal lung function potential as a young adult may develop chronic bronchitis at the same age as a heavy smoker who achieved maximal lung growth.[4] The findings in Hertfordshire and Mysore suggest that the effects of poor growth and smoking on lung function are additive and not synergistic, although measures of early body weight may be poor indicators of lung growth. To test this more rigorously it will be necessary to relate early growth to the longitudinal rate of decline in FEV_1 in smokers and non-smokers.

Thinking on the pathogenesis of emphysema has been dominated by a destructive model involving protease–antiprotease balance.[59] Developmental models, such as those produced in animals, may be more relevant.[60]

Summary

The hypothesis that lower respiratory tract infection during infancy causes chronic bronchitis in adult life is supported by the similar geographical distribution of the two disorders. Follow-up studies have shown that low growth rates in utero and during infancy, and early respiratory infection, both predict abnormal lung function and chronic bronchitis in adult life. Airway growth in utero may therefore have an important effect on chronic bronchitis. Infection of the lower respiratory tract in infancy may also have persisting deleterious effects or may simply identify children in whom airway growth has been constrained in utero. The effects of cigarette smoking add to those that are initiated in early life.

References

1 Orie NGM, Sluiter HJ, eds. *Bronchitis – an international symposium*. Groningen, The Netherlands: Assen Royal Vengorium, 1961.

2 Holland WW, Halil T, Bennett AE, Elliott A. Factors influencing the onset of chronic respiratory disease. *Br Med J* 1969; **ii**: 205–208.

3 Reid DD. The beginnings of bronchitis. *Proceedings of the Royal Society of Medicine* 1969; **62**: 311–316.

4 Samet JM, Tager IB, Speizer FE. The relationship between respiratory illness in childhood and chronic air-flow obstruction in adulthood. *Am Rev Respir Dis* 1983; **127**: 508–523.

5 Phelan PD. Does adult chronic obstructive lung disease really begin in childhood? *Br J Dis Chest* 1984; **78**: 1–9.

6 Strachan DP. Do chesty children become chesty adults? *Arch Dis Child* 1990; **65**: 161–162.

7 Reid DD, Fletcher CM. International studies in chronic respiratory disease. *Br Med Bull* 1971; **27**: 59–64.

8 Osmond C, Barker DJP, Slattery JM. Risk of death from cardiovascular disease and chronic bronchitis determined by place of birth in England and Wales. *J Epidemiol Community Health* 1990; **44**: 139–141.

9 Kattan M, Keens TG, Lapierre JG, Levison H, Bryan AC, Reilly BJ. Pulmonary function abnormalities in symptom-free children after bronchiolitis. *Pediatrics* 1977; **59**: 683–688.

10 Gurwitz D, Mindorff C, Levison H. Increased incidence of bronchial reactivity in children with a history of bronchiolitis. *Pediatrics* 1981; **98**: 551–555.

11 Pullan CR, Hey EN. Wheezing, asthma and pulmonary dysfunction 10 years after infection with respiratory syncytial virus in infancy. *Br Med J* 1982; **284**: 1665–1669.

12 Mok JYQ, Simpson H. Outcome for acute bronchitis, bronchiolitis, and pneumonia in infancy. *Arch Dis Child* 1984; **59**: 306–309.

13 Kiernan KE, Colley JRT, Douglas JWB, Reid DD. Chronic cough in young adults in relation to smoking habits, childhood environment and chest illness. *Respiration* 1976; **33**: 236–244.

14 Britten N, Davies JMC, Colley JRT. Early respiratory experience and subsequent cough and peak expiratory flow rate in 36 year old men and women. *Br Med J* 1987; **294**: 1317–1320.

15 Mann SL, Wadsworth MEJ, Colley JRT. Accumulation of factors influencing respiratory illness in members of a national birth cohort and their offspring. *J Epidemiol Community Health* 1992; **46**: 286–292.

16 Gardner MJ, Winter PD, Barker DJP. *Atlas of mortality from selected diseases in England and Wales, 1968–78*. Chichester: John Wiley, 1984.

17 Barker DJP, Osmond C. Childhood respiratory infection and adult chronic bronchitis in England and Wales. *Br Med J* 1986; **293**: 1271–1275.

18 Registrar General. *Statistical review of England and Wales. Part I: tables, medical*. London: HMSO, 1880 and following years.

19 Boyd JT. Climate, air pollution and mortality. *Br J Prev Soc Med* 1960; **14**: 123–135.

20 Colley JRT. Respiratory disease in childhood. *Br Med Bull* 1971; **27**: 9–14.

21 Downham MAPS, Scott R, Sims DG, Webb JKG, Gardner PS. Breast-feeding protects against respiratory syncytial virus infections. *Br Med J* 1976; **ii**: 274–276.

22 Leeder SR, Corkhill R, Irwig LM, Holland WW, Colley JRT. Influence of family factors on the incidence of lower respiratory illness during the first year of life. *Br J Prev Soc Med* 1976; **30**: 203–212.

23 Pullan CR, Toms GL, Martin AJ, Gardner PS, Webb JKG, Appleton DR. Breast-feeding and respiratory syncytial virus infection. *Br Med J* 1980; **281**: 1034–1036.

24 Ogston SA, Florey C du V, Walker CHM. The Tayside infant morbidity and mortality study: effect on health of using gas for cooking. *Br Med J* 1985; **290**: 957–960.

25 Lambert PM, Reid DD. Smoking, air pollution, and bronchitis in Britain. *Lancet* 1970; **i**: 853–857.

26 Barker DJP, Godfrey KM, Fall C, Osmond C, Winter PD, Shaheen SO. Relation of birth weight and childhood respiratory infection to adult lung function and death from chronic obstructive airways disease. *Br Med J* 1991; **303**: 671–675.

27 Shaheen SO, Barker DJP, Shiell AW, Crocker FJ, Wield GA, Holgate ST. The relationship

between pneumonia in early childhood and impaired lung function in late adult life. *Am J Respir Crit Care Med* 1994; **149**: 616–619.

28 Bucher U, Reid L. Development of the intrasegmental bronchial tree: the pattern of branching and development of cartilage at various stages of intra-uterine life. *Thorax* 1961; **16**: 207–218.

29 Rona RJ, Gulliford MC, Chinn S. Effects of prematurity and intrauterine growth on respiratory health and lung function in childhood. *Br Med J* 1993; **306**: 817–820.

30 Chan KN, Noble-Jamieson CM, Elliman A, Bryan EM, Silverman M. Lung function in children of low birth weight. *Arch Dis Child* 1989; **64**: 1284–1293.

31 Matthes JWA, Lewis PA, Davies DP, Bethel JA. Birthweight at term and lung function in adolescence: no evidence for a programmed effect. *Arch Dis Child* 1995; **73**: 231–234.

32 Stein CE, Kumaran K, Fall CHD, Shaheen SO, Osmond C, Barker DJP. Relation of fetal growth to adult lung function in South India. *Thorax* 1997; **52**: 895–899.

33 Behera D, Jindal SK, Malhotra HS. Ventilatory function in non smoking rural Indian women using different cooking fuels. *Respiration* 1994; **61**: 89–92.

34 Taussig LM. The conundrum of wheezing and airway hyperreactivity in infancy. *Pediatr Pulmonol* 1992; **13**: 1–3.

35 Martinez FD, Morgan WJ, Wright AL, Holberg C, Taussig LM. Initial airway function is a risk factor for recurrent wheezing respiratory illnesses during the first three years of life. *Am Rev Respir Dis* 1991; **143**: 312–316.

36 Shaheen SO, Barker DJP. Early lung growth and chronic airflow obstruction. *Thorax* 1994; **49**: 533–536.

37 Wigglesworth JS, Desai R. Is fetal respiratory function a major determinant of perinatal survival? *Lancet* 1982; **i**: 264–267.

38 Wigglesworth JS, Desai R. Use of DNA estimation for growth assessment in normal and hypoplastic fetal lungs. *Arch Dis Child* 1981; **56**: 601–605.

39 Langston C, Kida K, Reed M, Thurlbeck WM. Human lung growth in late gestation and in the neonate. *Am Rev Respir Dis* 1984; **129**: 607–613.

40 Hislop AA, Wigglesworth JS, Desai R. Alveolar development in the human fetus and infant. *Early Hum Dev* 1986; **13**: 1–11.

41 Dunnill MS. Postnatal growth of the lung. *Thorax* 1962; **17**: 329–333.

42 Davies G, Reid L. Growth of the alveoli and pulmonary arteries in childhood. *Thorax* 1970; **25**: 669–681.

43 Thurlbeck WM. Postnatal human lung growth. *Thorax* 1982; **37**: 564–571.

44 Pagtakhan RD, Bjelland JC, Landau LI, Loughlin G, Kaltenborn W, Seeley G, et al. Sex differences in growth patterns of the airways and lung parenchyma in children. *J Appl Physiol* 1984; **56**: 1204–1210.

45 Tepper RS, Morgan WJ, Cota K, Wright A, Taussig LM. Physiologic growth and development of the lung during the first year of life. *Am Rev Respir Dis* 1986; **134**: 513–519.

46 Dockery DW, Berkey CS, Ware JH, Speizer FE, Ferris BG. Distribution of forced vital capacity and forced expiratory volume in one second in children 6 to 11 years of age. *Am Rev Respir Dis* 1983; **128**: 405–412.

47 Chan KN, Wong YC, Silverman M. Relationship between infant lung mechanics and childhood lung function in children of very low birthweight. *Pediatr Pulmonol* 1990; **8**: 74–81.

48 Brody JS, Vaccaro C. Postnatal formation of alveoli: interstitial events and physiologic consequences. *Fed Proc* 1979; **38**: 215–223.

49 Hardy JB, Mellits ED. Does maternal smoking during pregnancy have a long-term effect on the child? *Lancet* 1972; **12**: 1332–1336.

50 Colley JRT, Holland WW, Corkhill RT. Influence of passive smoking and parental phlegm on pneumonia and bronchitis in early childhood. *Lancet* 1974; **2**: 1031–1034.

51 Harlap S, Davies AM. Infant admissions to hospital and maternal smoking. *Lancet* 1974; **1**: 529–532.

52 Lieberman E, Torday J, Barbieri R, Cohen A, Van Vunakis H, Weiss ST. Association of intrauterine cigarette smoke exposure with indices of fetal lung maturation. *Obstet Gynecol* 1992; **79**: 564–570.

53 Hibbert ME, Couriel JM, Landau LI. Changes in lung, airway and chest wall function in boys and girls between 8 and 12 years. *J Appl Physiol* 1984; **57**: 304–308.

54 Gold DR, Tager IB, Weiss ST, Tosteson TD, Speizer FE. Acute lower respiratory illness in childhood as a predictor of lung function and chronic respiratory symptoms. *Am Rev Respir Dis* 1989; **140**: 877–884.

55 Glezen WP, Denny FW. Epidemiology of acute lower respiratory disease in children. *N Engl J Med* 1973; **288**: 498–505.

56 Breese Hall C. Respiratory syncytial virus. In: Feigin RD, Cherry JD, eds. *Textbook of pediatric infectious diseases*. Philadelphia: WB Saunders, 1981; 1247–1266.

57 Burrows B. Natural history of chronic airflow obstruction. In: Hensley MJ, Saunders NA, eds. *Clinical epidemiology of chronic obstructive pulmonary disease. Lung biology in health and disease*. New York: Marcel Dekker, 1989; 99–107.

58 Green M, Mead J, Turner JM. Variability of maximum expiratory flow-volume curves. *J Appl Physiol* 1974; **37**: 67–74.

59 Janoff A. State of the art. Elastases and emphysema: current assessment of the protease–antiprotease hypothesis. *Am Rev Respir Dis* 1985; **132**: 417–433.

60 O'Dell BL, Kilburn KH, McKenzie WN, Thurston RJ. The lung of the copper-deficient rat. A model for developmental pulmonary emphysema. *Am J Pathol* 1978; **91**: 413–432.

8

The undernourished baby

Although the growth of a fetus is influenced by its genes, studies in humans and animals suggest that it is usually limited by the nutrients and oxygen it receives.[1,2] The mother seems to exert a stronger effect on fetal growth than the father. Among half-siblings, related only through one parent, those with the same mother have similar birthweights, the correlation coefficient being 0.58. The birthweights of half-siblings with the same father are, however, dissimilar, the correlation coefficient being only 0.1.[3] Other studies of relatives have shown that first cousins related through the mother tend to have similar birthweights whereas paternal first cousins do not.[4] Penrose[5] analysed the birthweights of relatives and concluded that 62% of the variation between individuals was the result of the intrauterine environment, 20% was the result of maternal genes and 18% of fetal genes. A study of babies born after ovum donation showed that while their birthweights were strongly related to the weight of the recipient mother (Fig. 8.1), they were unrelated to the weight of the woman who

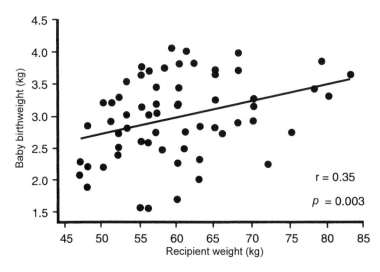

Fig. 8.1 Birthweight of babies born after ovum donation according to weight of the recipient mother.

donated the egg.[6] These and other findings, together with studies in domestic animals, suggest that birth size is essentially controlled by the mother rather than the genetic inheritance from both parents.[7–10]

MATERNAL–FETAL CONFLICT

Haig and others have suggested that the relation between mother and fetus can usefully be viewed as genetic conflict.[11, 12] The effects of natural selection on genes expressed in fetuses may be opposed by the effects of natural selection on genes expressed in mothers. Fetal genes will be selected to increase the transfer of nutrients to the fetus so that it grows larger. Maternal genes will be selected to limit transfer to the fetus to protect the mother, and to ensure her survival and that of her children, born and unborn. What is best for the fetus need not be best for its mother, or so it seems.

The theory of parent–child conflict proposes that children are selected to demand more resources from parents than parents are selected to give. Three sets of genes have different interests: the mother's genes, the fetus' genes derived from the mother, and the fetus' genes derived from the father. If the genes of the fetus make excessive demands on the mother, it will prejudice the mother's ability to pass her genes on to other offspring. It is argued that genes derived from the father have been selected to take more resources from the mother's tissues than the genes derived from the mother.[13] The conflict between the maternal and paternal genomes over the nutritional demands that the fetus imposes on its mother may explain why genes derived from one parent can 'imprint', or override, the expression of those derived from the other.[14] An example of 'genomic imprinting' is that of the genes for insulin-like growth factor II; in the mouse, only those derived from the father are expressed.[15, 16]

An interesting example of the conflict of interests between mother and baby comes from the breeding habits of southern elephant seals.[17] They come ashore to breed on the island of South Georgia and nourish their pups only from the reserves of fat and protein stored in their bodies on arrival at the beaches. The proportion of the food reserves made available to the pups may be critical to both mother and child. Mothers that expend a large proportion on their pups may compromise their survival to the next breeding season or reduce their subsequent reproductive output. On the other hand pups that are small and thin have reduced chances of survival to breeding age. The production of small pups by smaller mothers may be a compromise between the future reproductive success of the mother and the survival of the pup. Male pups are heavier at birth than females and the smallest elephant seal mothers only give birth to females, which suggests that they abort male pups. This may be an advantage if they are unable to raise a male pup to a viable size without jeopardising their own survival and reproductive success.

When animals breed before they are mature maternal–fetal conflict may be enhanced. James has suggested that whereas the hormonal responses to pregnancy in adult women seem geared to optimising the flow of nutrients to the fetus, the opposite seems to occur when adolescent girls are pregnant.[18] Paradoxically, feeding young pregnant adolescent lambs leads to a selective channelling of nutrients to the mother who thrives at the expense of the fetus.

In Walton & Hammond's[19] well known experiments, in which Shetland and Shire horses were crossed, the foals were smaller at birth when the Shetland pony was the mother than when the Shire horse was the mother. As the genetic composition of the two crosses was similar, this implied that the Shetland mother had constrained the growth of the fetus. Similar results were obtained when South Devon cattle, the largest breed of cattle in the British Isles, were crossed with Dexter cattle, the smallest breed.[20] The results of these cross-breeding experiments are supported by recent embryo transfer experiments. The size at birth of animal embryos removed from their mothers' uteri is related to the size of the uterus into which they are transferred.[21]

The Ounsteds[22] examined a group of mothers who had growth-retarded babies. They found that the mothers were similar in height and other characteristics to a group of controls. Their earlier children, however, had lower mean birthweight. This suggested that these mothers had constrained the intrauterine growth of all their children. Further studies showed that the mothers themselves had had low mean birthweight.

INTERGENERATIONAL CONSTRAINTS ON FETAL GROWTH

Other studies have shown that the birthweights of mothers are related to those of their children and even their children's children.[23–28] Women who were small for gestational age at birth are at twice the risk of having a small for gestational age baby and their babies are more likely to die in the perinatal period.[28, 29] Women who had low birthweight also tend to have thin babies. The father's birthweight has no effect on ponderal index,[30] though it influences placental weight. These observations have led to the conclusion that mothers constrain fetal growth and that the degree of constraint they exert is set when they themselves are in utero.[31] 'Maternal constraint' is thought to reflect the limited capacity of the mother to deliver nutrients to her fetus.[32] Sisters, who experience a common level of constraint in utero, exert a similar level of constraint on their own fetuses. Although low birthweight is a feature of the families of mothers who have growth-retarded babies, it is not a feature of the families of the fathers. Studies of babies who are unusually large at birth have shown, however, that large birthweight is common in the families of both parents. One interpretation of this is that the father influences the fetal growth trajectory only when maternal constraint is relaxed.[31] We do not know the mechanisms by which a mother's poor fetal growth impairs the fetal growth of her offspring but one possibility is that a reduced uterine vasculature is laid down in utero and this impairs placentation in the next generation.

Fifty years ago Mussey wrote: 'It must be borne in mind that the diet of a given generation may affect the offspring several generations hence'.[33] This has been demonstrated experimentally in animals. Stewart and colleagues undernourished a colony of rats with a protein-deficient diet over 12 generations. When they refed them with a normal diet it took three generations before fetal growth and development were restored to normal.[34] Similarly the adverse effects of exercise in pregnancy on fetal growth in rats are evident in the second generation.[35] It follows that in humans who move from poorly nourished to well nourished communities, Indian migrants to Europe for example, it will take more than one generation before fetal growth increases to the level of the host country.[36]

The realisation that a mother's physiological capacity to nourish her fetus was established when she herself was in utero is not new. Edward Mellanby wrote:

It is certain that the significance of correct nutrition in child-bearing does not begin in pregnancy itself or even in the adult female before pregnancy. It looms large as soon as a female child is born and indeed in its intrauterine life.[37]

Hence the fetus adapts its rate of growth, and the lifelong structure and function of its body, not only to its mother, but to the environment its grandmother provided for its mother. Sensitivity to more than one generation allows the fetus to adapt to the level of nutrition which has prevailed over many years rather than only to that at the time of its conception. This may be important in places where there is periodic famine.

Mother's height, smoking and fetal growth

Mother's height is related to birthweight: short women have small babies.[8] Teleologically this form of constraint can be viewed as a way of ensuring that the fetus cannot outgrow the size of the mother's pelvis and birth canal. Mother's skeletal size is not, however, related to the long-term changes in the physiology and metabolism of the fetus which are described in this book.[38, 39] Similarly while mother's cigarette smoking is associated with reduced birthweight it does not appear to be associated with long-term changes (p. 71). Consistent with this neither mother's height, smoking habits or age are related to cord blood insulin concentrations whereas mother's dietary intakes of carbohydrate and protein are strongly associated with cord blood concentrations of insulin and its precursors.[40] Discussion of maternal constraint in this chapter will therefore focus on other influences that determine delivery of nutrients to the fetus.

FETAL ADAPTATIONS TO UNDERNUTRITION

The supply of nutrients to the fetus is the major influence that regulates its growth. It depends on the mother's body composition and size, her nutrient stores, what she eats during pregnancy, transport of nutrients to the placenta and transfer across it. This long and vulnerable series of steps is known as the fetal supply line. Clearly the fetus will become undernourished when its demand for nutrients exceeds its supply. Either the supply may be low, for example when the mother is thin or starving or when the placenta fails, or demand may be high because the fetus is growing rapidly.

Early in development the embryo comprises two groups of cells, the inner cell mass which becomes the fetus and the outer cell mass which becomes the placenta. Experiments in animals indicate that the allocation of cells between the two masses is influenced by nutrition and by hormones.[41, 42] Cell allocation alters the trajectory of growth that is established around this time and which thereafter 'tracks' through gestation (Ch. 2, p. 16). Better periconceptual nutrition is thought to raise the growth trajectory.[43] The growth trajectory is also higher in males. A high growth trajectory, established in early gestation when the fetus' absolute requirement for nutrients is small, leads to an increased demand for nutrients in late gestation, when requirements are relatively large and when the progressive reduction in the ratio of placental to fetal size reduces placental reserve capacity.[44] The observations on sheep (Fig. 2.4) of Harding and colleagues illustrate how the fetus' ability to sustain growth during a period of undernutrition depend on its previous growth rate, more rapidly growing fetuses with a high demand for nutrients being less able to sustain growth.[45, 46]

Because the fetus' requirements for nutrients are small in early gestation it is often assumed that undernutrition will not influence growth until late gestation, when substrate supply becomes inadequate to meet increasing fetal demand for tissue building blocks. This is not, however, the case. When, for example, female pigs are fed low protein diets from the time of mating the weight and length of their fetuses are already reduced at mid-gestation.[47] This indicates that fetal undernutrition affects fetal growth through mechanisms other than lack of substrate supply to growing tissues.

In common with other living things the human fetus is plastic, able to adapt to undernutrition. Its responses to undernutrition include metabolic changes, redistribution of blood flow and changes in the production of fetal and placental hormones which control growth.[48] They are shown in Figure 8.2. Its

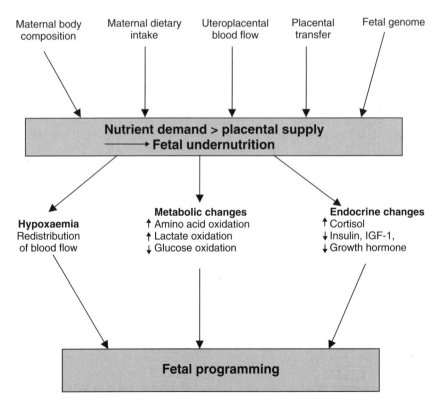

Fig. 8.2 Fetal adaptations to undernutrition: a framework.

immediate metabolic response to undernutrition is catabolism: it consumes its own substrates to provide energy.[47] More prolonged undernutrition leads to a slowing in growth rate. This enhances the fetuses' ability to survive by reducing the use of substrates and lowering the metabolic rate. Slowing of growth in late gestation leads to disproportion in organ size since organs and tissues that are growing rapidly at the time are affected the most. For example, undernutrition in late gestation may lead to reduced growth of the kidney which is developing rapidly at that time. Reduced replication of kidney cells may permanently reduce cell numbers, because after birth there seems to be no capacity for renal cell division to 'catch-up'.[49, 50]

Animal studies show that a variety of different patterns of fetal growth result in similar birth size. For example, a fetus that grows slowly throughout gestation may have the same size at birth as a fetus whose growth was arrested for a period and then 'caught up'. Different patterns of fetal growth will have different effects on the relative size of different organs at birth, even though overall body size may be the same. This emphasises the severe limitation of birthweight as a measure of fetal growth.

While slowing its rate of growth the fetus may protect tissues that are important for immediate survival, the brain especially. One way in which the brain can be protected is by redistribution of blood flow to favour it.[51, 52] This adaptation is known to occur in many mammals but in humans it may have exaggerated costs for other tissues, notably the liver and other abdominal viscera, because of the large size of the brain.

It is becoming increasingly clear that nutrition has profound effects on fetal hormones, and on the hormonal and metabolic interactions between the fetus, placenta and mother on whose coordination fetal growth depends.[47] Fetal insulin and the insulin-like growth factors (IGFs) are thought to have a central role in the regulation of growth and respond rapidly to changes in fetal nutrition (Fig. 2.5).[53] If a mother decreases her food intake, fetal insulin, IGF-1 and glucose concentrations fall, possibly through the effect of decreased maternal growth hormone and IGF. This leads to reduced transfer of amino acids and glucose from mother to fetus, and ultimately to reduced rates of fetal growth.[54] In late gestation and after birth the fetus' growth hormone and IGF axis take over, from insulin, a central role in driving linear growth. Whereas undernutrition leads to a fall in the concentrations of hormones that control fetal growth it leads to a rise in cortisol, whose main effects are on cell differentiation (Fig. 2.5).[48]

The differing effects of undernutrition at different stages of gestation may be summarised as follows.[39]

Early pregnancy

As has been described already the concentrations of nutrients in the earliest stages of pregnancy influence growth of the embryo. Animal studies have shown that birth size can be profoundly changed by a brief period of in vitro culture before implantation. Suboptimal nutrition before implantation retards growth and development, the one-cell embryo being particularly sensitive. The early embryo is selective in its use of nutrients and respires pyruvate, lactate, and amino acids such as glutamine rather than glucose.[43] Before implantation it switches to a glucose-based metabolism, and low glucose concentrations retard its growth and development.[55] Paradoxically, perhaps, high glucose concentrations, which accompany maternal diabetes, also delay embryonic growth. This effect contrasts with the accelerated growth associated with high glucose concentrations in late pregnancy.

Mid-pregnancy

The placenta grows faster than the fetus in mid-pregnancy and nutrient deficiency may therefore affect fetal growth by changing the interaction between the fetus and the placenta. Whereas maternal undernutrition restricts growth of fetus and placenta, mild undernutrition may lead to increased placental but not fetal size (p. 70).[56] This placental overgrowth may be an adaptation to sustain nutrient supply from the mother. Localised placental hypertrophy can also be induced experimentally in sheep by reducing the number of implantation sites. Owens & Robinson[57] have shown that the compensatory growth at the remaining sites occurs before there is noticeable retardation of fetal growth, and may be a sensitive, early response to reduced nutrient supply.

During undernutrition fetal growth may be sacrificed to maintain placental function. In animals oxygen, glucose and amino acids may be redistributed, so that the placenta reduces its consumption of oxygen and glucose while maintaining a large output of lactate to the fetus.[58] The lactate is partly derived from amino acids of fetal origin, and the fetus may waste and be thin at birth.[58] There is evidence for similar metabolic changes in growth-retarded human fetuses, in whom wasting has been observed by ultrasonography.[59–61]

Late pregnancy

In late gestation undernutrition results in immediate slowing of fetal growth. Acute undernutrition causes prompt slowing of fetal growth associated with fetal catabolism,[45] but fetal growth rapidly resumes when nutrition is restored. In contrast, prolonged undernutrition may irreversibly slow the rate of fetal growth in lambs and lead to reduced length at birth.[62] The basis of this irreversibility is uncertain, but it is reflected in the clinical observation that children with intrauterine growth retardation who show postnatal growth failure are those with evidence of more prolonged intrauterine growth retardation.[63]

Genes and fetal adaptations

Little is known about the genes which underlie the fetal cardiovascular, metabolic and hormonal adaptations to undernutrition. Genes which allow the fetus to successfully adapt to undernutrition are likely to be favoured by natural selection even though they may lead to disease and premature death in post-reproductive life. The fundamental role of genetic information is to enable the cell and organism to maintain homeostasis in the face of environmental changes, that is to maintain the intracellular concentrations necessary for survival, while the supply of these from external sources fluctuates. Common genetic variation results in different individuals in a population having differing ability to maintain homeostasis under different environmental challenges.

In response to poor nutrient availability in utero some fetuses will fail to make appropriate homeostatic responses and will die; some will make responses that will allow growth to continue at the same rate; others will make homeostatic responses that will ensure survival but the growth rates of some tissues and systems will slow. This last group will be at risk of coronary heart disease and other disorders in adult life.

MATERNAL NUTRITION AND BIRTHWEIGHT

Fetal nutrition must be distinguished from maternal nutrition. Experience in famine, described later in this chapter, shows that even extreme restrictions in mother's food intake during pregnancy have only modest effects on birthweight. From this it cannot be concluded that fetal growth is not regulated by its nutrient supply. Rather it suggests that maternal nutrient intakes during pregnancy have relatively small effects on birth size, which may depend more on mother's nutritional state before pregnancy, that is on the turnover of her protein and fatty acid stores in her muscle and fat. Birthweight is a crude measure of fetal growth: babies of the same weight may, for example, be short and fat or long and thin, and may be markedly different in organ size and structure, physiology and metabolism. The next sections describe what is known about the effects of maternal diet and body composition on birth size, body proportions at birth, and placental growth.

Mother's body size before pregnancy

A mother's body size before pregnancy is the most important determinant of the size of her baby. Figure 8.3 illustrates the remarkable variety of body form among young women in one part of England. The variety of body form around the world is much greater and is changing rapidly. This must have profound consequences for fetal growth. Whereas in western countries women like the one in the middle are slim by choice, around the world most women with low body weight in relation to their height have been chronically undernourished since childhood. Women who have low body weight before pregnancy have small babies.[64–67] Chronic undernutrition also influences birthweight through its effect on maternal stature, independent of body weight.[8, 68] It may also be associated with deficiencies in specific nutrients which influence fetal growth, including vitamins A, C, and D, folate, iron and zinc.[69]

Among chronically undernourished mothers, high weight gain during pregnancy partly offsets the effects of low weight before pregnancy, although the babies' weights still tend to remain below average.[70, 71] The mother stores fat in the first half of pregnancy and mobilises it in the second under the influence of placental growth hormone and other hormones. In this way she spares glucose for the fetus by switching to fat as her primary energy source. Observations on weight gain in obese women point to the importance of pre-pregnant weight in determining birthweight. Those who gain little weight during pregnancy, or even lose weight, still have babies of average or above average weight.[70–74]

The young women in Figure 8.3 differ not only in their body weight but also in their distribution of body fat. They differ considerably in the relative

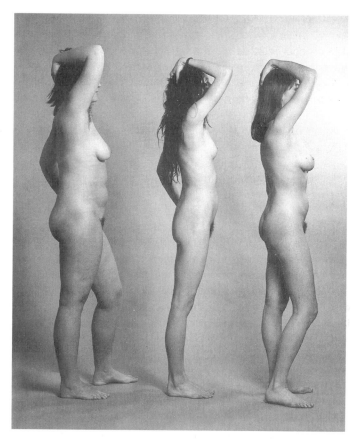

Fig. 8.3 Variations in body fat in normal young women. (Courtesy of the photographer, Helen Garnett.)

thickness of their skinfolds at different sites, including the upper arm (triceps and biceps), below the shoulder (subscapular), and above the hip (suprailiac). They also have varying amounts of abdominal fat shown by the circumference of their waists in relation to the circumference of their hips. The woman on the left has the highest 'waist:hip' ratio. The distribution of body fat is determined by the total amount of fat, reflected in the body mass index, and by other influences including fetal growth. Chapter 6 (p. 111) describes how people who had low birthweight tend to store fat centrally, having a high ratio of subscapular to triceps skinfold thickness and a high waist:hip ratio. Differences in the proportions of fat in different parts of the body are known to be linked to differences in metabolism and hormonal profile. Deposition of fat on the abdomen, for example, is associated with resistance to insulin and an altered balance of sex hormones,[75] and fat at different sites on the body makes varying amounts of oestrogen. The effects that the hormonal and metabolic variations which are linked to body fat distribution have on the fetus are largely unknown.

Weight gain and diet during pregnancy

In Europe mothers gain around 12 kg (26 lb) in weight during pregnancy. The maternal component of this averages 7.7 kg (17 lb) and comprises increases in fat, extracellular fluid, uterine and breast tissue. Maternal fat stores of around 3 kg (7 lb) are mostly laid down during the first half of pregnancy and provide an energy store for the fetus in late gestation. The extracellular fluid volume is increased by 3 litres. Half of this increase is due to expansion of the plasma volume which, together with a fall in the peripheral resistance and increase in heart rate, leads to an increase in cardiac output. The cardiac output increases by 40% during the first trimester. Plasma volume increases more if the fetus is large and the mother's cardiovascular adaptations, which determine the perfusion of the placenta, are important determinants of fetal nutrition. We know little about the effects of the mother's body composition and nutrition before pregnancy on these adaptations.[76]

In western countries, except in extreme circumstances, maternal undernutrition during pregnancy, reflected in low maternal weight gain, leads to only modest reductions in birthweight.[77-80] Indeed the weak relationship between maternal weight gain in pregnancy and birth size has contributed to the myth that, in affluent populations, nutrition has little effect on fetal growth.[81] This myth arises from failure to understand the importance of maternal body composition, itself determined by nutrition, failure to distinguish fetal from maternal nutrition, and the use of crude indicators of fetal growth such as birthweight.

During the past 50 years numerous studies have examined whether the quality of the diet eaten by a pregnant woman influences the birthweight of the baby. The results have been various and contradictory.[82] The relationship between calorie intake in pregnancy and birthweight, found in observational studies and trials, is of varying size and generally less than had been expected.[83] In one of the best known studies, in Aberdeen, Scotland, the diets of primagravid women were recorded by weighed food intakes and food diaries during the 7th month of pregnancy.[84] Calorie intake was associated with birthweight in that women who consumed less than 1800 calories per day had babies who weighed 240 g (0.5 lb) less than those of mothers who ate 3000 and more calories, but this is a small effect.

The Dutch 'hunger winter' lasted for 5 months and daily calorie intakes fell below 1000. Babies exposed to the famine during the first half of gestation, who were born after the famine was lifted, had normal birthweight. Those exposed during the second half of gestation had lower birthweight, being 327 g (0.7 lb) lighter than babies born before the famine.[85, 86] The effect of the famine in Wuppertal, Germany, during 1945–46 was less. Calorie intake was reduced to around 2400 a day and birthweight was reduced by around 185 g (0.4 lb).[87] The exceptionally severe famine in Leningrad (now St Petersburg) during 1941–43 led to a 530 g (1.2 lb) fall in mean birthweight.[88] The German blockade of Leningrad between September 1941 and January 1944 prevented supplies from reaching the city for 900 days. During the siege approximately 1 million Leningrad citizens died from a total population of 2.4 million. Most of these deaths occurred during the 'hunger winter' of November 1941 to February 1942 when the siege was in full force and the average daily ration was about 300 calories, composed almost entirely of carbohydrate. Nearly 50% of all term infants exposed to famine during the second half of gestation weighed less than 2.5 kg (5.5 lb).

In some trials supplementation of the mother's diet has led to an increase in mean birthweight, though generally of small size. One trial of protein-calorie supplementation, among poorly nourished mothers in New York City, produced a fall in mean birthweight.[89] This unexpected result led to a re-analysis of all reported supplementation trials.[90] Supplements with a low percentage of calories as protein were found to have increased birthweight whereas supplements with a high protein density reduced birthweight.

A number of studies support the idea that the inconsistency in the results of different trials could be the result of differing effects in women whose nutritional status differed before pregnancy. Underweight women with high calorie intakes during pregnancy have babies of similar size to those of overweight women with low calorie intakes. A trial among Asian women living in England suggested that the babies of women whose triceps skinfold thickness did not increase in mid-pregnancy benefited most from protein and energy supplementation.[91] In the Gambia, energy supplementation increased birthweight only during the wet season, a time when food is scarce and women work hard planting crops.[92] In the New York study, only the babies of mothers who smoked cigarettes benefited;[89] whether this reflected the different diets of smokers and non-smokers is not known.

MATERNAL NUTRITION AND BODY PROPORTIONS AT BIRTH

Animal studies show that fetal undernutrition at different times in gestation may lead to newborns with different overall body size or with similar body size but marked differences in the proportional size of different organs (Ch. 2). In sheep, for example, undernutrition in late pregnancy increases the weight of the heart without altering body size. Chronic nutritional deprivation sustained from early pregnancy is associated with proportionate growth failure in head size, length and weight.[9, 44] Undernutrition in mid- or late gestation is associated with disproportionate growth, reflected in thinness or shortness at birth (p. 16). This is, of course, an oversimplification. Though thinness at birth may result from failure of nutrient supply in late pregnancy, this failure may originate from influences affecting placental development in early gestation.[93] The guinea pig fetus becomes thin only if the mother is continuously undernourished from early or mid-pregnancy to term, while it will become short if the mother is undernourished in early or mid pregnancy only. Chapters 3–6 showed that physiological disorders in adult life are linked not only to birthweight but to body proportions at birth. Babies who are thin at birth (Fig. 3.9) develop different disorders from babies who are short or have low birthweight in relation to head circumference (Fig. 3.10). This suggests that undernutrition at different stages of gestation has different long-term effects.

There is limited information about the maternal influences that determine different body proportions at birth. Figure 8.4 shows that the babies of mothers who had low birthweight tend to be thin irrespective of the mother's current body size.[30, 94] In that particular study maternal stature had no additional effect, though Kramer and colleagues have found that taller mothers tend to have longer, thinner babies.[94] The father's birthweight did not influence ponderal

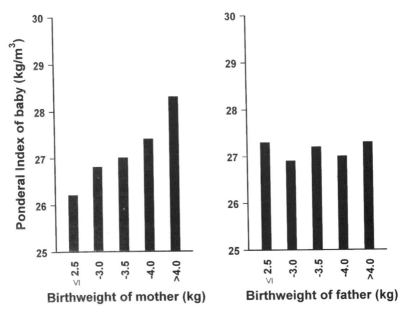

Fig. 8.4 Ponderal index at birth of 492 term babies according to the birthweight of their mothers and fathers.

index but taller fathers have longer, thinner babies.[30] Low dairy protein intake in late pregnancy is also associated with thinness at birth.[30] Other studies have shown that reduced protein intake in pregnancy is associated with shortness at birth.[95]

Dutch babies exposed to wartime famine in mid–late gestation were either thin or had low birthweight in relation to their head size.[86, 96] Table 8.1 shows the characteristics of 2414 babies born in the Wilhelmina Gasthuis Hospital, Amsterdam, at that time. The period of famine was clearly delineated, for it began abruptly in late November 1944 and ended with liberation by the Allied Forces in early May 1945. Official rations varied between 400 and 800 calories per day in the first months of 1945. In Table 8.1 babies are

Table 8.1 Body size of 2414 babies born around the time of the Dutch famine

		Exposed to famine			
Birth size	Born before famine $n = 764$	In late pregnancy $n = 307$	In mid-pregnancy $n = 297$	In early pregnancy $n = 217$	Conceived after famine $n = 829$
Birthweight, g	3373	3133	3217	3470	3413
Crown-to-heel length, cm	50.5	49.4	49.8	50.9	50.5
Head circumference, cm	32.9	32.3	32.1	32.8	33.2
Placental area, cm²	291	266	271	267	275
Ponderal index, kg/m³	26.1	25.8	26.0	26.2	26.5
Head circumference/weight	9.9	10.4	10.1	9.6	9.9
Mother's weight in late pregnancy, kg	63.5	61.9	59.9	63.0	65.1

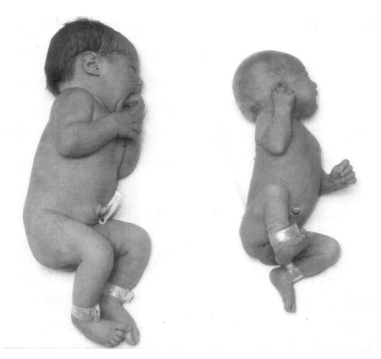

Fig. 8.5 The newborn baby on the right is proportionately smaller than the baby on the left.

classified as being exposed to famine in utero if the average maternal daily food ration during any 13-week period of gestation was below 1000 calories. They are divided into those exposed only in late gestation, whose mothers were already pregnant when the famine began, and those exposed in mid- or early gestation. When compared with babies born before the famine, or conceived after it, the babies of mothers exposed to famine in mid- or late pregnancy had lower birthweights, lengths, head circumferences and were thinner. The increase in the babies' head-to-birthweight ratios suggests that brain- sparing adaptations occurred. Paradoxically, the babies who were conceived during the famine were heavier and longer. This is difficult to interpret because many women would have been infertile during the famine and the nutrition of those who conceived improved sharply in late pregnancy, after liberation, as is shown by mothers' weights in late pregnancy (Table 8.1).

An important difference between fetal growth in the developing countries and that in western countries is that proportionate growth retardation (Fig. 8.5) is common in the developing countries whereas disproportionate, or 'asymmetrical', growth retardation prevails in western countries.[9] Babies with proportionate growth retardation seem to be more prone to neurodevelopmental impairment, whereas those with disproportionate growth retardation seem to be more at risk of perinatal death.[97–99]

MATERNAL NUTRITION AND THE PLACENTA

The fetus can become undernourished in spite of an adequate nutrient supply from the mother if transport across the placenta is inadequate. This may result from poor implantation or breakdown of feedback control between the fetus and placenta. Some complications of pregnancy, including pre-eclampsia, are associated with reduced placental size.

Maternal undernutrition has variable effects on placental growth. In general it has little effect in early and late gestation; in mid-gestation its effects vary. Some animal studies have shown that maternal undernutrition in mid-pregnancy reduces placental weight.[100, 101] Others have shown increased placental weight (in sheep), or an increase in the ratio of placental to fetal weight (in guinea-pigs).[56, 102, 103] The findings in sheep are not readily reproducible and McCrabb and colleagues suggested that this might be the result of different maternal nutritional reserves before conception.[103] Subsequently Robinson and colleagues in Adelaide showed that good nutrition around the time of conception followed by a restricted diet in mid-pregnancy stimulated placental growth in sheep, whereas mid-pregnancy undernutrition in an already poorly nourished ewe restricted placental growth.[104] These observations on the effect of a changing plane of nutrition during pregnancy are consistent with empirical practices in sheep farming whereby ewes are moved from rich pasture to poor pasture after mating. If they are then returned to rich pasture in late pregnancy the lambs are heavier than those whose mothers were on rich pasture throughout. These surprising observations inevitably raise questions about the effects of nausea and anorexia in human pregnancy.

In humans there is some evidence that high food intakes in mid-pregnancy may also suppress placental growth. A study of the diets of an unselected group of pregnant women suggested that high intakes of carbohydrates in mid-pregnancy, especially simple carbohydrates such as are found in soft drinks, suppressed placental growth.[105] This was especially marked if high carbohydrate intake in mid-pregnancy was followed by low dairy protein intake in late pregnancy. Differential effects of carbohydrates on placental size were also found in a recent trial. In this instance, however, 'aboriginal' carbohydrates, which are associated with a lower blood sugar after ingestion led to reduced placental and fetal size.[106]

In contrast to the apparent suppressive effect of carbohydrate Beischer and colleagues showed that anaemia during pregnancy was associated with increased placental size.[107] In a study of 8684 pregnant women in Oxford, those whose haemoglobin concentrations fell to lower values during pregnancy had larger placentas.[108] Subsequent studies showed that among women with low haemoglobin placental volume was already increased at 18 weeks of pregnancy.[109] Furthermore, Wheeler and colleagues showed that maternal haemoglobin concentrations between 9 and 11 weeks of pregnancy were inversely related to the maternal serum concentrations of chorionic gonadotrophin and placental lactogen, hormones synthesised by the placenta.[110] The associations between maternal haemoglobin and placental size and function are not explained by the effects of haemodilution. They may reflect the effects of a reduced oxygen content in maternal blood. Hypoxia may stimulate blood vessel formation in the growing placenta by increasing the expression of angiogenic growth factors such as vascular endothelial growth factor (VEGF).

The mild hypoxaemia associated with life at high altitude is also associated with an increase in the ratio of placental to fetal weight.[111, 112] Clapp & Rizk have shown that if mothers exercise vigorously in early pregnancy the volume of the placenta in mid-pregnancy is increased.[113] Cigarette smoking suppresses both placental and fetal growth but suppression of the placenta is less and the ratio of placental to fetal weight at birth is therefore increased.[111] These effects may also be mediated by hypoxia, though other influences must also affect the ratio of placental to fetal weight, which is raised if the mother has a high body mass.[114]

Further evidence that the placental enlargement may be an adaptive response to lack of oxygen or nutrients comes from a study of babies that were unusually small (below the 10th centile) for their gestational age.[115] Their ratio of placental to birthweight was higher than that of babies whose size was appropriate to their gestational age.

Long-term effects of placental growth

Placental size and the ratio of placental weight to birthweight are associated with important long-term outcomes. Figure 8.6 shows that there is a U-shaped relation between death rates from coronary heart disease among men and the ratio of placental weight to birthweight. Either a high or a low ratio is associated with increased death rates.[116] Babies with a placenta that is disproportionately large in relation to their birthweight are known to be at increased risk of raised blood pressure (Table 4.6),[117, 118] impaired glucose tolerance,[119] and raised plasma fibrinogen concentrations.[120] These associations, however, are not consistently found. In Aberdeen for example, raised blood pressure was

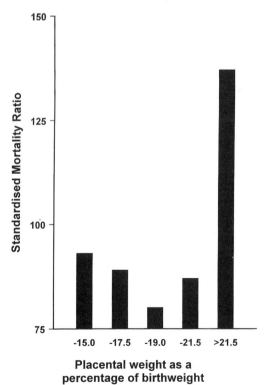

Fig. 8.6 Standardised mortality ratios for coronary heart disease according to the ratio of placental weight to birthweight in 1320 men.

associated with low placental weight[121] and in the Sheffield study death from stroke was associated with a low placental weight in relation to head size at birth.[116] Other studies have failed to find any associations between blood pressure and placental size.[122] One explanation for this is that placental responses to maternal undernutrition vary according to the stage of gestation at which undernutrition occurs and the nutrition of the mother before pregnancy.

LONG-TERM EFFECTS OF FETAL UNDERNUTRITION ON CORONARY HEART DISEASE

A theme of this book is that fetal adaptations to undernutrition tend to be permanent. Persistent changes in the production of the hormones that control growth, or in the sensitivity of tissues to them, may permanently program metabolism.[39, 123] For example, the fetus may acquire a persisting deficiency in insulin production or may become resistant to insulin. After birth insulin deficiency and resistance are manifest through effects on glucose metabolism. As described in Chapter 6 non-insulin-dependent diabetes may originate in this way. Other findings described in this book suggest that adaptive stressor responses including those mediated by the hypothalamic-pituitary-adrenal and sympatho-adrenal axes may persist into adult life and underlie the association between restricted fetal growth and the metabolic syndrome (pp. 73, 75, 105).

Intrauterine growth retardation in humans is associated with alterations in growth hormone similar to those seen during postnatal fasting. There is hypersecretion of growth hormone but evidence of tissue resistance to it.[124] Gluckman and colleagues proposed that babies who are short at birth and grow slowly in infancy may have persisting defects in their growth hormone and IGF axes; either growth hormone deficiency or resistance.[39] The offspring of undernourished rats are known to have a marked delay in postnatal catch-up growth which is associated with a delay in the development of responsivity to growth hormone. The Hertfordshire and Sheffield studies have shown that babies who are short at birth, with a small liver, as measured by the abdominal circumference, and who fail to gain weight in infancy, have raised plasma concentrations of low density lipoprotein cholesterol and plasma fibrinogen as adults (Ch. 5) and raised death rates from coronary heart disease (Ch. 3). Adults with growth hormone deficiency have an increased mortality from cardiovascular disease, low serum high density lipoprotein and raised triglyceride concentrations, increased body mass and raised blood pressure.[125, 126] Administration of growth hormone to normal subjects stimulates the low density lipoprotein cholesterol receptor in the liver and lowers serum cholesterol concentrations by 25%.[127] One may therefore speculate that persisting alterations in circulating growth hormone concentrations or in tissue sensitivity to the hormone may be a mechanism in the pathogenesis of coronary heart disease.

A FRAMEWORK

Figure 8.7 brings together some of the ideas and findings about mechanisms discussed in this book, and offers a framework within which the links between

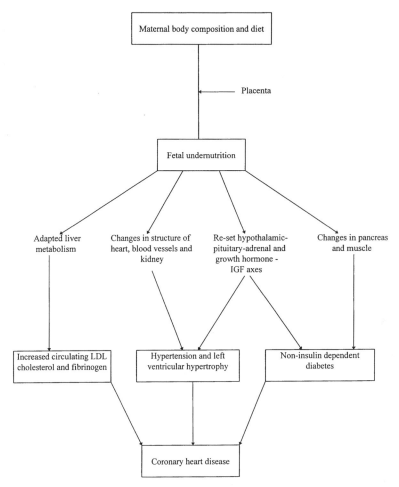

Fig. 8.7   A framework of possible mechanisms linking fetal undernutrition and coronary heart disease.

fetal undernutrition and coronary heart disease can be explored. It is a working hypothesis and will need to be re-evaluated as more information becomes available.

Summary

The growth of a baby is constrained by the nutrients and oxygen it receives from the mother. A mother's ability to nourish her baby is established during her own fetal life and by her nutritional experiences in childhood and adolescence, which determine her body weight. Mother's diet in pregnancy has little effect on the baby's size at birth but nevertheless programs the baby. The fetus adapts to undernutrition by changing its metabolism, altering its production of hormones and the sensitivity of tissues to them, redistributing its blood flow and slowing its growth rate. In some circumstances the placenta may enlarge. Adaptations to undernutrition that occur during development can permanently alter the structure and function of the body.

References

1 McCance RA, Widdowson EM. The determinants of growth and form. *Proc R Soc Lond B* 1974; **185**: 1–17.

2 Gluckman PD, Breier BH, Oliver M, Harding J, Bassett N. Fetal growth in late gestation – a constrained pattern of growth. *Acta Paediatr Scand Suppl* 1990; **367**: 105–110.

3 Morton NE. The inheritance of human birth weight. *Ann Hum Genet* 1955; **20**: 123–134.

4 Robson EB. Birth weight in cousins. *Ann Hum Genet* 1955; **19**: 262–268.

5 Penrose LS. Some recent trends in human genetics. *Caryologia* 1954; **6(Suppl)**: 521–530.

6 Brooks AA, Johnson MR, Steer PJ, Pawson ME, Abdalla HI. Birth weight: nature or nurture? *Early Hum Dev* 1995; **42**: 29–35.

7 Lush JL, Hetzer HO, Culbertson CC. Factors affecting birth weights of swine. *Genetics* 1934; **19**: 329–343.

8 Cawley RH, McKeown T, Record RG. Parental stature and birth weight. *Ann Hum Genet* 1954; **6**: 448–456.

9 Kline J, Stein Z, Susser M. *Conception to birth – epidemiology of prenatal development.* New York: Oxford University Press, 1989.

10 Roberts DF. The genetics of human growth. In: Falkner F, Tanner JM, eds. *Human growth, vol 3, Methodology: ecological, genetic and nutritional effects on growth.* New York: Plenum Press, 1986.

11 Trivers RL. Parent–offspring conflict. *Am Zool* 1974; **14**: 249–264.

12 Moore T, Haig D. Genomic imprinting in mammalian development: a parental tug of war. *Trends Genet* 1991; **7**: 45–49.

13 Haig D, Graham C. Genomic imprinting and the strange case of the insulin-like growth factor II receptor. *Cell* 1991; **64**: 1045–1046.

14 Lyle R. Gametic imprinting in development and disease. *J Endocrinol* 1997; **155**: 1–12.

15 Hall JG. Genomic imprinting: review and relevance to human diseases. *Am J Hum Genet* 1990; **46**: 857–873.

16 De Chiara TM, Robertson EJ, Efstratiadis A. Parental imprinting of the mouse insulin-like growth factor II gene. *Cell* 1991; **64**: 849–859.

17 Fedak MA, Arnbom T, Boyd IL. The relation between the size of southern elephant seal mothers, the growth of their pups, and the use of maternal energy, fat, and protein during lactation. *Physiol Zool* 1996; **69**: 887–911.

18 James WPT. Long-term fetal programming of body composition and longevity. *Nutr Rev* 1997; **55**: S41–S43.

19 Walton A, Hammond J. The maternal effects on growth and conformation in Shire horse–Shetland pony crosses. *Proc Roy Soc Lond B* 1938; **125**: 311–335.

20 Joubert DM, Hammond J. A crossbreeding experiment with cattle, with special reference to the maternal effect in South Devon–Dexter crosses. *J Agric Sci* 1958; **51**: 325–341.

21 Snow MHL. Effects of genome on fetal size at birth. In: Sharp F, Fraser RB, Milner RDG, eds. *Fetal growth Proceedings of the 20th Study Group.* London: Royal College of Obstetricians and Gynaecologists, 1989; 1–11.

22 Ounsted M, Ounsted C. Maternal regulation of intra-uterine growth. *Nature* 1966; **212**: 995–997.

23 Hackman E, Emanuel I, van Belle G, Daling J. Maternal birth weight and subsequent pregnancy outcome. *J Am Med Assoc* 1983; **250**: 2016–2019.

24 Klebanoff MA, Graubard B, Kessel SS, Berendes HW. Low birth weight across generations. *J Am Med Assoc* 1984; **252**: 2423–2427.

25 Carr-Hill R, Campbell DM, Hall MH, Meredith A. Is birth weight determined genetically? *Br Med J* 1987; **295**: 687–689.

26 Alberman E, Emanuel I, Filakti H, Evans SJW. The contrasting effects of parental birthweight and gestational age on the birthweight of offspring. *Paediatric and Perinatal Epidemiology* 1992; **6**: 134–144.

27 Emanuel I, Filakti H, Alberman E, Evans SJW. Intergenerational studies of human birthweight from the 1958 birth cohort. I. Evidence for a multigenerational effect. *Br J Obstet Gynaecol* 1992; **99**: 67–74.

28 Klebanoff MA, Meirik O, Berendes HW. Second-generation consequences of small-for-dates birth. *Pediatrics* 1989; **84**: 343–347.

29 Skjaerven R, Wilcox AJ, Oyen N, Magnus P. Mothers' birth weight and survival of their

offspring: population based study. *Br Med J* 1997; **314**: 1376–1380.

30 Godfrey KM, Barker DJP, Robinson S, Osmond C. Maternal birthweight and diet in pregnancy in relation to the infant's thinness at birth. *Br J Obstet Gynaecol* 1997; **104**: 663–667.

31 Ounsted M, Scott A, Ounsted C. Transmission through the female line of a mechanism constraining human fetal growth. *Ann Hum Biol* 1986; **13**: 143–151.

32 Gluckman P, Harding J. The regulation of fetal growth. In: Hernandez M, Argente J, eds. *Human growth: basic and clinical aspects*. Elsevier, 1992; 253–259.

33 Mussey RD. Nutrition and human reproduction: an historical review. *Am J Obstet Gynecol* 1949; **57**: 1037–1048.

34 Stewart RJC, Sheppard H, Preece R, Waterlow JC. The effect of rehabilitation at different stages of development of rats marginally malnourished for ten to twelve generations. *Br J Nutr* 1980; **43**: 403–412.

35 Pinto ML, Shetty PS. Influence of exercise-induced maternal stress on fetal outcome in Wistar rats: inter-generational effects. *Br J Nutr* 1995; **73**: 645–653.

36 Dhawan S. Birth weights of infants of first generation Asian women in Britain compared with second generation Asian women. *Br Med J* 1995; **311**: 86–88.

37 Mellanby E. Nutrition and child-bearing. *Lancet* 1933; **2**: 1131–1137.

38 Forsen T, Eriksson JG, Tuomilehto J, Teramo K, Osmond C, Barker DJP. Mother's weight in pregnancy and coronary heart disease in a cohort of Finnish men: follow up study. *Br Med J* 1997; **315**: 837–840.

39 Barker DJP, Gluckman PD, Godfrey KM, Harding JE, Owens JA, Robinson JS. Fetal nutrition and cardiovascular disease in adult life. *Lancet* 1993; **341**: 938–941.

40 Godfrey KM, Robinson S, Hales CN, Barker DJP, Osmond C, Taylor KP. Nutrition in pregnancy and the concentrations of proinsulin, 32–33 split proinsulin, insulin, and C-peptide in cord plasma. *Diabet Med* 1996; **13**: 868–873.

41 Kleeman DO, Walker SK, Seamark RF. Enhanced fetal growth in sheep administered progesterone during the first three days of pregnancy. *J Reprod Fertil* 1994; **102**: 411–417.

42 Walker SK, Hartwich KM, Seamark RF. The production of unusually large offspring following embryo manipulation: concepts and challenges. *Theriogenology* 1996; **45**: 111–120.

43 Leese HJ. The energy metabolism of the pre-implantation embryo. In: Heyner S, Wiley L, eds. *Early embryo development and paracrine relationships*. New York: Alan R. Liss, 1990; 67–78.

44 Woods DL. The constraint of maternal nutrition on the trajectory of fetal growth in humans. In: Bruton MN, ed. *Alternative life-history styles of animals*. Dordrecht: Kluwer Academic, 1989; 459–464.

45 Harding J, Liu L, Evans P, Oliver M, Gluckman P. Intrauterine feeding of the growth retarded fetus: can we help? *Early Hum Dev* 1992; **29**: 193–197.

46 Widdowson EM, McCance RA. The effect of finite periods of undernutrition at different ages on the composition and subsequent development of the rat. *Proc Roy Soc Lond B* 1963; **158**: 329–342.

47 Harding JE, Johnston BM. Nutrition and fetal growth. *Reprod Fertil Dev* 1995; **7**: 539–547.

48 Fowden AL. Endocrine regulation of fetal growth. *Reprod Fertil Dev* 1995; **7**: 351–363.

49 Widdowson EM. Immediate and long-term consequences of being large or small at birth: a comparative approach. In: Elliott K, Knight J, eds. *Size at birth. Ciba Symposium 27*. Amsterdam: Elsevier, 1974; 65–82.

50 Hinchliffe SA, Lynch MRJ, Sargent PH, Howard CV, Van Velzen D. The effect of intrauterine growth retardation on the development of renal nephrons. *Br J Obstet Gynaecol* 1992; **99**: 296–301.

51 Campbell AGM, Dawes GS, Fishman AP, Hyman AI. Regional redistribution of blood flow in the mature fetal lamb. *Circulation Research* 1967; **21**: 229–235.

52 Rudolph AM. The fetal circulation and its response to stress. *J Dev Physiol* 1984; **6**: 11–19.

53 Fowden AL. The role of insulin in prenatal growth. *J Dev Physiol* 1989; **12**: 173–182.

54 Oliver MH, Harding JE, Breier BH, Evans PC, Gluckman PD. Glucose but not a mixed amino acid infusion regulates plasma insulin-like growth factor-1 concentrations in fetal sheep. *Pediatr Res* 1993; **34**: 62–65.

55 Gott AL, Hardy K, Winston RML, Leese HJ. Non-invasive measurement of pyruvate and

glucose uptake and lactate production by single human preimplantation embryos. *Hum Reproduction* 1990; **5**: 104–108.

56 McCrabb GJ, Egan AR, Hosking BJ. Maternal undernutrition during mid-pregnancy in sheep. Placental size and its relationship to calcium transfer during late pregnancy. *Br J Nutr* 1991; **65**: 157–168.

57 Owens JA, Robinson JS. The effect of experimental manipulation of placental growth and development. In: Cockburn F, ed. *Fetal and neonatal growth*. Chichester: John Wiley, 1988; 49–77.

58 Owens JA, Falconer J, Robinson JS. Effect of restriction of placental growth on fetal and utero-placental metabolism. *J Dev Physiol* 1987; **9**: 225–238.

59 Divon MY, Chamberlain PF, Sipos L, Manning FA, Platt LD. Identification of the small for gestational age fetus with the use of gestational age-independent indices of fetal growth. *Am J Obstet Gynecol* 1986; **155**: 1197–1201.

60 Soothill PW, Nicolaides KH, Campbell S. Prenatal asphyxia, hyperlacticaemia, hypoglycaemia and erythroblastosis in growth retarded fetus. *Br Med J* 1987; **294**: 1051–1053.

61 Cetin I, Corbetta C, Sereni LP, Marconi AM, Bozzetti P, Pardi G, et al. Umbilical amino acid concentrations in normal and growth-retarded fetuses sampled in utero by cordocentesis. *Am J Obstet Gynecol* 1990; **162**: 253–261.

62 Mellor DJ, Murray L. Effects on the rate of increase in fetal girth of refeeding ewes after short periods of severe undernutrition during late pregnancy. *Res Vet Sci* 1982; **32**: 377–382.

63 Fancourt R, Campbell S, Harvey D, Norman AP. Follow-up study of small-for-dates babies. *Br Med J* 1976; **i**: 1435–1437.

64 Tompkins WT, Wiehl DG, Mitchell RM. The underweight patient as an increased obstetric hazard. *Am J Obstet Gynecol* 1955; **69**: 114–123.

65 Love EJ, Kinch RAH. Factors influencing the birth weight in normal pregnancy. *Am J Obstet Gynecol* 1965; **91**: 342–349.

66 Edwards LE, Alton IR, Barrada MI, Hakanson EY. Pregnancy in the underweight woman. Course, outcome, and growth patterns of the infant. *Am J Obstet Gynecol* 1979; **135**: 297–302.

67 Naeye RL, Blanc W, Paul C. Effects of maternal nutrition on the human fetus. *Pediatrics* 1973; **52**: 494–503.

68 Baird D. The influence of social and economic factors on stillbirths and neonatal deaths. *Journal of Obstetrics and Gynaecology of the British Empire* 1945; **52**: 339–366.

69 Backstrand JR, Allen LH. The timing and etiology of undernutrition. In: Boulton J, Laron Z, Rey J, eds. *Long-term consequences of early feeding*. Philadelphia: Lippincott-Raven, 1995.

70 Eastman NJ, Jackson E. Weight relationships in pregnancy. I. The bearing of maternal weight gain and pre-pregnancy weight on birth weight in full term pregnancies. *Obstet Gynecol Surv* 1968; **23**: 1003–1025.

71 Rosso P. Nutrition and maternal–fetal exchange. *Am J Clin Nutr* 1981; **34**: 744–755.

72 Simpson JW, Lawless RW, Mitchell AC. Responsibility of the obstetrician to the fetus. *Obstet Gynecol* 1975; **45**: 481–487.

73 Edwards LE, Dickes WF, Alton IR, Hakanson EY. Pregnancy in the massively obese: course, outcome, and obesity prognosis of the infant. *Am J Obstet Gynecol* 1978; **131**: 479–483.

74 Abrams BF, Laros RK. Prepregnancy weight, weight gain, and birth weight. *Am J Obstet Gynecol* 1986; **154**: 503–509.

75 Bjorntorp P. Adipose tissue distribution and function. *Int J Obesity* 1991; **15**: 67–81.

76 Capeless EL, Clapp JF. Cardiovascular changes in early phase of pregnancy. *Am J Obstet Gynecol* 1989; **161**: 1449–1453.

77 Susser M. Maternal weight gain, infant birthweight and diet: causal sequences. *Am J Clin Nutr* 1991; **53**: 1384–1396.

78 Niswander K, Jackson EC. Physical characteristics of the gravida and their association with birth weight and perinatal death. *Am J Obstet Gynecol* 1974; **119**: 306–313.

79 Gormican A, Valentine J, Satter E. Relationships of maternal weight gain, prepregnancy weight, and infant birthweight. *J Am Diet Assoc* 1980; **77**: 662–667.

80 Hytten FE, Chamberlain G. *Clinical physiology in obstetrics*. Oxford: Blackwell Scientific, 1980.

81 Editorial: Maternal nutrition and low birth-weight. *Lancet* 1975; **ii**: 445.

82 Rosso P. *Nutrition and metabolism in pregnancy – mother and fetus.* New York: Oxford University Press, 1990.

83 Lechtig A, Klein RE. Pre-natal nutrition and birth weight: is there a causal association. In: Dobbing J, ed. *Maternal nutrition in pregnancy – eating for two?* London: Academic Press, 1981; 131–174.

84 Thomson AM. Diet in pregnancy. 3. Diet in relation to the course and outcome of pregnancy. *Br J Nutr* 1959; **13**: 509–525.

85 Smith CA. The effect of wartime starvation in Holland upon pregnancy and its product. *Am J Obstet Gynecol* 1947; **53**: 599–608.

86 Stein Z, Susser M, Saenger G, Marolla F. *Famine and human development: The Dutch hunger winter of 1944/45.* New York: Oxford University Press, 1975.

87 Dean RFA. The size of the baby at birth and the yield of breast milk. In: Anonymous. *Studies of undernutrition. Wuppertal 1946–9.* London: HMSO, 1951; 346–378.

88 Antonov AN. Children born during the siege of Leningrad in 1942. *J Pediatr* 1947; **30**: 250–259.

89 Rush D, Stein Z, Susser M. A randomized controlled trial of prenatal nutritional supplementation in New York City. *Pediatrics* 1980; **65**: 683–697.

90 Rush D. Effects of changes in maternal energy and protein intake during pregnancy, with special reference to fetal growth. In: Sharp F, Fraser RB, Milner RDG, eds. *Fetal growth.* London: Royal College of Obstetricians and Gynaecologists, 1989; 203–233.

91 Viegas OAC, Scott PH, Cole TJ, Eaton P, Needham PG, Wharton BA. Dietary protein energy supplementation of pregnant Asian mothers at Sorrento, Birmingham. II: Selective during third trimester only. *Br Med J* 1982; **285**: 592–595.

92 Prentice AM, Whitehead RG, Watkinson M, Lamb WH, Cole TJ. Prenatal dietary supplementation of African women and birth-weight. *Lancet* 1983; **ii**: 489–492.

93 Robinson JS, Owens JA, de Barro T, Lok F, Chidzanja S. Maternal nutrition and fetal growth. In: Ward RHT, Smith SK, Donnai D, eds. *Early fetal growth and development.* London: Royal College of Obstetricians and Gynaecologists, 1994; 317–334.

94 Kramer MS, Olivier M, McLean FH, Dougherty GE, Willis DM, Usher RH. Determinants of fetal growth and body proportionality. *Pediatrics* 1990; **86**: 18–26.

95 Burke BS, Harding VV, Stuart HC. Nutrition studies during pregnancy IV. Relation of protein content of mothers diet during pregnancy to birth length, birth weight, and condition of infant at birth. *J Pediatr* 1948; **32**: 506–515.

96 Stein Z, Susser M. The Dutch Famine 1944–45 and the reproductive process. I. Effects on six indices at birth. *Pediatr Res* 1975; **9**: 70–76.

97 Walther FJ, Ramaekers LHJ. Neonatal morbidity of SGA infants in relation to their nutritional status at birth. *Acta Paediatr Scand* 1982; **71**: 437–440.

98 Villar J, Smeriglio V, Martorell R, Brown CH, Klein RE. Heterogeneous growth and mental development of intrauterine growth-retarded infants during the first 3 years of life. *Pediatrics* 1984; **74**: 783–791.

99 Haas JD, Balcazar H, Caulfield L. Variation in early neonatal mortality for different types of fetal growth retardation. *Am J Phys Anthropol* 1987; **73**: 467–473.

100 Everitt GC. Maternal undernutrition and retarded foetal development in Merino sheep. *Nature* 1964; **201**: 1341–1342.

101 Wallace AM. The growth of lambs before and after birth in relation to the level of nutrition. *J Agric Sci* 1984; **38**: 243–302.

102 Faichney GJ, White GA. Effects of maternal nutritional status on fetal and placental growth and on fetal urea synthesis in sheep. *Aust J Biol Sci* 1987; **40**: 365–377.

103 McCrabb GJ, Egan AR, Hosking BJ. Maternal undernutrition during mid pregnancy in sheep; variable effects on placental growth. *J Agric Sci* 1992; **118**: 127–132.

104 DeBarro TM, Owens J, Earl CR, Robinson JS. Nutrition during early/mid pregnancy interacts with mating weight to affect placental weight in sheep. *Australian Society for Reproductive Biology, Adelaide* 1992; (Abstract).

105 Godfrey K, Robinson S, Barker DJP, Osmond C, Cox V. Maternal nutrition in early and late pregnancy in relation to placental and fetal growth. *Br Med J* 1996; **312**: 410–414.

106 Clapp J, Ridzon S, Lopez B, Appleby-Wineberg S, Tomaselli J, Little K. Diet, exercise, and feto-placental growth. *J Soc Gynecol Invest* 1996; **3**: 273A (Abstract).

107 Beischer NA, Sivasamboo R, Vohra S, Silpisornkosal S, Reid S. Placental hypertrophy in

severe pregnancy anaemia. *Journal of Obstetrics and Gynaecology of the British Commonwealth* 1970; **77**: 398–409.

108 Godfrey KM, Redman CWG, Barker DJP, Osmond C. The effect of maternal anaemia and iron deficiency on the ratio of fetal weight to placental weight. *Br J Obstet Gynaecol* 1991; **98**: 886–891.

109 Howe D, Wheeler T. Maternal iron stores and placental growth. *J Physiol* 1993; **467**: 290 (Abstract).

110 Wheeler T, Sollero C, Alderman S, Landen J, Anthony F, Osmond C. Relation between maternal haemoglobin and placental hormone concentrations in early pregnancy. *Lancet* 1994; **343**: 511–513.

111 Meyer MB. Effects of maternal smoking and altitude on birth weight and gestation. In: Reed DM, Stanley FJ, eds. *The epidemiology of prematurity*. Baltimore: Urban and Schwarzenberg, 1977; 81–104.

112 Mayhew TM, Jackson MR, Haas JD. Oxygen diffusive conductances of human placentae from term pregnancies at low and high altitudes. *Placenta* 1990; **11**: 493–503.

113 Clapp JF, Rizk KH. Effect of recreational exercise on midtrimester placental growth. *Am J Obstet Gynecol* 1992; **167**: 1518–1521.

114 Williams LA, Evans SF, Newnham JP. Factors influencing the relative growths of the fetus and the placenta. *Australian Perinatal Society* 1996; A46 (Abstract).

115 Lao TT, Wong WM. Placental ratio and intrauterine growth retardation. *Br J Obstet Gynaecol* 1996; **103**: 924–926.

116 Martyn CN, Barker DJP, Osmond C. Mothers' pelvic size, fetal growth, and death from stroke and coronary heart disease in men in the UK. *Lancet* 1996; **348**: 1264–1268.

117 Barker DJP, Bull AR, Osmond C, Simmonds SJ. Fetal and placental size and risk of hypertension in adult life. *Br Med J* 1990; **301**: 259–262.

118 Moore VM, Miller AG, Boulton TJC, Cockington RA, Hamilton Craig I, Magarey AM, et al. Placental weight, birth measurements, and blood pressure at age 8 years. *Arch Dis Child* 1996; **74**: 538–541.

119 Phipps K, Barker DJP, Hales CN, Fall CHD, Osmond C, Clark PMS. Fetal growth and impaired glucose tolerance in men and women. *Diabetologia* 1993; **36**: 225–228.

120 Barker DJP, Meade TW, Fall CHD, Lee A, Osmond C, Phipps K, et al. Relation of fetal and infant growth to plasma fibrinogen and factor VII concentrations in adult life. *Br Med J* 1992; **304**: 148–152.

121 Campbell DM, Hall MH, Barker DJP, Cross J, Shiell AW, Godfrey KM. Diet in pregnancy and the offspring's blood pressure 40 years later. *Br J Obstet Gynaecol* 1996; **103**: 273–280.

122 Whincup PH, Cook DG, Papacosta O. Do maternal and intrauterine factors influence blood pressure in childhood? *Arch Dis Child* 1992; **67**: 1423–1429.

123 Hales CN, Barker DJP. Type 2 (non-insulin-dependent) diabetes mellitus: the thrifty phenotype hypothesis. *Diabetologia* 1992; **35**: 595–601.

124 de Zegher F, Francois I, van Helvoirt M, van der Berghe G. Small as fetus and short as child: from endogenous to exogenous growth hormone. *J Clin Endocrinol Metab* 1997; **82**: 2021–2026.

125 Rosen T, Bengtsson BA. Premature mortality due to cardiovascular disease in hypopituitarism. *Lancet* 1990; **336**: 285–288.

126 Rosen T, Eden S, Larson G, Wilhelmsen L, Bengtsson BA. Cardiovascular risk factors in adult patients with growth hormone deficiency. *Acta Endocrinol* 1993; **129**: 195–200.

127 Rudling M, Norstedt G, Olivecrona H, Reihner E, Gustafsson J, Angelin B. Importance of growth hormone for the induction of hepatic low density lipoprotein receptors. *Proc Natl Acad Sci* 1992; **89**: 6983–6987.

9

Childhood infections and disease in later life

Persistent effects of lower respiratory tract infection during infancy are immediately apparent. Bronchiolitis, bronchitis and pneumonia are often followed by cough, wheeze, and impaired lung function which persist through childhood. Effects of other infections in early childhood, however, are not immediately apparent. There may be a prolonged latent period before disorders develop in middle or late life. 'Shingles' (herpes zoster), a disease of later life caused by infection with the chickenpox virus during childhood, is a familiar example.

This chapter examines a group of diseases whose aetiology has not been explained by events occurring around the time of clinical presentation. The epidemiology of these diseases is consistent with their being, in various ways, delayed consequences of childhood infection. Disease may be initiated through either the intensity of exposure to common infections in early childhood, as is thought to underlie appendicitis and asthma, or through persistence of organisms or damage caused by them, as may underlie Paget's disease of bone, Parkinson's disease, and motor neuron disease; or through infection by a common microorganism occurring at an unusual age with unusual consequences, as may underlie multiple sclerosis.

ACUTE APPENDICITIS

Time trends

Acute appendicitis occurs at all ages but is most common during childhood and adolescence. A striking feature of the epidemiology of the disease is its time trends. Average annual mortality rates for appendicitis in England and Wales have fallen since early in this century when the disease was first recognised as an entity by the Registrar General (Fig. 11.6).[1] In medical journals at the beginning of the century there was considerable correspondence about the disease and general agreement that it increased sharply in Britain around 1890–95. The disease was recognised and described long before that but was seemingly rare.[2] Anecdotal evidence and analysis of hospital records suggest that the rise began abruptly.[3-5] There is evidence of a similarly abrupt rise in Germany, in the French army, and in Russia.[6-8]

151

It is probable that during the first two decades of the century incidence rates rose more steeply than death rates because case fatality fell sharply. The rise may, however, have been exaggerated by wider recognition of the disease. Probably the constant mortality during the 1920s reflected rising incidence and falling case fatality.[1, 9, 10] There are no incidence data for the general population but National Health Insurance statistics for Scotland during 1931–35 indicate a remarkably high annual incidence of around 55 per 10 000. Thus over a 10-year period 5% of the population developed acute appendicitis.[9]

During the 1930s death rates began to fall. Examination of age-specific trends by single year, rather than the 5-year averages shown in Figure 11.6, shows that in all age groups except the very elderly death rates were already declining when the Second World War began (Fig. 9.1). From 1940 onwards the rate of fall did not change greatly, and the decline continued almost without interruption through the postwar years. In the USA there was also a decline in mortality during the 1930s.[9] Hospital discharge rates in Britain, general practitioner consultation rates, and a local survey confirm that the postwar decline in mortality reflected a large and continuing decline in incidence.[11–14] A postwar decline in incidence has also been recorded in other European countries and in the USA.[15–18]

The upsurge of the disease from around 1895 may have been exaggerated by more widespread recognition. Its decline, as reflected in mortality, may have been accelerated by changing diagnostic practices in patients with abdominal pain, changing criteria for appendicectomy and falling case fatality. Nevertheless the overall pattern is clear: a steep rise which began abruptly around 1895 and a steep fall from the 1930s onwards.

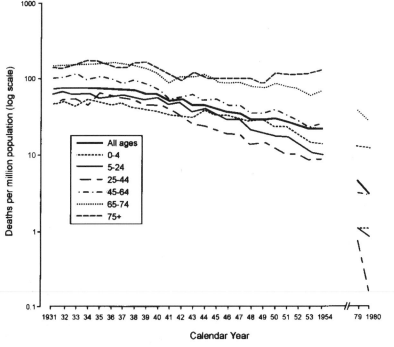

Fig. 9.1 Age-specific annual death rates for appendicitis 1931–54 and 1979–80 in England and Wales.

Social class

When appendicitis first appeared in Britain it was noted to be more common among the children of the rich.[5] These observations were supported by the higher mortality in social classes I and II.[9] Among recruits into the army in the Second World War there were astonishing differences in appendicectomy rates according to social origins.[19] These must have reflected differences in access to medical care as well as incidence of the disease. Since the Second World War the social class gradient in appendicectomy has disappeared.[18]

Geography

In 1910, Owen Williams[20] reviewed the world distribution of the disease. His findings, later extended by Murray[3] and Rendle Short,[4] showed that although it occurred throughout the world it was predominantly a disease of industrialised countries. In non-industrialised countries it was seen only among European residents. More recently, although it remains rare in some areas such as rural sub-Saharan Africa, acute appendicitis is now commonly seen in some parts of non-industrialised countries, and findings among Inuit communities support the idea that it has arisen in these areas in association with changes in the way of life.[21]

Diet

In 1920 Rendle Short[4] reviewed the rise of appendicitis in Britain during the previous 20 years and the international differences in its frequency. He concluded that the disease had arisen as a result of 'the relatively less quantity of cellulose eaten on account of the wider use of imported foods'. From this conclusion arose the 'dietary fibre hypothesis' which Burkitt and Trowell later extended to include a range of diseases commonly seen in western societies.[22–24] Figure 9.2, showing trends in consumption of cereal and vegetable fibre, meat and sugar since 1880, is based on national estimates of food supplies and consumption in Britain.[25, 26] Consumption of meat, sugar, and vegetable fibre increased whereas cereal fibre consumption decreased. These trends were interrupted by the Second World War when introduction of food rationing in 1942 led to a sharp fall in intakes of meat and sugar and a rise in fibre intake, especially cereal fibre which was present in large amounts in the wheat flour used from 1942 to 1953.

Clearly the decline in appendicitis from 1930 onwards does not correlate with changes in fibre, meat, or sugar. Moreover, the information in Figure 9.1 gives little support to the conclusion that the decline was initiated by the major changes in the British diet during the Second World War.[27, 28] Nor does Figure 9.1 suggest that a decline which had already begun was accelerated during wartime.

If the large rise in incidence, from rarity to around 50 cases per 10 000 population per year, was the effect of changing levels of consumption of a particular food, the new levels must be associated with a high risk, both absolute and relative to that in the population before the change. Given the variations among individual diets which still exist within the population, a food associated at certain levels of consumption with a high risk of disease should be readily

9

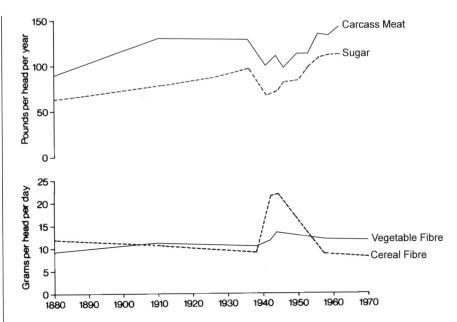

Fig. 9.2 Trends in United Kingdom food supplies from 1880.

identified by comparison of the diets of cases of appendicitis with those of controls. This has not proved to be so: the results of case-control studies have been inconclusive.[29–31]

If changes in consumption of a food caused the upsurge of appendicitis, the 1880 consumption levels must be regarded as thresholds above which (for fibre) or below which (for meat or sugar) the disease is rarely induced. Such an interpretation, however, is not consistent with the trends during and after the Second World War. At that time both cereal and vegetable fibre consumption were appreciably above the 1880 levels, and meat and sugar consumption fell to levels close to those in 1880. Given a latent period of no more than a few years, at least in children, these dietary changes would be predicted to cause a sharp drop in appendicitis in the 1940s, followed by a rise in incidence in the 1950s when food rationing ceased. There is no evidence that this occurred.

It may be concluded that dietary changes during the past century do not offer a sufficient explanation for either the rise or the decline of appendicitis in Britain. In particular, a close dependence on dietary fibre intake, postulated 60 years ago, and the origin of the hypothesis linking fibre to a range of 'western diseases', does not withstand critical examination of trends. Nevertheless, although dietary changes do not explain the changing incidence of the disease, comparisons of food consumption and rates of acute appendicitis in different areas of Britain and Ireland do suggest that green vegetables may protect against the disease, possibly by changing the bacterial flora of the appendix.[32]

The hygiene hypothesis: an explanation for the rise and fall of appendicitis

The structure of the appendix is similar to that of other parts of the gut. It has a muscular coat, and a thick submucosal layer distended with lymphatic tissue which tends to encroach on the lumen and make it somewhat small. This lymphatic tissue resembles the tonsil, and may protect the ecosystem of the large intestine from bacteria and viruses. Residue from the small intestine may be diverted into the appendix and sampled by the lymphoid tissue, which may then respond by secreting specific antibodies.[33] In 1932 Aschoff[8] showed that the ultimate event in appendicitis was invasion of the distal appendicular wall by organisms habitually present among the enteric flora. This remains the general view,[34] and debate centres on the preceding pathological changes. In 1946 Bohrod[35] argued that the initiating event in appendicitis was lymphoid hyperplasia in the appendicular wall and consequent obstruction of the proximal lumen. He pointed out that this would explain the remarkably constant age distribution of the disease in different times and places, because the bulk of lymphoid tissue in the appendicular wall in relation to luminal size is maximal during childhood and adolescence and declines thereafter.

The appendicitis epidemic in Britain started at the time when infections had begun to decline steeply, in consequence of improved living standards and sanitation.[36] It may be postulated that decreased incidence of infection among infants and young children, especially in wealthier families, changed their patterns of immunity so that they responded to later enteric or respiratory infections with lymphoid hyperplasia – which included the lymphoid tissue in the wall of the appendix.

The so-called 'hygiene hypothesis' is able to explain the international distribution of appendicitis. Countries where it is common are characterised by lower incidences of infectious disease. The rising incidence of appendicitis among the more affluent, urbanised communities within non-industrialised countries is explained by the improvement in the hygienic conditions of these communities.

Epidemiological studies in Britain and Hong Kong suggest that the provision of domestic hot water systems may be the critical improvement in hygiene which triggers the rise in acute appendicitis.[18, 37] Reduction in domestic overcrowding may contribute but seems less important.[38] Studies in Anglesey suggest that appendicitis rates depend more on the provision of hot water systems and fixed baths than on other household amenities such as piped water and water closets.[39] It is interesting that in Northern Ireland in 1956, before widespread poliomyelitis immunisation, the antibody status of children was not related to whether the house had a piped water supply. There was, however, a strong association between seropositivity and absence of a hot water system, independent of social class.[40] Reduction in the number of months for which infants are breast fed could be another influence that initiated the rise in appendicitis. A study in Naples, Italy, found that children with acute appendicitis had been breast fed for a shorter period than controls, which may indicate a lessened immune competence.[41] Breast fed infants respond to infection more mildly than bottle fed ones, which could program their immune system advantageously.

The 'hygiene hypothesis' proposes two phases in the incidence of appendicitis.[1] When hygiene begins to improve in a community, levels of infection in infants fall. This alters the response to enteric infection encountered at later ages, leading perhaps to more vigorous lymphoid hyperplasia in the appendicular wall with consequent luminal obstruction. As hygiene continues to improve, however, exposure to enteric infections which trigger acute appendicitis is reduced further, and appendicitis declines. The hygiene hypothesis illustrates how the incidence of a disease may rise and fall in response to one continuing environmental change. This is important because when 'western diseases' such as appendicitis appear in response to industrialisation and the accompanying changes in way of life, it is often argued that their prevention depends upon a return to practices of the past. This theme is developed in Chapter 11.

ASTHMA

The sharp increase in the prevalence of asthma, eczema and hay fever in industrialised countries over the past 30 years is largely unexplained.[42] Inevitably, given current concepts of disease causation, attempted explanations have focused on influences in the external environment such as air pollution; but the demonstrable effects of these are small. It is likely that an increase in the prevalence of atopy underlies the rise in these diseases. Atopy is characterised by exaggerated Th2 cell responses to common allergens with production of raised concentrations of allergen-specific IgE.

Strachan found that people with hay fever, or a history of infant eczema, tended to have fewer older siblings than other people,[43] an observation confirmed in other studies.[44] He proposed that atopy had increased because of a fall in exposure to infections in early childhood, which in some way protect against atopy. Children with more older siblings will have more exposure to infections at an early age and hence will be protected. These ideas are similar to those invoked to explain the rise in appendicitis. Direct evidence that childhood infection may prevent atopy has come from a study in Guinea-Bissau, West Africa. Young adults who had measles during childhood were found to be less likely to be atopic than those who had been vaccinated and had not had the disease.[45,46] Among Italian military students those who were seropositive for hepatitis A were less likely to be atopic.[47] Perhaps there is a range of childhood infections which protect against atopy.

There is also evidence that atopic disease may be linked to fetal growth. Babies who develop atopy in infancy have an altered T lymphocyte phenotype at birth.[48] Babies with above average birthweight and those born after a prolonged gestation of 41 or more weeks have been found to be at increased risk of developing atopic skin disease in childhood, though this does not seem to be a consistent finding.[49] In adults, however, higher birthweight and large head circumference at birth, together with prolonged gestation, are associated with raised serum concentrations of IgE, a marker of atopy.[50] The suggestion is that a rapidly growing fetus that becomes undernourished in late gestation may sacrifice development of tissues undergoing rapid growth at that time, which include the thymus, to sustain brain growth. This could permanently change the balance of the Th1 and Th2 cell populations in the thymus in favour of Th2 cells and so lead to atopy. A study of 16 year old children in New Zealand recently confirmed the association between a large head circumference at birth and the risk of asthma.[51]

This disorder is characterised by progressive skeletal deformity. The subclinical form, identified by radiological changes in the bones, is remarkably common in elderly people. In Britain death rates from Paget's disease have declined steeply during the last 40 years. If rates are analysed so that they show the mortality experience of successive generations, or cohorts, those born from around 1880 onwards had progressively lower death rates at any particular age. Generation analysis of mortality from Paget's disease in Scotland and among white people in the USA reveals a similar pattern, although the US rates are lower through-out.[52] If mortality from Paget's disease is accepted as an indicator of incidence, then an inference is that successive generations have been less and less exposed to some aetiological influence. Generation effects of this kind are seen when a disease originates from an environmental influence that acts in early life but is manifest at different ages in later life after a long latent period. If the level of exposure to the causative agent changes, the effect is seen in succeeding generations. In contrast where diseases originate after a short latent period, following exposure to an environmental agent that affects all ages, changing exposure will lead to a synchronous change in disease in all age-groups. Both coronary heart disease and stroke show generation effects, which are discussed further in Chapter 11.

Although isolated case reports have come from many parts of the world, clinical observations suggest that the disease is common only in Europe, North America, Australia, and New Zealand.[53] Perhaps the most remarkable feature of the disease's geography is the variation in rates within Europe (Fig. 9.3). The disease is commonest in Britain, where 4.6% of people over the age of 55 years have the disease in subclinical form. The prevalence in France is around half that in Britain, and beyond France the frequency declines to the south, east and north-east. The disease is rare in Scandinavia and Ireland.[54] Within Britain there is a localised area of high prevalence within the county of Lancashire[55] and within Spain there is a focus of high prevalence in La Cabrera.[56]

Within the USA comparison of a northern city, New York, with Atlanta, in the south, showed a marked difference, with prevalences among white people being 3.9% in New York and only 0.9% in Atlanta (Table 9.1).[57, 58] Markedly lower rates in the southern city were also seen among black people. It is interesting that the prevalences in black Americans were similar to those among white people, because the disease has rarely been reported in Africa, outside of South Africa where prevalences in white and black people are also similar.[59, 60] Findings in Australia (Table 9.2) parallel those in the USA. The prevalence among British-born immigrants (4.0%) was intermediate between the British rate (5.0%) and the rate among native-born Australians (3.2%).[61] Taken together with the localised geographical distribution of the disease within Europe, these two sets of observations among communities that have migrated point strongly to the importance of environmental influences in the aetiology of the disease. The generational effects suggest that these influences act early in life.

Many hypotheses about environmental causes of Paget's disease, for example, bacterial infection, a toxin, or fluorine poisoning, have arisen and been discarded. Current interest centres on the discovery that the nuclei of osteoclast

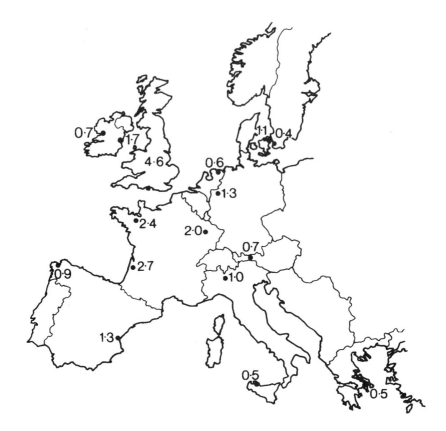

Fig. 9.3 Prevalence (%) of Paget's disease among men and women aged 55 years and over in European towns.

cells in pagetoid bone contain inclusion bodies whose appearance resembles paramyxovirus nucleocapsides.[62, 63] This raises the possibility that the disease is the result of infection with a 'slow virus', which is acquired in childhood and in later life initiates malfunctioning of osteoclast cells – currently thought to be the primary pathological disorder in the disease. Interest is centred on two particular paramyxoviruses: measles virus and respiratory syncytial virus. We do not know why these common childhood infections might in some circumstances persist and cause Paget's disease in later life, but there is an obvious parallel with the chickenpox virus and herpes zoster.

Table 9.1 Prevalence of Paget's disease by ethnic group in two American cities

City	Ethnic group	No. of radiographs	Age-standardised prevalence, %		
			Men	Women	Both sexes
New York	Black	950	3.3 (12)	2.0 (12)	2.6 (24)
New York	White	1082	5.2 (30)	2.5 (13)	3.9 (43)
Atlanta	Black	1111	1.9 (11)	0.6 (3)	1.2 (14)
Atlanta	White	1563	0.9 (7)	0.8 (6)	0.9 (13)

Figures in parentheses are numbers of cases.

Table 9.2 Prevalence of Paget's disease in Australia and the United Kingdom by place of birth and place of residence

Place of birth	Place of residence	Age-standard prevalence, %		
		Men	Women	Both sexes
UK	UK	6.2	3.9	5.0
UK	Australia	5.7	2.3	4.0
Australia	Australia	3.5	2.8	3.2

NEUROLOGICAL DISEASE

The continuing story of research into Paget's disease illustrates how, in the search for the causes of some chronic adult diseases, attention is being redirected from the role of exposure to noxious influences in the adult environment to the role of infection during childhood. The new ideas on the causes of appendicitis and asthma illustrate how the intensity of infection in early childhood may be important in determining susceptibility to disease. Martyn has developed ideas about intensity and age at infection in relation to three neurological diseases: Parkinson's disease, motor neuron disease and multiple sclerosis.[64] As with Paget's disease the time trends and geography of these diseases are compatible with the hypothesis that they are delayed consequences of childhood infection, and clinical and laboratory evidence is suggestive.

Parkinson's disease

This common extrapyramidal movement disorder is associated with loss of neurons in the substantia nigra in the brain stem. In most cases the cause is unknown. In 1963 Poskanzer & Schwab reviewed the records of nearly 1000 patients seen at the Massachusetts General since 1920.[65] They discovered that patients seen in recent years were, on average, 27 years older than those seen during 1920–24. They proposed that Parkinsonism is a delayed consequence of exposure to encephalitis lethargica which occurred as a pandemic during 1919–26. During the pandemic the incidence of this disease was highest in adolescents and young adults. Poskanzer & Schwab argued that while people who experienced an overt encephalitic illness developed Parkinsonism immediately, those who had only a mild, subclinical infection with the virus might only develop the disease in later life, when the loss of neurons that occur with age compound loss caused by the infection.

Data from countries other than the USA were consistent with an increase in Parkinson's disease following the encephalitis lethargica pandemic.[66–68] Analysis of death rates from Parkinson's disease in England and Wales since 1950 shows that while they are falling in people under 80 years they are rising in people over 80. A generation, or cohort, analysis shows that the generation born around the turn of the century were two to three times more likely to die from Parkinson's disease than people born earlier or 20 years later.[64] This was the generation who were adolescents or young adults during the encephalitis lethargica pandemic. If encephalitis lethargica did indeed initiate

Parkinson's disease, projections show that in Britain the number of cases is at its peak and will now begin to decline.

MOTOR NEURON DISEASE

In motor neuron disease there is a progressive loss of neurons, which usually begins in late adult life and leads to death within a few years. The aetiology is unknown, but its clinical similarity to poliomyelitis long ago raised the possibility that it was a delayed consequence of exposure to the poliovirus. Although few patients with the disease have suffered from paralytic poliomyelitis earlier in their lives, the illness which follows poliovirus infection may be no more than a mild aseptic meningitis. Primates infected with the virus may have neuronal lesions even if they exhibit no signs of illness.

Because of its high fatality death rates from motor neuron disease are similar to its incidence. Figure 9.4 shows the similarity between the distribution of death rates in England and Wales and notification rates from poliomyelitis in the past.[69] The correlation coefficient is 0.42 and the relation is specific. Correlation coefficients between motor neuron disease and other notifiable infectious diseases are either very small or negative.

Poliomyelitis is unique amongst infectious diseases in that it becomes commoner rather than rarer as hygiene and social conditions improve. In poor conditions the virus is ubiquitous and infection occurs in the first few months after birth, when the infant is still protected by maternal antibody and the virus does not invade beyond the gastrointestinal tract. As conditions improve, the age of first infection with the virus increases; the virus invades the central nervous system and paralytic poliomyelitis occurs. Over the first 50 years of this century there were steep increases in paralytic poliomyelitis in Europe and North America (Fig. 11.6). Studies in Britain and the USA show that motor neuron disease is now behaving in the same way.[70, 71] If the poliomyelitis hypothesis is correct motor neuron disease will continue to increase for the next 10–15 years until the first cohorts of people immunised against poliomyelitis reach the age when it occurs. Thereafter there will be a continuing decline, which will be seen first in younger people.

Multiple sclerosis

Multiple sclerosis is one of the commonest neurological diseases. Patches of demyelination occurring over many years lead to focal lesions of the nervous system. A striking feature of the disease is the tendency to remissions and relapses. The disease is common in temperate regions but rare in the tropics: frequency increases with increasing distance from the equator.[64] People who move from a country where the disease is common to one where it is rare generally have a reduced rate of the disease. However, people who make the opposite journey, from a country where the disease is rare to one where it is common retain their low risk of disease.[72, 73] One explanation of this latter observation is that there is a protective influence which operates in places where the disease is rare and confers lifelong immunity. Since studies examining the effect of age

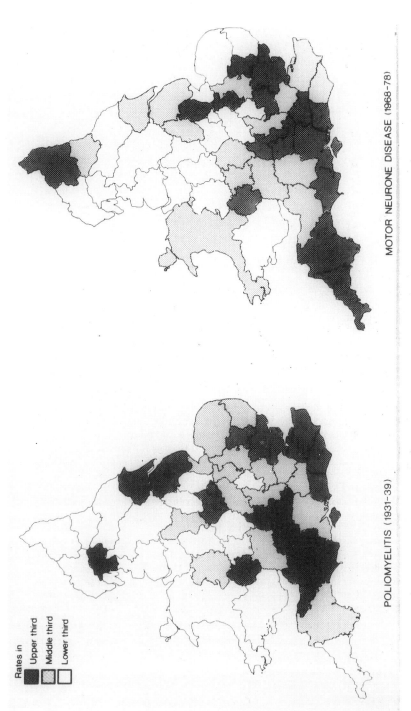

Rates in

■ Upper third
▨ Middle third
□ Lower third

MOTOR NEURONE DISEASE (1968–78)

POLIOMYELITIS (1931–39)

Fig. 9.4 Standardised mortality ratios for motor neuron disease (1968–78) and poliomyelitis (1931–39) in areas of England and Wales grouped by notification rates for poliomyelitis.

at migration suggest that an individual's risk of the disease is established in the first two decades of life this protective influence seems to act at that time.

The epidemiology of multiple sclerosis would be explained if the disease was a rare sequel to exposure to a common microorganism, a sequel which occurs when first exposure to the organism is at an older age than usual. The hepatitis B virus illustrates how the long-term consequences of childhood infection may vary according to the age at which infection occurs. Infection with the virus during early childhood often results in a chronic carrier state, but rarely causes hepatitis. When infection is delayed to adult life the carrier state is rare but hepatitis common.

Several studies have shown that people with multiple sclerosis contracted the common childhood infections at a later age than usual.[74] Recent interest has focused on the Epstein–Barr virus,[75, 76] whose effects are known to depend on the age at which first infection occurs. Infection in early childhood, as is usual in tropical countries, is not associated with disease. If infection is delayed until adolescence or later, as occurs in temperate countries, infectious mononucleosis commonly results. A recent study in Denmark showed that people infected with the Epstein–Barr virus at a later age had a threefold increase in risk of developing multiple sclerosis.[77]

The evidence linking the Epstein–Barr virus with multiple sclerosis is circumstantial, as is that linking encephalitis lethargica with Parkinson's disease and poliomyelitis with motor neuron disease. The epidemiological evidence now needs to be developed in the laboratory.

Summary

The epidemiological features of a number of diseases suggest that they may be delayed consequences of infections during childhood, though as yet the evidence is largely circumstantial. Improvements in hygiene and housing over the past century have reduced the intensity of exposure to common enteric and respiratory infections during early childhood. This may permanently alter the immune system in ways which predispose to the later development of acute appendicitis and asthma.

Reduction in exposure to infection also delays first infections with certain microorganisms until later childhood or adolescence. Age at infection is known to influence the short- and long-term outcome of infection; and multiple sclerosis may be the consequence of late infection with the Epstein–Barr virus. Three diseases of old age, Paget's disease of bone, Parkinson's disease and motor neuron disease may be delayed consequences of childhood infection with, respectively, the measles virus, the virus causing encephalitis lethargica and the poliovirus. Either the viruses persist or lesions caused by them become unmasked by ageing.

References

1 Barker DJP. Acute appendicitis and dietary fibre: an alternative hypothesis. *Br Med J* 1985; **290**: 1125–1127.
2 Fitz RH. Perforating inflammation of the vermiform appendix: with special reference to its early diagnosis and treatment. *Am J Med Sci* 1886; **92**: 321–346.
3 Murray RW. The geographical distribution of appendicitis. *Lancet* 1914; **ii**: 227–230.
4 Rendle Short A. The causation of appendicitis. *Br J Surg* 1920; **8**: 171–188.

5 Spencer AM. Aetiology of acute appendicitis. *Br Med J* 1938; **i**: 227–230.

6 Special correspondence. *Br Med J* 1903; **i**: 1373.

7 Gazeta dos Hospitaes. Quoted in *Br Med J* 1908; **ii**: 191.

8 Aschoff L, (translated by Pether GC). *Appendicitis, its aetiology and pathology*. London: Constable, 1932.

9 Young M, Russell WT. *Appendicitis, a statistical study. Medical Research Council Special Report Series No 233*. London, 1939.

10 Boyce FF. *Acute appendicitis and its complications*. New York: Oxford University Press, 1949.

11 *Report on the hospital in-patient enquiry*. London: HMSO, 1957.

12 *Mortality statistics from general practice, studies on medical and population subjects, Nos 14 and 26*. London: HMSO, 1958.

13 Donnan SPB, Lambert PM. Appendicitis: incidence and mortality. *Population trends* 1976; **5**: 26–28.

14 Raguveer-Saran MK, Keddie NC. The falling incidence of appendicitis. *Br J Surg* 1980; **67**: 681.

15 Castleton KB, Puestow CB, Sauer D. Is appendicitis decreasing in frequency? *Arch Surg* 1959; **78**: 794–801.

16 Palumbo LT. Appendicitis – is it on the wane? *Am J Surg* 1959; **98**: 702–703.

17 Arnbjornsson E, Asp NG, Westin SI. Decreasing incidence of acute appendicitis, with special reference to the consumption of dietary fiber. *Acta Chir Scand* 1982; **148**: 461–464.

18 Barker DJP, Osmond C, Golding J, Wadsworth MEJ. Acute appendicitis and bathrooms in three samples of British children. *Br Med J* 1988; **296**: 956–958.

19 Lunn-Rockliffe WEC. Army recruits and appendicitis. *Br Med J* 1942; **i**: 623

20 Williams OT. The distribution of appendicitis, with some observations on its relation to diet. *Br Med J* 1910; **ii**: 2016–2021.

21 Schaefer O. Aetiology of appendicitis. *Br Med J* 1979; **i**: 1215.

22 Burkitt DP. The aetiology of appendicitis. *Br J Surg* 1971; **58**: 695–699.

23 Trowell HC, Burkitt DP. *Western diseases; their emergence and prevention*. London: Edward Arnold, 1981.

24 Burkitt DP. *Dietary fibre*. London: Applied Science, 1983.

25 Greaves JP, Hollingsworth DF. Trends in food consumption in the United Kingdom. *World Rev Nutr Diet* 1966; **6**: 34–89.

26 Southgate DAT, Bingham S, Robertson J. Dietary fibre in the British diet. *Nature* 1978; **274**: 51–52.

27 Rendle Short A. *The causation of appendicitis*. Bristol: John Wright, 1946.

28 Donnan SPB. Aetiology of appendicitis. *Br Med J* 1979; **i**: 1215.

29 Cove-Smith J, Langman MJS. Appendicitis and dietary fibre. *Gut* 1975; **16**: 409.

30 Arnbjornsson E. Acute appendicitis and dietary fiber. *Arch Surg* 1983; **118**: 868–870.

31 Nelson M, Morris J, Barker DJP, Simmonds S. A case control study of acute appendicitis and diet in children. *J Epidemiol Community Health* 1986; **41**: 316–318.

32 Barker DJP, Morris J. Acute appendicitis, bathrooms and diet in Britain and Ireland. *Br Med J* 1988; **296**: 953–955.

33 Read NW. Pathophysiological mechanisms in the appendix. In: *The aetiology of acute appendicitis (Scientific Report No 7)*. Southampton: MRC Environmental Epidemiology Unit, 1986; 23–26.

34 Pieper R, Kager L, Weintraub A, Lindberg AA, Nord CE. The role of bacteroides fragilis in the pathogenesis of acute appendicitis. *Acta Chir Scand* 1982; **148**: 39–44.

35 Bohrod MG. The pathogenesis of acute appendicitis. *Am J Clin Pathol* 1946; **16**: 752–760.

36 McKeown T, Lowe CR. *An introduction to social medicine*. Oxford: Blackwell, 1974.

37 Donnan SPB. Appendicitis in Hong Kong. In: *The aetiology of acute appendicitis (Scientific Report No 7)*. Southampton: MRC Environmental Epidemiology Unit, 1986; 16–19.

38 Coggon D, Barker DJP, Cruddas M, Oliver RHP. Housing and appendicitis in Anglesey. *J Epidemiol Community Health* 1991; **45**: 244–246.

39 Barker DJP, Morris JA, Simmonds SJ, Oliver RHP. Appendicitis epidemic following introduction of piped water to Anglesey. *J Epidemiol Community Health* 1988; **42**: 144–148.

40 Backett EM. Social patterns of antibody to poliovirus. *Lancet* 1957; **i**: 778–783.

41 Pisacane A, de Luca U, Impagliazzo N, Russo M, de Caprio C, Caracciolo G. Breast feeding and acute appendicitis. *Br Med J* 1995; **310**: 836–837.

42 Shaheen SO. Discovering the causes of atopy: patterns of childhood infection and fetal growth may be implicated. *Br Med J* 1997; **314**: 987–988.

43 Strachan DP. Hay fever, hygiene, and household size. *Br Med J* 1989; **299**: 1259–1260.

44 Strachan DP. Allergy and family size: a riddle worth solving. *Clin Exp Allergy* 1997; **27**: 235–236.

45 Shaheen SO, Aaby P, Hall AJ, Barker DJP, Heyes CB, Shiell AW, et al. Measles and atopy in Guinea-Bissau. *Lancet* 1996; **347**: 1792–1796.

46 Shaheen SO, Aaby P, Hall AJ, Barker DJP, Heyes CB, Shiell AW, et al. Cell-mediated immunity after measles infection in Guinea-Bissau: historical cohort study. *Br Med J* 1996; **313**: 969–974.

47 Matricardi PM, Rosmini F, Ferrigno L, Nisini R, Rapicetta M, Chionne P, et al. Cross sectional retrospective study of prevalence of atopy among Italian military students with antibodies against hepatitis A virus. *Br Med J* 1997; **314**: 999–1003.

48 Miles EA, Warner JA, Lane AC, Jones AC, Colwell BM, Warner JO. Altered T lymphocyte phenotype at birth in babies born to atopic parents. *Pediatr Allergy Immunol* 1994; **5**: 202–208.

49 Strachan DP, Harkins LS, Johnston DA, Anderson HR. Childhood antecedents of allergic sensitization in young British adults. *J Allergy Clin Immunol* 1997; **99**: 6–12.

50 Godfrey KM, Barker DJP, Osmond C. Disproportionate fetal growth and raised IgE concentration in adult life. *Clin Exp Allergy* 1994; **24**: 641–648.

51 Fergusson DM, Crane J, Beasley R, Horwood LJ. Perinatal factors and atopic disease in childhood. *Clin Exp Allergy* 1997; **27**: 1394–1401.

52 Barker DJP. The epidemiology of Paget's disease of bone. *Br Med Bull* 1984; **40**: 396–400.

53 Barry HC. *Paget's disease of bone*. Edinburgh: Livingstone, 1969.

54 Detheridge FM, Guyer PB, Barker DJP. European distribution of Paget's disease of bone. *Br Med J* 1982; **285**: 1005–1008.

55 Barker DJP, Chamberlain AT, Guyer PB, Gardner MJ. Paget's disease of bone: the Lancashire focus. *Br Med J* 1980; **1**: 1105–1107.

56 Piga AM, Lopez-Abente G, Ibanez AE, Vadillo AG, Lanza MG, Jodra VM. Risk factors for Paget's disease: a new hypothesis. *Int J Epidemiol* 1988; **17**: 198–201.

57 Guyer PB, Chamberlain AT. Paget's disease of bone in two American cities. *Br Med J* 1980; **280**: 985.

58 Rosenbaum HD, Hanson DJ. Geographic variation in the prevalence of Paget's disease of bone. *Radiology* 1969; **92**: 959–963.

59 Van Meerdervoort HFP, Richter GG. Paget's disease of bone in South African blacks. *S Afr Med J* 1976; **50**: 1897–1899.

60 Guyer PB, Chamberlain AT. Paget's disease of bone in South Africa. *Clin Radiol* 1988; **39**: 51–52.

61 Gardner MJ, Guyer PB, Barker DJP. Radiological prevalence of Paget's disease of bone in British migrants to Australia. *Br Med J* 1978; **i**: 1655–1657.

62 Rebel A, Basle M, Pouplard A, Kouyoumdjian S, Filmon R, Lepatezour A. Viral antigens in osteoclasts from Paget's disease of bone. *Lancet* 1980; **ii**: 344–346.

63 Singer FR, Mills BG. The etiology of Paget's disease of bone. *Clin Orthop* 1977; **127**: 37–42.

64 Martyn CN. Infection in childhood and neurological diseases in adult life. *Br Med Bull* 1997; **53**: 24–39.

65 Poskanzer DC, Schwab RS. Cohort analysis of Parkinson's syndrome: evidence for a single etiology related to subclinical infection about 1920. *J Chron Dis* 1963; **16**: 961–973.

66 Brown EL, Knox EG. Epidemiological approach to Parkinson's disease. *Lancet* 1972; **i**: 974–976.

67 Marmot MG. Parkinson's disease and encephalitis: the cohort hypothesis re-examined. In: Rose FC, ed. *Clinical Neuroepidemiology*. Tunbridge Wells: Pitman Medical, 1980; 391–401.

68 Ben-Shlomo Y, Finnan F, Allwright S, Davey Smith G. The epidemiology of Parkinson's disease in the Republic of Ireland: observations from routine data sources. *Ir Med J* 1993; **86**: 190–192.

69 Martyn CN, Barker DJP, Osmond C. Motoneuron disease and past poliomyelitis in England and Wales. *Lancet* 1988; **1**: 1319–1322.

70 Buckley J, Warlow C, Smith P, Hilton-Jones D, Irvine S, Tew JR. Motor neuron disease in England and Wales 1959–1979. *J Neurol Neurosurg Psychiatry* 1983; **46**: 197–205.

71 Lilienfeld DE, Ehland J, Godbold J, Landrigen PJ, Marsh G, et al. Rising mortality from motoneuron disease in the USA, 1962–1984. *Lancet* 1989; **i**: 710–713.

72 Kahana E, Zilber N, Abramson JH, Biton V, Leibowitz Y, Abramsky O. Multiple sclerosis: genetic versus environmental aetiology; epidemiology in Israel updated. *J Neurol* 1994; **241**: 341–346.

73 Elian M, Nightingale S, Dean G. Multiple sclerosis among United Kingdom-born children of immigrants from the Indian subcontinent, Africa and the West Indies. *J Neurol Neurosurg Psychiatry* 1990; **53**: 906–911.

74 Alter M, Cendrowski W. Multiple sclerosis and childhood infections. *Neurology* 1976; **26**: 201–204.

75 Warner HB, Carp RI. Multiple sclerosis and Epstein–Barr virus. *Lancet* 1981; **i**: 1290.

76 Martyn CN, Cruddas M, Compston DAS. Symptomatic Epstein–Barr virus infection and multiple sclerosis. *J Neurol Neurosurg Psychiatry* 1993; **56**: 167–168.

77 Haahr S, Koch-Henriksen N, Moller-Larsen A, Eriksen LS, Andersen HMK. Increased risk of multiple sclerosis after late Epstein–Barr virus infection. *Multiple Sclerosis* 1995; **1**: 73–77.

10

Preventing chronic disease: lessons from the past

We have a winding sheet in our mother's womb that grows with us from our conception and we come into the world wound up in that winding sheet for we come to seek a grave. We celebrate our own funeral with cries even at our birth as though our three score and ten years of life were spent in our mother's labour and our circle made up in the first point thereof. (John Donne 1572–1631).

Chapter 8 outlined the scientific agenda which now has to be explored if we are to understand how the fetus is nourished, and how its nourishment may be improved. It may be a few years before understanding progresses to the point where effective advice can be given to women before and during pregnancy. Meanwhile, history gives an insight into the social conditions which have affected the well-being of mothers and their babies and, in consequence, may have changed the life expectancy of their children.

THREE LANCASHIRE TOWNS

In Lancashire, England, the cotton industry was harsh to mothers and their babies.[1] Figure 10.1 shows women employed in a mill in Preston, who worked during pregnancy and returned soon after delivery.[2]

Many women returned to full time work just a few days after having had a baby and there was growing concern that this was contributing towards the high infant death rate in Preston. In 1886 Dr James Rigby produced a critical enquiry on the subject. He described a day in the life of a young mother. She would, he said, have to get up at 5.30 am, wrap the baby in a shawl and take it to a nurse who would care for it during the day. These baby-minders had little concern for the children in their care and often drugged them heavily. At 8.30 the mother would rush back from the mill to breast feed her baby and would probably snatch a piece of bread for herself on the way back. At midday she would rush back to feed the baby and then work on until 5.30 pm. This went on day after day until mother and baby were completely debilitated.[2]

Burnley is one of three Lancashire towns, Burnley, Nelson and Colne, situated side by side on the western slope of the Pennine Hills (Fig. 10.2). The towns developed in the last century as centres for cotton weaving. Most of

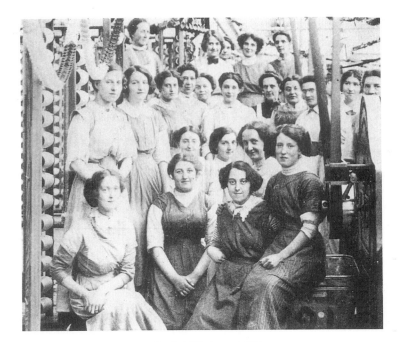

Fig. 10.1 Women weavers at Tulketh Mill about 1917.

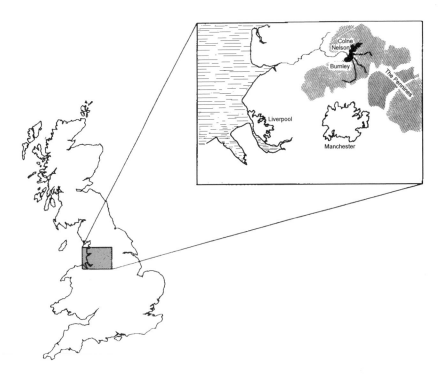

Fig. 10.2 Map of Great Britain showing the location of Burnley, Nelson and Colne.

Burnley is in the valley where the rivers Brun and Calder meet. Nelson and Colne lie above it. For the six miles from the centre of Burnley through Nelson

Table 10.1 Three Lancashire towns: standardised mortality ratios for causes of death at ages 55–74 years in 1968–78 (both sexes)

Causes of death	Nelson	Colne	Burnley
All causes	*100*	*109*	*121*
Coronary heart disease	106	119	120
Chronic bronchitis	134	132	188
Pneumonia	108	125	174
Stroke	101	121	120
Lung cancer	81	83	100
Other cancers	90	106	101
Other causes	97	93	117

to Colne, there is hardly a break in the line of houses. For many years there have been large differences in the death rates in the towns.[1] In Burnley adult mortality rates are among the highest for any of the large towns in England and Wales, the standardised mortality ratio (SMR) for all causes being 121 (Table 10.1). In Colne mortality is only 9% above the national average (SMR = 109) whereas in Nelson, situated between the others, mortality is average (SMR = 100). Table 10.1 gives figures for a recent 11-year period for which national death rates were analysed in unusual detail. Of the excess mortality in Burnley, 80% is certified as being the result of coronary heart disease, chronic bronchitis, stroke or bronchopneumonia. Mortality from cancer in the towns is around the national average, and mortality from lung cancer, an index of cigarette smoking, is average or below average.

The close proximity of the towns precludes explaining the large differences in mortality in terms of environmental influences such as climate. It is also unlikely that there are important differences in medical care, since the hospital services for all the towns are centred on Burnley. Could socioeconomic differences between the towns play a role? Recent census data show that all three towns are among the poorer towns in England and Wales, as indicated by the high percentage of manual workers, poor housing, and low income.[3] Socioeconomic differences between Nelson and Burnley are, however, small and less than the differences from the national average (Table 10.2). It is of interest that Nelson has the greatest excess of manual workers but nevertheless has a death rate from all causes that is equal to the national average.

The present similarity of the towns belies the large differences that formerly existed and led to large differences in mortality among infants and young children. Table 10.3 shows infant mortality rates in the towns for four periods from 1896 to 1925.[4,5] Throughout this time rates rose from Nelson to Colne to Burnley. Rates in Burnley were considerably above the average for England and Wales, and were consistently among the highest of any town. Data for 1911–13 distinguish neonatal and postneonatal deaths; rates rose between Nelson and Burnley for both neonatal and postneonatal deaths, and for deaths from the three main groups of causes, that is, diarrhoea, bronchitis and pneumonia, and the so-called 'group of five' diseases. The 'group of five' diseases were premature birth, congenital defects, birth injury, lack of breast milk, and marasmus; the most common of these were premature birth and congenital defects. Differences in mortality between the towns persisted through early childhood to 5 years of age. The birth rate also rose from Nelson to Colne to Burnley.

Table 10.2 Three Lancashire towns: socioeconomic indices in 1971 compared with those in England and Wales

	Nelson	Colne	Burnley	England and Wales
Employed men in social classes, %				
I	2	3	3	5
II	13	14	13	18
III, non-manual	8	10	10	12
III, manual	48	47	45	38
IV	18	16	20	18
V	11	11	10	9
Households with exclusive use of all amenities *, %	67	72	63	82
People living more than one person per room, %	14	10	14	12
Households in dwellings of less than five rooms, %	55	44	51	36
Households owning a car, %	40	36	34	52
Infant mortality per 1000, 1968–72	20	19	22	18
Total population	31 249	18 940	76 513	

* Hot water, fixed bath, inside lavatory.

Table 10.3 Three Lancashire towns: infant mortality rates per 1000 births from 1896 to 1925: Infant and child mortality and birth rate from 1911 to 1913

	Nelson	Colne	Burnley	England and Wales
1896 to 1925				
Infant mortality per 1000 births				
1896–98	154	170	197	155
1907–10	107	130	171	113
1911–13	87	130	177	111
1921–25	79	109	114	76
1911 to 1913				
Infant mortality per 1000 births				
Neonatal	38	37	49	
Postneonatal	49	93	128	
Cause				
Group of five diseases*	35	33	53	
Bronchitis and pneumonia	17	25	26	
Diarrhoea	16	30	48	
Mortality at age 1–5 years per 1000 survivors at age 1 year	58	85	96	
Birth rate per 1000 population	18	21	23	

* See text.

Social conditions in the past

We have an unusually detailed knowledge of social conditions in the towns at the beginning of the century because they were described in a report of the Local Government Board in 1914.[5] The generation whose infancy is described in this report belong to those whose recent death rates are shown in Table 10.1. In all three towns the level of employment was high, and wages were relatively good. The staple industry was cotton weaving, and the industry employed 40% of all the women and girls aged 10 years and over. Many of the women who worked in the weaving mills of Burnley and Colne were from the second or third generation of Lancashire industrial workers. Nelson, however, had developed more recently and had an eightfold increase in population between 1871 and 1911. Most of the people in Nelson were immigrants from adjacent areas, especially from rural parts of Yorkshire:

This fact has an important bearing on the question of infantile mortality, owing to the general good health and the habits of cleanliness and thrift characteristic of these immigrants from rural districts.[5]

The women were described as 'sturdier and healthier' than those in Burnley.

There were no creches at the mills. Usually the return of the mother to work was soon followed by complete weaning and the infant, together with other children in the family below school age, was placed in the care of an untrained 'minder' who was paid by the mother.

In view of the fact that so many mothers are anxious, for the sake of the wages, to get back to employment in the mills as soon as possible after childbirth, a large proportion of children born in Burnley are deprived of the advantages of breast feeding after the first few weeks of life . . . In Colne and still more in Nelson breast feeding is usually continued longer than in Burnley.[5]

Most houses in the towns were built of stone. In Nelson, however, houses were newer and had more rooms (Table 10.4), and so were less crowded. The worst houses were the back-to-back houses in the oldest parts of Burnley and Colne, which were small, had no means of ventilation to the outside air, and lacked facilities for the storage of food and milk. Infant mortality was much higher in such houses: 248 per 1000 in the back-to-back houses of Colne during 1912, for example, compared with 80 in the so called 'through' houses. Much of this excess mortality was the result of diarrhoea. Resettlement of families from back-to-back houses to 'through' houses was accompanied by a fall in infant mortality to around the average for 'through' houses, showing that high mortality was a consequence of the structure of the houses rather than of the habits of those who occupied them.

Sanitary conditions in Nelson were better than those in the other two towns. In Nelson the women kept the streets outside their houses clean: 'more water being said to be used for this purpose in Nelson than in any other town in

Table 10.4 Three Lancashire towns: housing conditions, mean family size, and total population, 1911

	Nelson	Colne	Burnley	England and Wales
Percentage of population in dwellings of less than four rooms	5.6	15.1	13.6	19.4
Percentage of population living more than two persons to a room	3.7	6.6	9.5	9.1
Percentage (no.) of dwellings back-to-back or single room	0.6 (52)	17.0 (1000)	9.9 (2371)	—
Mean family size	4.3	4.3	4.4	4.4
Total population	39 479	25 689	106 322	

Lancashire'. In Nelson communal pits, used for disposal of household refuse, were small and covered and were 'in striking contrast' to the large open pits in Burnley and Colne, which favoured the breeding of flies. Refuse collected from the pits and bins in Nelson and Colne was destroyed, whereas in Burnley around half was put on to 'tips', which were also sites for breeding flies. In Nelson, and to a lesser extent Colne, the manure pits around stables and cow-sheds were disinfected in summer to prevent flies breeding. Sanitary regulations for the production and sale of milk were more strictly enforced in Nelson.

Summary

The past differences in infant mortality among the three towns can be linked to differences in the health and physique of mothers, infant feeding practices, housing, and sanitation. They were not related to differences in income or occupation. The children born to the 'sturdier and healthier' mothers in Nelson, more of whom were breast fed, now have lower death rates from cardiovascular disease. After birth these children lived in better, less crowded houses and now have lower death rates from chronic bronchitis.

Mothers in Nelson had better health and physique because it was a newer town. The people were recent migrants from nearby rural areas rather than second or third generation industrial workers. The effects of life in towns in reducing the fitness of successive generations was described by Charles Booth in his *Life and labour of the people in London*, based on surveys carried out in London from 1886 onwards.[6]

LONDON

For more than a hundred years, people living in the cities and large towns of Britain have had higher death rates than people living in small towns and villages.[7, 8] London is an exception. During 1980–85, for example, standardised mortality ratios for all causes in London, expressed in relation to a national average of 100, were 96 among men and 93 among women. These low standardised mortality ratios resulted largely from low rates of cardiovascular disease.[7] SMRs for coronary heart disease were 90 in men and 87 in women; SMRs for stroke were 78 in each sex. Londoners' low cardiovascular death rates have never been explained.

During 1968–78 standardised mortality ratios in London for coronary heart disease and stroke combined were 87 in men and 83 in women. In none of the 33 London boroughs was cardiovascular mortality above the national average in either sex. London's low cardiovascular mortality contrasts with above average mortality from diseases associated with poor socioeconomic conditions, cigarette smoking, and alcohol consumption. Standardised mortality ratios were 105 for chronic bronchitis in men and 111 in women; 114 and 127 for lung cancer; 101 and 103 for cirrhosis of the liver; and 115 and 130 for suicide. In only four of the 33 boroughs were lung cancer death rates below the national average, the lowest standardised mortality ratio being 92. Thus the lifestyle of Londoners does not seem especially healthy and is not consistent with their low death rates from cardiovascular disease.

In the early years of this century London had low rates of maternal and neonatal mortality. Maternal mortality during 1911–14, for example, was 3.1

per 1000 births compared with 4.0 in England and Wales. Neonatal mortality was 33 per 1000 births compared with 39. In the past, maternal mortality was low in places where women had good physique, nutrition, and health, and neonatal mortality was low where few babies had low birthweight.[9, 10] The low maternal and neonatal mortality in London therefore implies that, at the beginning of this century, its women had good physique, health, and nutrition, which is surprising. It conflicts with the picture of London presented by novelists, and with detailed descriptions of life in London given by the surveys which Charles Booth carried out from 1886 onwards. Writing of the London poor, he said:

Their life is the life of savages with vicissitudes of extreme hardship and occasional excess. Their food is of the coarsest description, and their only luxury is drink.[6]

Amid this savagery, pregnancy, childbirth, and early infancy were unusually safe for both the mother and the baby. Why?

Social conditions in the past

Young women in London had remarkably low death rates at the beginning of the century. These low rates contrasted with the high rates in girls under 15. Figure 10.3 shows age specific death rates among women in London during 1901–10, expressed as a percentage of the rates in England and Wales.[7] Among girls under 5 years of age London rates were above the national average, and 20% above in girls aged 2–3 years. With increasing age the rates for girls and women fell sharply so that from 15 to 34 years they were well below the average, 17% below in girls aged 20–24. Among older women rates rose and were again above the average. Among men the overall pattern was similar to that in women, with lower rates in young adults; however only at ages 15–24 were

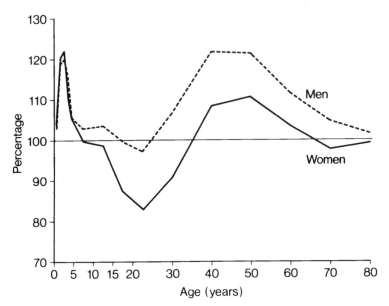

Fig. 10.3 Age-specific death rates in London, 1901–10, expressed as a percentage of national rates for England and Wales.

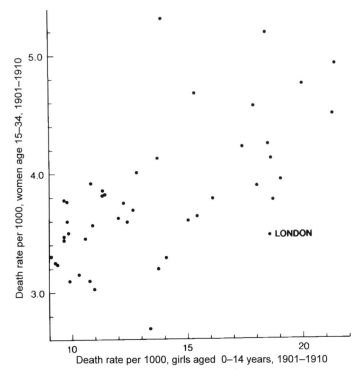

Death rate per 1000, women age 15–34, 1901–1910

Death rate per 1000, girls aged 0–14 years, 1901–1910

Fig. 10.4 Death rates among girls under 15 years and women aged 15–34 years in the counties of England and Wales 1901–10.

London rates below the national average. Analysis of death rates for the previous decade, 1891–1900, shows a similar pattern.[11]

Figure 10.4 compares death rates in girls under 15 years of age in the counties of England and Wales with death rates in young women aged 15–34 years. As expected the rates are related. Counties with lower death rates in girls, which are mostly in the south and east of the country, have lower rates in young women, and vice versa. London is exceptional. The low death rate in young women is disproportionate to the high rate in girls.

The main causes of death of young women in London, and the relation of London death rates to national rates, are shown in Table 10.5. London women had low death rates from tuberculosis and other infectious diseases, and low mortality during childbirth. Analysis of death rates during the previous decade, 1891–1900, shows a similar pattern, with low death rates for tuberculosis and the major infectious diseases, and from childbirth, and high rates for cancer and violent death.[11]

At this time the death rates of London children from common infections, including measles and whooping cough, were the highest of any county in England and Wales. Booth described London children in the poorer classes as 'underfed, ill-clad, badly lodged, and poorly born'.[12] They lived where

the main streets, narrow at best, branch off into others narrower still; and these again into a labyrinth of blind alleys, courts and lanes; all dirty, foul-smelling, and littered with garbage of every kind. The houses are old, damp and dilapidated.[13]

Table 10.5 Leading causes of death among women aged 15–34 years in London, 1901–10

Cause of death	Death rate per million		London rates as percentage of England and Wales
	London	England and Wales	
Tuberculosis	1231	1485	83
Childbirth	288	386	75
Pneumonia	202	236	85
Cancer	131	97	134
Violence	130	120	108
Enteric fever	71	98	72
Septic diseases	69	40	174
Rheumatic fever	57	65	87
All other causes	1300	1381	94

Two possible explanations for the good health of young women in London are migration and domestic service.[7] Dwindling rural industries, the depression of agriculture, and low wages in the villages encouraged young people to migrate to the towns. Those in the southern counties went in large numbers to London, attracted by the opportunities for employment and the high wages. The usual age of migration was between 15 and 30 years, and more young women than young men went to London, largely because of the demand for domestic servants. This was reflected in the relative excess of young women in London's population which persisted through the 18th and 19th centuries.[14]

Booth described migration into London (Fig. 10.5):

The countrymen drawn in (to London) are mainly the cream of the youth of the villages, travelling not so often vaguely in search of work as definitely to seek a known economic advantage . . . It is the result of the conditions of life in great towns, and especially in this the greatest town of all, that muscular strength and energy get gradually used up; the second generation of Londoners is of lower physique and has less power of persistent work than the first; and the third generation (where it exists) is lower than the second . . . London is to a great extent nourished by the literal consumption of bone and sinew from the country; by the absorption every year of large numbers of persons of stronger physique, who leaven the whole mass, largely direct the industries, raise the standard of health and comfort, and keep up the rate of growth of the great city only to give place in their turn to a fresh set of recruits, after London life for one or two generations has reduced them to the level of those among whom they live.[13]

Mothers and babies in London at that time were described by Burnett:[15]

The child of the well-fed, well-worked, cheerful, happy woman, living in a sunlit airy habitation, is at birth the finest specimen of its kind. On the other hand what a miserable sight do the newborn babies of our courts and alleys, and of the pampered, tight-laced, high-heeled, lazy, lounging, carriage-possessing women of the higher classes present! The extremes meet: the poor blanched creature, half-starved, over-worked, shut up in some close sunless dwelling, brings forth fruit very like that of her pale-faced, over-fed, under-worked sofa-loving sister of the mansion and of the palace . . . Clearly then we may take it for granted that the development of the fruit within the womb can be modified for good and for ill.

Figure 10.6 shows that, although many girls in the north of England, especially Lancashire, were employed in industry from a young age, girls in

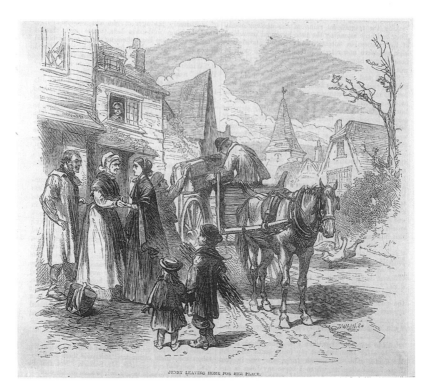

JENNY LEAVING HOME FOR HER PLACE.

Fig. 10.5 Girls leaving the country to go into service were among 'the cream of the youth of the villages, travelling . . . definitely to seek a known economic advantage'.[13] They made up over a fifth of the young women in London at the 1911 census. (Mary Evans Picture Library, with permission.)

London escaped this. Their usual employment was in domestic service. Of the young women in employment in London, 30% were in domestic service at the time of the 1911 census. Women generally left domestic service when they married, and an unknown percentage of the young women who were married would have previously been in domestic service. Young women who went into domestic service would have had good nutrition in the years before their marriage and pregnancies.[16] The food given to domestic servants

was usually very good, and in all but very rare cases greatly superior to that obtainable by the other members of the working class families from which servants are drawn.[17]

When members of the Domestic Servants Society, formed in 1912, applied for health insurance, they were found to be more healthy than any other group of women workers.[18]

During routine examinations of London school children around the time of the First World War the girls were more likely than boys to be classed as having 'excellent nutrition'.[19] This contrasted with findings in industrial towns, where boys were fed better than girls. In Hull, for example, during 1913

the proportion of boys classed as enjoying 'good' nutrition far exceeded the proportion of girls so classed . . . by a factor of five among the 10 year old children.[20]

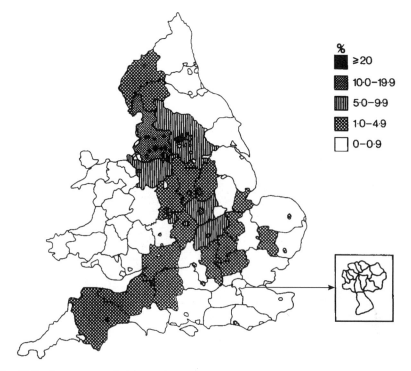

Fig. 10.6 Percentage of girls aged 10–14 years working in 1901 (not as domestic servants), administrative counties and county boroughs of England and Wales.

Rowntree wrote:

the women and children suffer from underfeeding to a much greater extent than the men. It is tacitly agreed that the man must have a certain minimum of food in order that he may be able to perform the muscular work demanded of him; and the provision of this minimum, in the case of families with small incomes, involves a degree of under-feeding for the women and children . . . [21]

Girls in London seemed to escape the unequal division of the family's food which occurred in industrial Britain because of the emphasis on male manual work.[22] Unequal division of food in favour of the man still occurs, however, around the world, in patrilineal societies, and in societies where veneration of ancestors is centred on men.

Summary

The health of young women in London at the beginning of the century was unusually good because many were born in the fertile agricultural counties of southern England or had mothers who were born in these counties. They therefore had good nutrition in fetal life and infancy. Among children in London there was no preferential feeding of boys. Girls who went into domestic service were unusually well fed in adolescence and as young adults. The children born to these young women today have low death rates from cardiovascular disease. After birth these children lived in poor, overcrowded houses and today have high death rates from chronic bronchitis.

Preventing chronic disease: lessons from the past

The studies of socioeconomic conditions in three Lancashire towns and London add little to the evidence that the prenatal and early postnatal environment have a major effect on cardiovascular disease and other disorders. This evidence rests on follow-up studies of thousands of people, described in this book. Lancashire and London do, however, give an insight into past social changes which may have determined patterns of mortality today. By directing attention to socioeconomic conditions that prevailed at the time of birth of people now falling ill and dying in later life, they allow conclusions which go beyond such general statements as that of the Black report on inequalities of health in Britain:[23] 'Much, we feel, can only be understood in terms of the more diffuse consequences of the class structure'.

The detailed descriptions of maternal and infant health and socioeconomic conditions in Lancashire and London early in this century have to be viewed against the backdrop of longer term changes in health. In England mortality began to decline around the middle of the 18th century. There were continued, though relatively small increases in life expectancy through the 19th century and steep increases in the early part of the 20th century. During the first two decades of this century life expectation in Britain increased by 12 years. There were similar trends elsewhere in Europe and in the USA.

A number of influences contributed to this remarkable extension of the lifespan, including the abolition of famine,[24] improvements in hygiene and sanitation towards the end of the last century,[22, 25] and advances in medical knowledge.[26] The dominant influence, however, seems to have been what Fogel has called 'the escape from hunger'.[27] It is estimated that towards the end of the 18th century the average calorie intake in England was similar to that in India today, while that in France was lower, similar to that in Rwanda today. At such low calorie intakes many people must have starved[28] and the capacity for work would be low, even allowing for the smaller body size and hence reduced energy requirements for basal metabolism. Improvements in the supply of food allowed France, Britain and other western European populations to become taller and heavier.[29] This increased their energy requirements, allowed more physical work and reset the population's balance between food supply and demand at a new and higher level.

Whether or not an adult, or a child or a fetus becomes undernourished depends on the balance between supply and demand. Levels of supply that are adequate to maintain equilibrium when demand is low (that is when people are small) are inadequate when demand is raised by increased body size, increased activity or infective disease. Booth's description (p. 175) shows how people, the 'cream of the youth,' arriving in London from the countryside became undernourished so that by the third generation their physique was reduced 'to the level of those among whom they live'. Elsewhere in Britain too, migration from the countryside into the expanding industrial towns seems to have been associated with a worsening of nutrition.[30] 'Take indifferently twenty well-fed husbandmen, and compare them with twenty industrial workers who have equal means of support' Thackrah wrote in 1832 'and the superiority of the agricultural peasants in health, vigour and size will be obvious'. We do not know in any detail how the diet in industrial towns at the turn of the century was deficient. There is, however, anecdotal evidence.

In a recent survey of elderly women in six areas of England, a woman who worked in rural Hertfordshire as an upstairs maid in the 1920s described her diet.[16]

We had four wonderful meals a day and it was comfort from the word go . . . An excellent breakfast of porridge, egg dishes or bacon. Lunch was always meat and vegetables and a pudding of sorts. Tea was bread and butter and cake, and supper was usually cold meat, bubble and squeak or a cheese dish. I must say when I got married I thought, 'Oh dear, I don't like this poverty', after living in so much comfort.

The daughter of a labourer growing up in Sheffield at the same time recalled:

I didn't go hungry but we'd no luxuries. Breakfast and tea would be bread and butter mostly. On a Sunday morning we had a bit of cooked bacon, when my dad was working, just a little bit like that and my dad's words were, 'Now then, little bits of bacon and big lumps of bread'.

The general picture given by studies such as this is of girls and young women in industrial areas eating fewer meals a day, and having less red meat, fruit and vegetables. One can postulate that this kind of undernutrition occurring in pregnancy, at a level of energy balance which was considerably higher than that which had prevailed in the past, altered the maternal–fetal relation in ways which were to the disadvantage of the fetus: the fetus's adaptations to this initiated coronary heart disease in later life. This theme is developed in Chapter 11. To what extent high rates of infection in infancy and childhood, of the kind experienced in Burnley, also played a role in initiating coronary heart disease is unknown but the lesson from London may be that to the well nourished fetus they were unimportant. They are likely, however, to have contributed to the development of chronic bronchitis (Ch. 7) and possibly to other non-cardiovascular disorders (Ch. 9).

The undernutrition of girls and young women in industrial Britain may have been compounded by preferential feeding of boy children and men in manual occupations, and by the conditions of their own occupations. In areas where there was little employment for women, notably many coal-mining areas, girls married young and had large families, which may have reduced further their nutritional state.

Summary

History suggests that today's inequalities in health are linked to poor maternal physique and nutrition in the past. It endorses the findings from follow-up studies of men and women, and experiments on animals, described in this book. To prevent disease in the next generation we need to direct our attention to the nutrition of mothers and their babies and to exposure to infection in early childhood.

References

1 Barker DJP, Osmond C. Inequalities in health in Britain: specific explanations in three Lancashire towns. Br Med J 1987; 294: 749–52.
2 Harris Museum and Art Gallery. The story of Preston. Preston: 1992.

3 Census Office. *Census of England and Wales 1901.* London: HMSO, 1917 and following censuses.

4 Local Government Board. Forty second annual report, 1912–13. In: *Supplement in continuation of the report of the medical officer of the board for 1912–13.* Second report on infant and child mortality. London: HMSO, 1913.

5 Local Government Board. Forty third annual report, 1913–14. In: *Supplement in continuation of the report of the medical officer of the board for 1913–14.* Third report on infant mortality dealing with infant mortality in Lancashire. London: HMSO, 1914.

6 Booth C. *Life and labour of the people in London.* First series: *Poverty.* Volume 1, *East central and south London.* London: Macmillan, 1902.

7 Barker DJP, Osmond C, Pannett B. Why Londoners have low death rates from ischaemic heart disease and stroke. *Br Med J* 1992; **305**: 1551–1554.

8 Registrar General. *Statistical review of England and Wales. Part I: tables, medical.* London: HMSO, 1880 and following years.

9 Campbell JM, Cameron D, Jones DM. High maternal mortality in certain areas. London: HMSO, 1932. (Ministry of Health reports on public health and medical subjects No. 68).

10 Local Government Board. Thirty-ninth annual report, 1909–10. In: *Supplement to the report of the board's medical officer. Supplement on infant and child mortality.* London: HMSO, 1910.

11 Registrar General of Births, Deaths and Marriages in England and Wales. *Supplement to the sixty fifth annual report. Part 1, Registration summary tables 1891–1900.* London, 1907.

12 Booth C. *Life and labour of the people in London.* First series: *Poverty.* Volume 3, *Blocks of buildings, schools and immigration.* London: Macmillan, 1902.

13 Booth C. *Life and labour of the people in London.* Second series: *Industry.* Volume, 5 *Part I: comparisons, Part II: survey and conclusions. Comparisons, survey and conclusions.* London: Macmillan, 1903.

14 Earle P. *A city full of people. Men and women of London 1650–1750.* London: Methuen, 1994.

15 Burnett JC. Prevention of hare-lip. *Homeopathic World* 1880; 437–451.

16 Fellague Ariouat J, Barker DJP. The diet of girls and young women at the beginning of the century. *Nutrition and Health* 1993; **9**: 15–23.

17 Booth C. *Life and labour of the people in London.* Second series: *Industry.* Volume 4. *Public professional and domestic service, unsuccessful classes, inmates of institutions.* London: Macmillan, 1903.

18 *The new survey of London life and labour. Volume II. London industries.* London: PS King, 1931.

19 London County Council. *Annual report of council 1915–19.* Volume III, *Public health.* London: LCC, 1919.

20 Wall R. *Some inequalities in the raising of boys and girls in nineteenth and twentieth-century England and Wales.* Cambridge: Cambridge Group for the History of Population and Social Structure, 1990.

21 Rowntree BS. *Poverty: a study of town life.* London: MacMillan, 1902.

22 Acheson ED. Tenth Boyd Orr Memorial Lecture. Food policy, nutrition and government. *Proc Nutr Soc* 1986; **45**: 131–138.

23 Townsend P, Davidson N. *Inequalities of health: the Black report.* Harmondsworth: Penguin, 1982.

24 Wrigley EA, Schofield RS. *The population history of England. 1541–1871: a reconstruction.* London: Edward Arnold, 1981.

25 McKeown T. *The modern rise of population.* London: Edward Arnold, 1976.

26 McKeown T, Lowe CR. *An introduction to social medicine.* Oxford: Blackwell, 1974.

27 Fogel RW. Second thoughts on the European escape from hunger. Famines, chronic malnutrition, and mortality. In: Osmani SR, ed. *Nutrition and Poverty.* Oxford: Clarendon Press, 1991.

28 Scrimshaw NS. The phenomenon of famine. *Annual Review of Nutrition* 1987; **7**:1–21.

29 Floud R, Wachter KW, Gregory A. *Height, health and history: nutritional status in the United Kingdom 1750–1980.* Cambridge: Cambridge University Press, 1990.

30 Thackrah CT. *The effects of arts, trades and professions and of civic states and the habits of living, on health and longevity: with suggestions for the removal of many of the agents which produce disease, and shorten the duration of life.* London: Longman, 1832.

11

Preventing chronic disease: the future

Man brings all that he has or can have into the world with him. Man is born like a garden ready planted and sown. (William Blake 1757–1827)

That events before birth are of lifelong importance has long been recognised by poets and prophets; psychiatrists are familiar with the importance of infancy through the theories of Freud. Recent discoveries in the USA have led anthropologists to similar conclusions. Around AD1000 a group of American Indians, who lived in what is now Illinois, changed from living as hunter-gatherers to farmers, growing maize. This change seems to have been accompanied by a worsening in their nutrition, and a lowering in the social status of women.[1] Examination of their skeletons, found buried in 'the Dickson Mounds', showed that those in whom the vertebral canal was narrow had died at a younger age.[2] The adult dimensions of the vertebral canal are established before 4 years of age: the dimensions of the thoracic part of the canal are established in utero. This led Clark to conclude that in prehistoric times impaired growth in utero led to a shortened lifespan as a result, he suggested, of impaired neuroendocrine and thymic development. Studies of teeth led to similar findings: those who had more enamel hypoplasia, a consequence of interrupted enamel matrix formation in early life, had shorter lives.[3] Impaired growth during childhood as opposed to fetal life and infancy was not related to longevity. Measures of skeletal size, established in childhood and adolescence, such as the length of the tibia, did not correlate with lifespan.

DEATH RATES IN GENERATIONS

In the past when tuberculosis and rheumatic fever were common, the proposition that health in childhood determined health in adult life was self-evident. In the 1920s records of annual death rates in Britain had accumulated over sufficient years to allow the link between childhood and adult disease rates to be examined statistically.[4] It was found that over the previous 80 years death rates at different ages had begun to fall at different times. Rates in the young began to fall earlier than those in the old. Derrick[5] showed that if death rates at each age were plotted by year of birth, that is, by generation, there was a remarkably regular pattern. Each succeeding generation displayed a lower mortality at all ages from childhood to old age. He concluded that 'each generation is endowed with a vitality peculiarly its own, which persistently manifests itself through the succeeding stages of its existence'.[5]

In the years up to the Second World War the existence of strong generation or 'cohort' effects on mortality was examined and confirmed.[6] Discussions of what caused them sought to apportion responsibility between genetic influences and the environment during childhood and adolescence. Seemingly uninformed by much knowledge of biology this statistical debate, which has been reviewed by Kuh & Davey Smith,[4] led to no conclusions. It did, however, establish the importance of generation effects in public health policy. Watt & Ecob[7] have recently re-emphasised this by comparing death rates in the two major cities in Scotland: Edinburgh, the capital, and the less affluent Glasgow. They found that in successive generations death rates in Glasgow were higher at all adult ages, and people in Glasgow experienced the same mortality rates as people in Edinburgh 3.6 years earlier in men and 3.9 years earlier in women.[7, 8]

For the same chronological age, Glaswegians are about four years older than people in Edinburgh. At any given age Glaswegians have more miles on the clock.

The existence of generation effects is important in relating the time trends of specific diseases to past trends in maternal and infant nutrition.

TRENDS IN DISEASE

The last chapter described how European populations began to 'escape' from chronic malnutrition in the 18th century. In the 19th century a succession of public health reforms further improved conditions for mothers and their babies.[9] Improvements in sanitation and housing, and reduction in family size and overcrowding, led to a fall in mortality from infectious diseases. In England and Wales infant mortality began to decline at the turn of the century, and fell almost without interruption from 152 per 1000 births in 1900 to 8 per 1000 live births in 1990. Neonatal and postneonatal death rates both fell, but the environment during infancy improved more rapidly than the intrauterine environment, and the proportion of deaths occurring in the neonatal period doubled.

To establish whether the improvements in fetal and infant nutrition and health that were reflected in the fall in infant mortality are now apparent in falling rates of adult disease, it is useful to divide adult diseases into three groups. These may be called diseases of poverty, diseases of affluence, and diseases of change.[10]

DISEASES OF POVERTY

The incidence of diseases associated with poor living standards, which include tuberculosis and rheumatic fever, has continued to decline during this century. Stroke and chronic bronchitis can be included with this group for they too are most common in the least affluent places and in people with the lowest incomes, and their incidence has fallen during the last 50 years.[11–14]

Stroke

Although stroke shares some of the epidemiological features of coronary heart disease, including a similar geographical distribution within the UK, the incidence of stroke has been falling in western countries for many years whereas, until recently, the incidence of coronary heart disease has been rising. Stroke is associated with low birthweight and placental weight in relation to head size at birth (p. 55). In the Sheffield study this pattern of fetal growth occurred when mothers had a 'flat' pelvis, a result of malnutrition in childhood.[15] In the Helsinki study it was associated with low maternal weight (unpublished). These observations have led to the hypothesis that stroke originates through malnutrition among girls and young women, which subsequently impairs their ability to sustain the growth of the placenta and fetus when they become pregnant. Preliminary data from Finland suggest that poor nutrition of the offspring in childhood may also play a role in the development of stroke (Fig. 11.10). The geographical distribution of stroke in Britain is similar to that of maternal and neonatal mortality in the early years of the century (Ch. 1). At that time maternal and neonatal mortality were highest in areas where women had poor physique, nutrition and health. The improvements in maternal health during this century should therefore be reflected in a later decline in death rates from stroke. Figure 11.1 shows the age-specific mortality from stroke for the period 1950–84.[14] Death rates declined continuously so that, by the end of the period, rates among men had halved and among women had fallen to three-eighths of

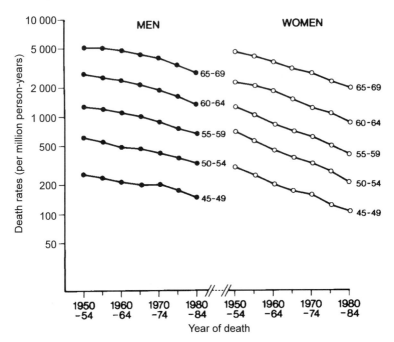

Fig. 11.1 Age-specific mortality from stroke in England and Wales; 1950–84 (ICD 8th revision, codes 431–438).

their 1950 levels. These data are consistent with generation effects, each successive generation having lower rates at each age than the one before. The fall in death rates from stroke began before the widespread use of antihypertensive therapy, though it now may be hastened by it.

Chronic bronchitis

This is linked to impaired lung growth in utero and during infancy and to infections of the lower respiratory tract during early childhood (Ch. 7). It follows that past improvements in maternal nutrition and health, improvements in housing, and reduction in family size and overcrowding should be reflected in a later decline in chronic bronchitis. In Britain age-specific mortality from chronic bronchitis has fallen progressively over the last 50 years.[11] Osmond[14] has shown that the trends are made up of two components: a 'cohort' value, summarising the mortality experience of a generation, and a 'period' value summarising the experience of all age groups at one point in time. Figures 11.2 and 11.3 show these two components in men and women.[13]

The 'cohort' component rises and falls and corresponds remarkably closely to that found for lung cancer. It may be attributed to the smoking habits of successive generations. These differed in men and women. The 'period' component, defined by year of death, declines steeply, age-specific death rates falling progressively from 1941. This pattern is quite different to that found for lung cancer, for which the period values were almost constant. It is consistent with chronic bronchitis being linked to early growth and infection whereas lung cancer is not (Fig. 7.4). The steeper fall among women than men is consistent with the smaller contribution of smoking to their mortality. Improved treatment after the advent of antibiotics could also have contributed to the period effect in both sexes.

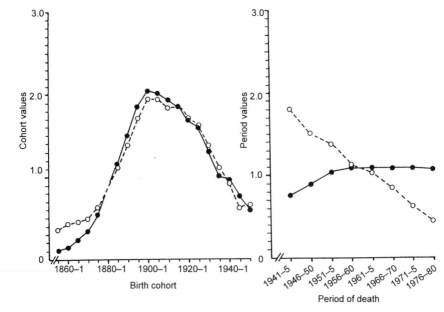

Fig. 11.2 Cohort and period of death values for chronic bronchitis and lung cancer in men aged over 25 years in England and Wales during 1941–80. O, bronchitisi; ●, lung cancer.

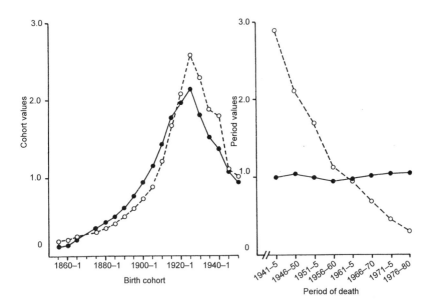

Fig. 11.3 Cohort and period of death values for chronic bronchitis and lung cancer in women aged over 25 in England and Wales during 1941–80. O, bronchitis; ●, lung cancer.

The Clean Air Act 1956 was not followed by a change in the rate of decline of chronic bronchitis. This suggests that chronic air pollution in adult life, as opposed to short episodes of high pollution, may be a less important cause of mortality from bronchitis than previously supposed. A survey of respiratory symptoms in a sample of British adults suggests that, in the absence of cigarette smoking, the influence of air pollution is small.[16]

DISEASES OF AFFLUENCE

The second group of diseases is associated with affluence. Such diseases are more common among more prosperous people living in more prosperous areas, and their incidence is rising. They include obesity, gallstones, renal stones, and cancers of the breast, ovary and prostate.[10, 11] There is evidence that obesity and the three reproductive cancers originate in utero. The findings for obesity were discussed in Chapter 6. Findings on the in utero origins of reproductive cancers, and of aspects of reproductive physiology, are described here.

Cancers of the breast and ovary

Cancers of the breast and ovary have been linked to high birthweight. Figure 11.4 shows the increase in the odds ratio for breast cancer across the range of birthweight among women taking part in the Nurses Study in the USA.[17] This trend is little influenced by adjusting for other variables, such as body mass and family history of breast cancer. Other data support a link between high birth-weight and breast cancer.[18] It has been suggested that high concentrations of oestrogen in pregnancy may play a role.[19]

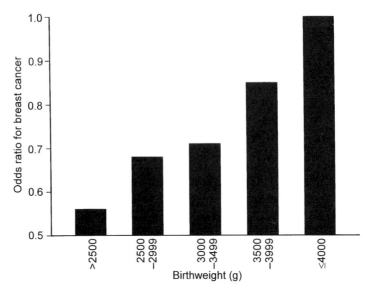

Fig. 11.4 Odds ratio for breast cancer by birthweight in the USA Nurses Study.

Figure 11.5 shows that in the Hertfordshire study rates of ovarian cancer increased, not with increasing birthweight, but with increasing weight at 1 year.[20] The suggested explanation is that hormonal or nutritional influences acting in utero imprint an altered pattern of gonadotrophin release. Experiments in rats (p. 30) show that the hypothalamus is imprinted by androgens during a sensitive perinatal phase. Low concentrations of androgen lead to cyclical release of gonadotrophins (the female pattern); high concentrations result in continuous secretion of gonadotrophin (the male pattern). In humans an

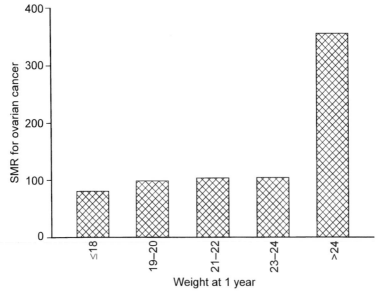

Fig. 11.5 Standardised mortality rate (SMR) of ovarian cancer by weight at 1 year in Hertfordshire.

altered pattern of gonadotrophin that increased oestrogen release would promote infant weight gain. In later life, it is suggested, it might induce malignant change in the ovary.

Aspects of reproductive physiology

Direct evidence that events in utero may imprint an altered pattern of gonadotrophin release, and thereby program disorders of the female reproductive tract, comes from a study of polycystic ovaries, a common disorder associated with menstrual irregularities, subfertility, hirsutism, acne and a spectrum of endocrine abnormalities including high plasma luteinising hormone (LH) concentrations, a high ratio of LH to follicle stimulating hormone (FSH), and excessive androgen production. In one of the two common forms of the disorder women are obese and androgenised, whereas in the other they are thin and have normal testosterone concentrations. The former group of women tend to have high birthweight and are born to heavy mothers.[21] The latter group, however, tend to be born after term. A possible explanation of why this latter group develop polycystic ovaries is that they have an altered hypothalamic–pituitary 'set point' for LH release as a result of their prolonged gestation. The human fetus produces large amounts of androgens which are converted to oestrogen by the placenta and pass to the maternal circulation. Placental failure associated with postmaturity could expose the fetal hypothalamus to increased concentrations of androgens or oestrogens and reset its responses to them.

The findings on polycystic ovary disease show how information on intrauterine development enables an heterogeneous disorder to be divided into aetiological subgroups. They also indicate that a woman's reproductive fitness may be programmed in utero. Further evidence comes from studies of age at menarche and at menopause. Table 11.1 shows the age at menarche in a national sample of British girls.[22] The girls who reached menarche at the youngest age were those who had low birthweight but put on weight rapidly in childhood. Conversely girls who were heavy at birth but light at the age of 7 years had a delayed menarche. Again the suggested link between fetal growth and age at menarche is in utero programming of the pattern of gonadotrophin release. Pulsatile release of LH and FSH is initiated in utero, continues through infancy, and thereafter ceases until it resumes at puberty.

Table 11.1 Age at menarche (years) according to birthweight and weight at 7 years, in 1471 girls born in 1946

Fifths of birth-weight kg (lb)	At 7 years of age kg (lb) fifths of weight					
	<20.1 (44)	–21.3 (47)	–22.7 (50)	–24.9 (55)	>24.9 (55)	All
<2.85 (6.3)	13.08	12.95	12.90	12.80	11.89	12.85
–3.18 (7.0)	12.93	12.96	12.83	12.93	12.25	12.81
–3.41 (7.5)	13.23	13.14	12.80	12.87	12.38	12.93
–3.75 (8.3)	13.14	13.08	12.92	12.73	12.60	12.84
>3.75 (8.3)	13.33	13.55	13.14	12.85	12.84	13.03
All	13.10	13.07	12.90	12.84	12.48	12.88

The opposing influences of intrauterine and childhood growth on the timing of menarche may permit better explanation of the secular trend in menarcheal age which has been observed since the last century.[23] The average age of menarche in the UK in 1840 was 16.5 years. It is now 12.8 years. However, this decline has now levelled and the downward trend is becoming an upward one. This reversal is difficult to explain on the basis of childhood nutrition and weight gain alone, but is compatible with opposing influences of improved fetal and childhood growth.

In Sheffield, women who were short at birth tended to have an early menopause.[24] Babies that are short tend to put on less weight during infancy and among women in Hertfordshire those who weighed 18 lb (8.2 kg) or less at 1 year of age experienced the menopause 1 year earlier than those who were heavier at 1 year.[24] An explanation of these findings is that when a female fetus sustains the growth of its brain at the expense of its body, it also impairs development of the ovaries. The number of primordial follicles is maximal during the 7th month of in utero life and thereafter declines. In adult life when the number falls below a critical level the menopause occurs.[25] Reduced ovarian growth in late gestation could lead to a smaller peak number of primordial follicles at birth, leading in turn to an earlier menopause. This has implications for health since early menopause is associated with increased risk of osteoporosis and cardiovascular disease.

A study in Belgium has extended the concept of in utero programming of the endocrine system to include the adrenarche. The androgenic hormone dehydroepiandrosterone sulphate (DHEAS)[26] is secreted by the fetal adrenal but after birth virtually disappears from the circulation until adrenarche, at around the age of 7 years. Comparing sibling pairs, Francois and de Zegher found that the child who was smaller for gestational age at birth had higher serum DHEAS than the normal sized sibling.[26] The long-term consequences of this exaggerated adrenarche are not known.

Prostate cancer

Ecological studies in England and Wales show that counties which have the tallest people have the highest rates of cancer of the breast, ovary and prostate, suggesting that promoted early growth is linked to all three hormonal cancers.[27] A small study of 21 prostate cancer cases in Sweden showed that there was a link with high birthweight.[28] This, however, was not confirmed in a larger Swedish study.[29] Prematurity and pre-eclampsia were, however, protective against the cancer. Because pre-eclampsia is associated with low circulating concentrations of sex hormones in the mother, Ekbom and colleagues concluded that these findings support a role for in utero exposure to sex steroids in the aetiology of prostate cancer.[29]

Other evidence that events in utero may program disorders of the male reproductive tract comes from the known association between low birthweight and hypogonadism and a recent study showing that men with low sperm counts had low birthweight.[30] Sperm production is limited by the number of Sertoli cells and the efficiency of spermatogenesis. Animal studies have shown that alteration in the number of Sertoli cells in early life determines testicular size and sperm output in adult life. There is currently concern that sperm counts in the general population are declining and toxic environmental agents that affect the testis in utero are suspected.[31] Altered exposure to endogenous hormones is an alternative explanation.

DISEASES OF CHANGE

The third group of diseases is at different times associated with poverty and affluence. It includes coronary heart disease, acute appendicitis, and duodenal ulcer. In the early part of this century these diseases were more common among the rich and their incidence rose. Later, they became more common among the poor and their incidence fell.

The term *western diseases* is used to describe a group of diseases that are common in industrialised countries, but uncommon elsewhere, whose incidence rises with the start of industrialisation.[32] As these diseases appear to be a consequence of industrialisation, it is argued that their prevention must depend on a return to practices of the past – for example resumption of a diet high in complex carbohydrates and low in animal fats. Yet 'western' diseases include both diseases of affluence and diseases of change, whose incidence has fallen whilst the environmental changes of industrialisation have persisted. Thyrotoxicosis serves as a model to examine how the incidence of a disease may rise and fall without a matching increase and decrease in exposure to an environmental influence.

Figure 11.6 shows death rates in England and Wales from a number of diseases of change, and includes death rates from thyrotoxicosis, which rose to a peak in the 1930s and thereafter declined. Most deaths from thyrotoxicosis occur in the elderly, among whom toxic multinodular goitre is the usual cause. Analyses of age-specific rates in successive generations show that rates rose

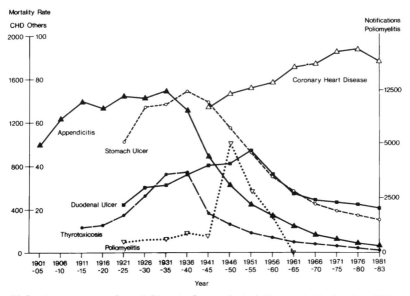

Fig. 11.6 Average annual mortality rate from selected diseases in England and Wales from 1901, and numbers of notifications of poliomyelitis, in 5-year periods. CHD, coronary heart disease.

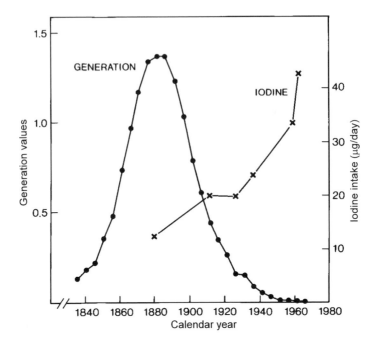

Fig. 11.7 Relative mortality from thyrotoxicosis in successive generations of women in England and Wales, according to year of birth, and estimated per capita daily iodine intake from milk, meat and fish.

progressively in people born after 1836, and reached a peak in those born between 1871 and 1886.[33] This is shown in Figure 11.7, which gives mortality in each generation according to their year of birth.

Figure 11.7 also shows the progressive increase in dietary iodine in Britain during this century, as a consequence of diversification of diet and availability of iodine in many foods including fish, meat, and milk.[34] Iodine deficiency during childhood was widespread among people born in Britain in the 1800s. Successive generations, however, were exposed to more iodine in adult life. There is evidence that people who are iodine-deficient in youth are less able to adapt to increased iodine intake in later life and tend to develop thyrotoxicosis.[35] This would explain the rise in deaths from thyrotoxicosis in the early part of this century (Fig. 11.6). Successive generations born after 1880 were exposed to more iodine in childhood, which would have lessened their susceptibility to iodine in adult life; accordingly thyrotoxicosis mortality fell from around 1940. This explanation of the time trends accounts for the apparent paradox that toxic nodular goitre is now common only in those areas of Britain where iodine deficiency used to be prevalent. The essential process thought to underlie the trends in the occurrence of toxic nodular goitre is a response to an environmental influence acting during early life which has a critical effect on the ability to adapt to subsequent exposure. The same process could determine trends in coronary heart disease.

Coronary heart disease

In the UK death certificates did not distinguish coronary heart disease from other forms of heart disease before 1940. Other evidence, however, shows that incidence and death rates for coronary heart disease rose steeply during the first part of the century. From 1940 death rates continued to rise and, in Britain, reached a plateau in the 1970s (Fig. 11.6). Since 1980 there has been a continuing decline. Similar patterns occurred in the USA, Canada, Australia, and New Zealand: following steep increases there were substantial falls – around one-quarter over 20 years in the USA.[36] Although during the increase coronary heart disease was more common in wealthier people, it is now more common among people with lower incomes living in less affluent areas. The time trends of the disease may therefore depend on two groups of environmental causes: the first acting in utero and infancy and associated with poor living standards, and the second associated with affluence and perhaps mediated through a high energy, high fat diet. The rise in the disease results from an increase in the second; its fall from reduction in the first.

Figures 11.8 and 11.9 show age-specific mortality from coronary heart disease, for the years 1950–84, plotted against year of birth. Among men the generation born around 1925 had the highest death rates at all ages so far attained. Among women the picture is similar, although the peak is less clearly defined at 1925. The occurrence of a worst affected generation is consistent with the hypothesis that coronary disease is determined by two sets of influences.

Although this hypothesis synthesises our new understanding of the role of fetal growth in coronary heart disease with more established ideas on the role of lifestyle, it is not necessary to invoke two sets of influences to explain the rise and fall of coronary heart disease or its changing rates in successive generations. Coronary heart disease does not seem to be associated with

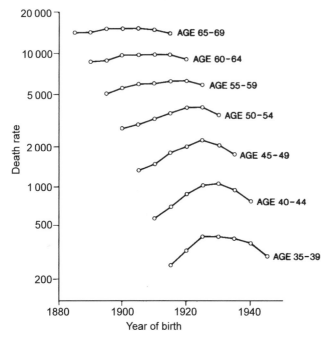

Fig. 11.8 Mortality rates from coronary heart disease in men in England and Wales during 1950–84.

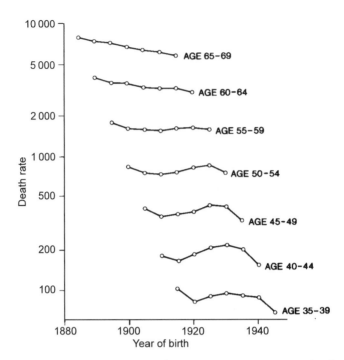

Fig. 11.9 Mortality rates from coronary heart disease in women in England and Wales during 1950–84.

proportionate or 'symmetrical' growth retardation, resulting from undernutrition in early gestation, but is associated with disproportionate growth retardation, which results from undernutrition in mid- or late gestation and leads to either thinness or stunting at birth. This is consistent with the different patterns of fetal growth that occur in different countries. An important difference between fetal growth in the less developed and that in western countries is that proportionate growth retardation is common in less developed countries, whereas disproportionate growth retardation prevails in western countries.[37] Table 11.2 shows the birth measurements of newborn babies who were included in the WHO study of lactational amenorrhoea (unpublished data). The babies in China have smaller heads and are shorter but fatter, as indicated by ponderal index, than babies in India or Sweden. The Chinese babies are proportionately small (Fig. 8.5). The babies in New Delhi are, however, thin as has been observed elsewhere in India.[38] These differences reflect marked differences in fetal nutrition.

Table 11.2 Mean birthweight, head circumference, length, and ponderal index of babies born at term in different countries

Country	Place	No. of babies	Birthweight, kg	Head circumference, cm	Length cm	Ponderal index, kg/m³
China	Chendu	543	3.33	33.5	49.1	28.1
India	New Delhi	550	2.97	34.2	49.7	24.2
Sweden	Uppsala	597	3.74	35.8	51.7	27.1

One can infer that in China mothers are chronically malnourished and the growth rate of babies is reduced from early gestation. This reduces their demand for nutrients in late gestation, and they are thereby protected from undernutrition at that time (p. 139) and are born fat.[39] They are not prone to coronary heart disease as adults, though they have raised blood pressure. In India mothers are less severely malnourished and the growth rate of babies is not reduced until mid-gestation. They have larger heads than Chinese babies, but undernutrition in late gestation makes them thin at birth or stunted. In Western communities mothers are better nourished and babies are large but fetal undernutrition in late gestation still occurs and may lead to thinness or reduced growth of the trunk with sparing of brain growth.

The hypothesis of this book is that coronary heart disease represents a stage of improving nutrition between chronic maternal malnutrition and nutrition at a plane that allows the mother to nourish her fetus adequately throughout gestation. This offers an economical interpretation of the time trends of coronary heart disease. Recent findings by Forsen, Eriksson and colleagues in Finland give the first direct support for it.[40] As described in Chapter 3 a follow-up study of men born in Helsinki during 1924–33 showed that death from coronary heart disease was associated with thinness at birth and low placental weight. Several studies have shown that thinness at birth is associated with insulin resistance which may be one of the mechanisms underlying its association with coronary heart disease. Table 11.3 shows that death rates from coronary heart disease among the Finnish men were also increased if the mother had a high body mass in late pregnancy. The highest death rates therefore occurred in men who were thin at birth and had a low placental weight but whose mothers had a high body mass index during pregnancy. Table 11.4 shows that the effect of mother's body mass index was, however, restricted to mothers whose height was below the average for the group (1.58 metres (62 inches)). The differences in death rates across Table 11.4 are large and highly statistically significant. It is remarkable that four simple measurements, the height and weight of the mother and the length and weight of the newborn baby, predict coronary heart disease so strongly.

The processes by which high body mass in women of short stature compound the increased risk of coronary heart disease that is associated with

Table 11.3 Standardised mortality ratios for coronary heart disease in Finnish men according to ponderal index at birth and mother's body mass index in late pregnancy.

Ponderal index of baby, kg/m³	Body mass index of mother, kg/m²					
	–24	–26	–28	–30	>30	All
–25	56 (6)	134 (20)	158 (17)	131 (7)	171 (7)	124 (57)
–27	88 (12)	87 (21)	123 (26)	104 (11)	131 (11)	104 (81)
–29	46 (5)	76 (17)	55 (13)	98 (12)	116 (16)	76 (63)
>29	38 (2)	61 (7)	45 (7)	68 (6)	72 (9)	58 (31)
All		62 (25)	89 (65)	89 (63)	97 (36)	111 (43)	89 (232)

Figures in parentheses are numbers of deaths.

Table 11.4 Standardised mortality ratios for coronary heart disease in Finnish men according to ponderal index at birth and mother's body mass index in late pregnancy

Ponderal index kg/m³	Body mass index of mother, kg/m²					
	−24	−26	−28	−30	>30	All
Mother's height below mean, ≤1.58 m (62 in)						
−25	55 (3)	106 (9)	168 (12)	170 (5)	224 (6)	131 (35)
−27	55 (3)	70 (8)	146 (17)	113 (6)	134 (6)	104 (40)
−29	26 (1)	54 (6)	31 (4)	137 (10)	149 (11)	75 (32)
>29	0 (0)	63 (3)	26 (2)	55 (3)	75 (4)	48 (12)
All	43 (7)	73 (26)	88 (35)	114 (24)	136 (27)	90 (119)
Mother's height above mean, >1.58 m (62 in)						
−25	57 (3)	170 (11)	138 (5)	83 (2)	71 (1)	115 (22)
−27	110 (9)	102 (13)	94 (9)	96 (5)	126 (5)	103 (41)
−29	57 (4)	97 (11)	85 (9)	40 (2)	79 (5)	77 (31)
>29	55 (2)	59 (4)	66 (5)	86 (3)	70 (5)	66 (19)
All	75 (18)	105 (39)	89 (28)	75 (12)	85 (16)	89 (113)

Figures in parentheses are numbers of deaths.

thinness at birth and insulin resistance are not known. The findings in India (p. 106) suggests that insulin deficiency may be one of them. Continuing studies in Finland should establish whether this is so. Meanwhile the findings in Finland illuminate the origins of the modern epidemic of coronary heart disease and its subsequent decline in many western countries. In chronically malnourished populations mothers are short and thin, and newborn babies are thin. Table 11.4 shows that rates of coronary heart disease will be low. The thinness of the newborn babies probably reflects the effects of maternal undernutrition over several generations, because a mother who herself had a low birthweight tends to have babies with low placental weights and low ponderal indices, regardless of her current height and weight (Fig. 8.4).[41] The immediate consequence of improved nutrition is that mothers' weights increase, though they remain short in stature. Table 11.4 shows that this will be associated with a steep increase in coronary heart disease. With continued improvements in nutrition in the population mothers become taller and heavier, maternal fatness no longer increases the risk of coronary heart disease, constraints on placental growth are relaxed and babies become fatter. Coronary heart disease therefore declines.

Chapter 6 described how the adverse effects of thinness at birth on glucose-insulin metabolism are compounded by the development of obesity in adult life, which is also a risk factor for coronary heart disease. The Finnish study includes data on child growth. Figure 11.10 shows that by the age of seven years the weight of the men who died of coronary heart disease and who were thin at birth, had 'caught-up'. Their body mass indices had become above the average and remained so throughout childhood (Eriksson, unpublished). This contrasts with the growth of men who died of stroke, whose body mass index remained below average throughout childhood. Table 11.5 shows that men in the lowest third of ponderal index at birth and the highest third of body mass in childhood had a four-fold increase in risk of coronary heart disease. These findings suggest that the disease is associated with poor nutrition in utero but good nutrition in childhood and later life.

The fundamental reason why epidemics of coronary heart disease accompany improving nutrition may be that whereas children and adults become better nourished over a short time, it takes several generations to improve the nutrition of the fetus, partly because of intergenerational constraints on placental growth. In the early phase of improving nutrition increased body mass in mothers, and in children and adults who were thin at birth, will lead to an increase in coronary heart disease.

Non-insulin-dependent diabetes

This is not strictly a 'western' disease because it is common in some developing countries including India.[42] Its incidence, however, rises steeply with industrialisation, and the highest known prevalences are in populations which have become 'westernised' unusually rapidly (p. 109). It is uncertain whether the prevalence has changed recently in the western world.[43] The disease is associated with undernutrition in utero and obesity in adult life (Ch. 6). One could therefore predict that its incidence will rise and fall as nutrition in a population improves. The initial rise will result from an increase in adult obesity, and the fall will occur when better fetal nutrition becomes reflected in better glucose/insulin metabolism in adult life. Table 6.3 showed how better growth in utero and during infancy protect against the effects of obesity on plasma glucose concentrations.

Findings which support this come from a survey of the Nauruan Islanders. A steep post-war rise in the prevalence of non-insulin-dependent diabetes was

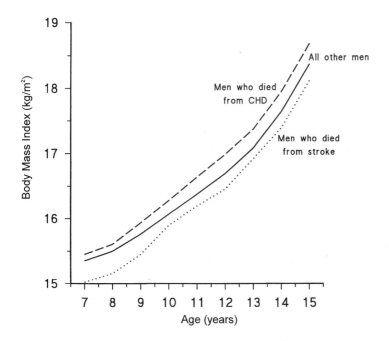

Fig. 11.10 Body mass index in childhood of 3 302 men in Finland.

Table 11.5 Hazard ratios for death from coronary heart disease among 3044 born at term

Ponderal index (kg/m³) at birth	Body mass index (kg/m²) at age 11 years		
	≤15.8	≤16.8	>16.8
≤25.9	2.2 (33)	2.9 (34)	4.0 (36)
–28	2.5 (30)	2.2 (31)	3.1 (42)
>28	1.0 (11)	1.0 (13)	2.0 (35)

associated with the rapid development of obesity in the population. The prevalence, however, is now falling.[44] This fall has occurred in people born after 1945, and has not been accompanied by change in the prevalence of obesity or other diabetes risk factors related to adult lifestyle. It is thought to reflect better fetal growth in post-war generations.

Poliomyelitis

Figure 11.6 shows the trend in notification rates for poliomyelitis in England and Wales. The disease was rare before this century but, as in other countries, it began to appear as hygienic and general living standards improved. This contrasts with the other common infectious diseases which declined at this time. There was a sharp rise in notifications of poliomyelitis after the Second World War which persisted until the introduction of large-scale immunisation. It is now known that the rise of poliomyelitis resulted from the increasing vulnerability of the central nervous system to poliovirus infection with increasing age. As hygiene, sanitation, and housing improved, the proportion of children escaping infection during the relatively safe period of infancy rose, and the number of cases of paralytic disease at later ages therefore rose in parallel.

Acute appendicitis

The outbreaks of appendicitis which have accompanied industrialisation in many parts of the world can similarly be explained as an age-dependent consequence of infection. The so-called 'hygiene hypothesis' for acute appendicitis was described in Chapter 9. In England and Wales death rates from appendicitis increased abruptly and steeply from around 1900 and then fell progressively from the 1930s onwards (Fig. 11.6). There is strong evidence that this trend reflected similar changes in incidence of the disease, and the same trends were recorded in other European countries and in the USA. The explanation of these trends is thought to lie in the reduced levels of enteric infection in young children brought about by better hygiene, making them more liable to develop appendicitis in response to infections at a later age. With continued improvements in hygiene exposure to infection throughout childhood and early adult life became less common. Acute appendicitis therefore declined.

Duodenal ulcer

Death rates from duodenal ulcer rose and fell in a similar way to those from acute appendicitis (Fig. 11.6). The distribution of duodenal ulcer with social class was similar to appendicitis; while it was increasing it was more common among the rich, but as it declined it became more common in poorer people. Recent findings of *Helicobacter* organisms in peptic ulcers suggest that the disease is spread through this infective agent.[45] The time trends point to age-dependent consequences of this infection.

WESTERN DISEASE AND RATES OF ENVIRONMENTAL CHANGE

Coronary heart disease, non-insulin-dependent diabetes, appendicitis, and duodenal ulcer seem to rise and fall in response to the environmental changes that accompany industrialisation. These diseases characterise the change from a rural to an industrial society, and there is increasing evidence that they originate in responses to the early environment, including adaptation to undernutrition during fetal life and the consequences of infection in childhood. Hitherto the search for causes of 'Western' diseases has concentrated on the adult environment. The importance of the fetal and infant environment in determining responses throughout life has been underestimated. Models of disease based on the effects of cigarette smoking, an influence in the adult environment which has been intensively studied, may have limited general application. Where differences in individuals' susceptibility to disease cannot be explained by differences in the adult environment, as is the case for coronary heart disease, they have often been attributed to genetic causes – especially if the disease has a familial tendency. Part of what was regarded as the genetic contribution to coronary heart disease and other disorders can now be attributed to the intrauterine or early postnatal environment.

Adaptations during early life may determine optimal rates of environmental change within populations. Appendicitis and duodenal ulcer became common at an early stage of improvements in hygiene. The size of epidemics of these diseases may depend on the speed with which hygiene improves throughout the population. The rise of appendicitis in Britain can be linked to the introduction of domestic hot water systems. The introduction of piped water supplies was spread over more than half a century, piped water not reaching some rural areas until after the Second World War. Swifter execution of sanitary health reforms started in the 19th century might have reduced the incidence of this and other diseases.

By contrast adaptations to undernutrition in utero may limit the extent of dietary change to which a generation can be exposed without adverse effects. People undernourished in utero are more susceptible to coronary heart disease and non-insulin-dependent diabetes[46, 47] if they become overweight in adult life. Figure 11.11, which is based on the Finnish data described in Chapter 3, shows the hazard ratios of coronary heart disease in men according to the height and weight of mothers. It seems that in the early phases of improving nutrition it is important to avoid an increase in women's body mass. The emphasis should be on increasing their stature and muscularity, which requires both improved nutrition and reduction in infection, especially enteric infections, during childhood. Protecting and improving the nutrition of girls and young women is therefore a priority during 'westernisation'. Yet in Britain

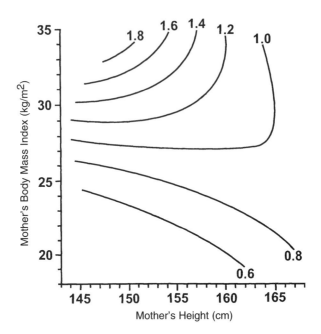

Fig. 11.11 Hazard ratios for coronary heart disease in Finnish men according to mother's body mass index and height.

though the industrial revolution brought high wages to adults children, especially girl children, continued to grow up undernourished and exposed to high rates of infection in poor, overcrowded homes.

Figure 11.12 shows the relative risk of coronary heart disease in Finnish men according to their ponderal index at birth and body mass in childhood. There are as yet no equivalent data for women. The figure uses body mass at age 11 years but body mass at any age from 7 to 16 years gives similar results. The effects of thinness at birth and a high body mass in childhood are additive. An important point illustrated in Figure 11.12 is that a boy who was thin at birth increases his risk of coronary heart disease by having even an average body mass index, while for a boy who had a high ponderal index even the highest body mass index has little effect on risk of the disease.

Steep increases in the incidence of 'western' diseases regularly follow industrialisation and the associated changes in diet and hygiene. Large-scale migration into cities in the less developed countries has changed people's diet, but poor hygiene persists. Elsewhere, as in China, improvements in hygiene have occurred with little change in the traditional diet, though it is becoming more plentiful. The message from the Finnish data, and other findings described in this book, seems clear. As populations escape from chronic malnutrition and high rates of infection in childhood there is an optimal vector for the consequent increases in height and body mass. For as long as fetal growth is constrained by low maternal weight and small placental size, for so long therefore that birthweight and ponderal index at birth remain low, it is important to avoid even modest levels of fatness in childhood and early adult life, since this will increase rates of coronary heart disease in that generation and, acting through the girls, in the next generation as well. The optimal levels of height

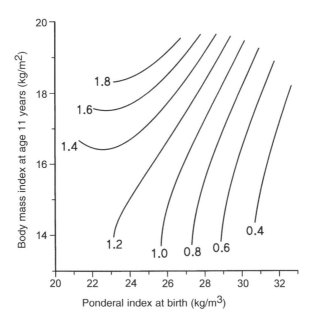

Fig. 11.12 Hazards ratios for coronary heart disease in Finnish men according to ponderal index at birth and mass index in childhood.

and weight among mothers, babies and children will presumably differ between populations with different habitual diets and metabolism. Data from populations other than Finland are now needed.

OTHER DISEASES WHICH ORIGINATE IN UTERO

This section briefly reviews a number of other common diseases for which there is evidence of in utero programming. They do not represent the extent and range of the effects of programming: fresh evidence linking in utero life with other diseases regularly appears.

Osteoporosis

Almost one in five of white North American women aged 50 years will have a hip fracture during their remaining lifetime, as will one in 17 men of the same age.[48] Low bone mass is a major risk factor for hip fracture, though there are other risk factors which either increase the risk of an old person falling, or affect the shape and architecture of bone.[49] Cooper and colleagues showed that the bone mass of young women at two common sites of osteoporotic fracture, the femoral neck and lumbar spine, was related to their weight at 1 year.[50] They found that this relation was also apparent among elderly men and women.[51] This finding suggests that skeletal development tracks from early life and that growth retardation in prenatal and early postnatal life may set in motion a series of pathological processes that lead eventually to osteoporotic fracture.

Bone mass is a function of bone size and mineral density. Growth is the most important determinant of size while density within the bony envelope is modified by a host of local factors including hormonal status and physical activity. Studies of the 24-hour growth hormone profiles of elderly men in Hertfordshire showed that peak growth hormone concentrations were related to bone density in the femoral neck,[52] which suggests that this aspect of growth hormone secretion is one of the influences which modify bone density through life. Median growth hormone concentrations in old age were related to weight at the age of 1 year. This particular aspect of the growth hormone secretory profile may therefore be programmed in utero or during infancy, initiating changes that lead ultimately to hip fracture.

Schizophrenia

The advent of new imaging techniques has revolutionised ideas about the cause of schizophrenia. 'Decades of scientifically unfounded psychological and social theories that blamed family and society have given way to increasingly compelling scientific evidence that schizophrenia is a brain disorder'.[53] Subtle reductions in cortical volume revealed by neuroimaging, together with necropsy observations of altered architecture in the cortex, have led to the conclusion that the disorder originates through defective migration of cells into the cortex during the second trimester of gestation.

Epidemiological evidence that schizophrenia originates in utero comes from the increased frequency of obstetric complications in the birth histories of patients,[54, 55] and delay in their motor and speech milestones during childhood.[56] There is preliminary evidence that both infection and undernutrition in utero may initiate the defects in early brain development that are subtly manifest in childhood but become dramatically evident in early adult life. In a study of people who were at risk of in utero exposure to the 1957 influenza epidemic, those at risk during the second trimester had higher rates of hospital admission for schizophrenia than those at risk during other trimesters or those not at risk.[57] The results of other similar studies have, however, been inconsistent.[53, 58] People exposed to the Dutch famine during the first 2 months of gestation had a twofold increase in risk of being hospitalised for schizophrenia.[59] A recent review of the time trends of schizophrenia suggests that it may be a 'disease of change', whose incidence rose in the early stages of industrialisation but is now declining.[60]

Depression

For many years depression in adult life has been thought to originate through parental indifference, abuse and other adverse influences in childhood. A study in Hertfordshire found that men and women who committed suicide, which is commonly the result of depression, had low weight gain in infancy.[61] While this could be due to adverse psychosocial influences in infancy there is nothing in the Hertfordshire records that supports this, and it raises the possibility that adult depression is initiated by in utero programming of hormonal axes which influence growth in infancy and mood in later life. Patients with depression have been found to have abnormal secretion of growth hormone and abnormalities in the hypothalamic–adrenal and hypothalamic–thyroid axes.[62] There is evidence that each of these axes are programmed in utero (Ch. 2).

Table 11.6 Indices of ageing related to infant weight in 717 elderly men and women

Weight at 1 year, lb (kg)	Hearing threshold, dBA	Grip strength, kg	Lens opacity score	Skin thickness, mm
≤18 (8.2)	33.6 (26)	29.8 (26)	2.67 (26)	1.20 (26)
–20 (9.1)	29.4 (134)	30.7 (134)	2.40 (133)	1.22 (134)
–22 (10.0)	29.3 (209)	31.1 (211)	2.33 (198)	1.24 (211)
–24 (10.9)	29.1 (194)	31.6 (194)	2.37 (187)	1.25 (194)
–26 (11.8)	26.5 (77)	32.6 (77)	2.33 (70)	1.25 (77)
>26 (11.8)	24.8 (41)	34.2 (41)	2.24 (41)	1.25 (41)
p value*	0.008	0.02	0.003	0.19
All	28.8	31.5	2.36	1.24

* Adjusted for age, sex, current social class, social class at birth and height.
Figures in parentheses are numbers of subjects.

Ageing

Among elderly men and women in Hertfordshire those who were heavy at 1 year of age had better hearing and grip strength, less opacification of the lens of the eye, and thicker skin (Table 11.6).[63] Better growth in infancy therefore seems linked to slower rates of ageing. Kirkwood has suggested that imperfect molecular repair and the consequent accumulation of tissue damage is one of the processes which underlies ageing.[64] This suggestion is supported by the premature ageing which occurs in Werner's syndrome, a genetically determined failure in DNA repair.[65] Aihie Sayer and colleagues have used this to explain the Hertfordshire findings.[63] She postulates that undernutrition in utero, leading to low weight gain in infancy, impairs the development of repair systems. Furthermore the particular associations found, shown in Table 11.6, suggest that undernutrition may affect tissues which contain a large proportion of long-lived molecules such as lens crystallins, collagen and elastin. In the relative absence of regeneration, molecular repair processes may be most critical to these tissues.

TODAY'S MOTHERS

The epidemiological evidence which links fetal nutrition and childhood infection with adult disease necessarily depends on studies of people born many years ago. People sometimes suggest that the fetal origins hypothesis is no longer relevant to the western world which, they imply, has completed the 'escape' from chronic malnutrition and endemic infection. They argue that the inequalities in disease in the western world, between rich and poor, between people living in one place and those in another, are largely a legacy of the past; and future generations will enjoy falling disease rates and a lessening of inequalities. There is, however, considerable evidence against this comfortable point of view.

Thin mothers

In Mysore, South India, it was the low birthweight babies born to the thin mothers who had the highest rates of coronary heart disease (Fig. 3.11). In the Dutch famine study (p. 101) it was people born to mothers with the lowest

Table 11.7 Fasting plasma insulin concentrations in men and women in Aberdeen, Scotland, according to their mother's body mass in pregnancy

	Body mass index of mother (kg/m²)				
	–23	–25	–27	>27	p for trend
Fasting insulin adjusted for sex and body mass, pmol/l	42	34	35	34	0.05

weights in late gestation who had the highest 2-hour plasma glucose concentrations. The actual weights of these thin mothers, however, were around 60 to 65 kg (132 to 143 lb) – far higher than the weights of the Indian mothers. Table 11.7 is a further illustration of how thin mothers in well-nourished communities adversely affect the glucose tolerance of their children. Among a group of middle-aged men and women born in Aberdeen, Scotland around 1950, those whose mothers had the lowest body mass indices in late pregnancy had raised fasting insulin concentrations, and were therefore more insulin-resistant (unpublished). These findings replicate those in China (Tables 6.7 and 6.8). The mothers in Beijing in 1950 were, not unexpectedly, thinner than the mothers in Aberdeen. Nevertheless the body mass indices of many pregnant European women today are within the range of the Chinese women (Table 6.8). The body mass of the young woman who is the central figure in Figure 8.3 was 16 and rose to 21 when she later became pregnant. Unlike the Chinese women her slenderness conforms to what is fashionable today and she is slim by choice.

The children of thin women have raised blood pressure as well as insulin resistance. However it seems to be thin skinfold thickness or low weight gain in pregnancy, rather than low body mass, that are associated with raised blood pressure. Jamaican women with thinner triceps skinfold thicknesses at 15 weeks of pregnancy and low weight gain in pregnancy had children with higher systolic blood pressure at the age of 10 years.[66] In the Gambia, low maternal pregnancy weight gain was associated with higher blood pressure in 8- and 9-year-old children.[67] In Birmingham, England, women whose triceps skinfold thickness was below the median (15 mm) in early pregnancy, and who had low weight gain in pregnancy, had children with raised blood pressure.[68] These associations were independent of the babies' birthweight, suggesting that blood pressure can be programmed by processes that do not involve differences in size at birth – a suggestion that is consistent with findings in animals.[69] Since triceps skinfold thickness changes little in early pregnancy[70] women who enter pregnancy poorly nourished may initiate these processes. One possibility is that they do so through impaired early placental growth (p. 135).

The only data that link maternal skinfold thickness to the blood pressures of adult offspring comes from Sheffield, where middle-aged men and women whose mothers had narrow hips, as measured by the diameter across the iliac crests, had raised blood pressure (Table 11.8). This again was independent of their size at birth. Pelvic diameters are measured by callipers and are influenced by skinfold thickness, which increases during pregnancy. The width across the iliac crests is influenced by the suprailiac skinfold. Since in other studies the mother's skeletal size, as measured by her height, is unrelated to her offspring's blood pressure, the association between narrow hips and offspring's blood pressure may reflect thinness rather than a small bony pelvis.

Table 11.8 Systolic blood pressure (mmHg) in men and women aged around 50 years in relation to the width of their mother's hips (intercristal diameter)

	Intercristal diameter, cm (in)				
	≤26 (10)	–27 (10.6)	–28 (11)	>28 (11)	p for trend
Systolic blood pressure	154	149	146	144	0.001
Diastolic blood pressure	88	86	84	85	0.05
No. of people	85	75	86	76	

Overweight mothers

The findings in Finland (Fig. 11.11 and Table 11.14) show the adverse effect on the offspring if a mother, especially one who is short in stature, has a high body mass in pregnancy. This effect is enhanced if the baby has a small placenta and is thin. We do not know the processes by which high maternal body mass compounds the increased risk of coronary heart disease that is associated with thinness at birth, though the findings in India (p. 106) suggest that insulin deficiency and consequent non-insulin-dependent diabetes may be one of them. Whatever the processes short, overweight young women are a feature of parts of the world, including Eastern Europe, Russia and Asia where epidemics of coronary heart disease are now occurring. The adverse effects of mother's body weight may not be limited to coronary heart disease and non-insulin-dependent diabetes. Women with polycystic ovary disease for example, are born to heavy mothers (p. 187).

Mother's diet in pregnancy

Campbell and colleagues showed that the blood pressures of men and women in Aberdeen were related to the balance of animal protein and carbohydrate in their mothers' diets in late pregnancy.[71] Most of the mothers ate less than 50 g of animal protein daily. Among them those with high carbohydrate intakes had offspring with raised systolic and diastolic blood pressure (Table 11.9). These findings are similar to those in experiments in rats.[69] In contrast, in the mothers whose animal protein intake exceeded 50 g daily those with low carbohydrate intakes had offspring with raised blood pressure. These effects of mother's diet on offspring's blood pressure did not depend on effects on birthweight, which was independently associated with blood pressure. This suggests that, as with the mother's skinfold thickness and weight gain, the mother's diet can program the offspring's blood pressure without changing size at birth. This does not necessarily imply that blood pressure can be programmed without altering fetal growth, since animal studies show that differing patterns of fetal growth may lead to similar size at birth (p. 134).

In Aberdeen the balance between animal protein and carbohydrate intake was also reflected in an altered placental weight. Figure 11.13 shows that where the mother's animal protein intake was less than 50 g a day, high carbohydrate intake was associated with reduced placental weight. This is consistent with findings in a recent study of maternal diet and placental growth.[72] Above an intake of 50 g of animal protein a day, low carbohydrate intake was associated with reduced placental weight. Animal protein and carbohydrate intakes may

Table 11.9 Systolic blood pressure (mmHg) of 253 men and women in Scotland according to their mother's intake of animal protein and carbohydrate in pregnancy

	Mean daily intake of animal protein (g)	
Mean daily intake of carbohydrate, g	≤50	>50
≤275	135	162
–350	137	139
>350	139	134
All	137	137
Unadjusted regression coefficient (mmHg per 100 g increase)	+ 2.7 (0.03)*	– 7.3 (0.03)
Regression coefficient adjusted for birthweight and mothers' blood pressure	+ 3.0 (0.02)	– 11.2 (0.004)

* Figures in parentheses are *p* values.

therefore program the offspring's blood pressure by reducing placental growth. They also influence ponderal index at birth, which may be mediated through altered placental growth.[41]

The protein intake of the Aberdeen mothers was also related to their offsprings' glucose-insulin metabolism. Low protein intake was associated with a raised fasting plasma insulin concentration, that is with insulin resistance, though this was a weaker relation than that with low maternal body mass. This is consistent with findings in people exposed in utero to the Dutch famine, whose mothers had low intakes of protein and whose reduced glucose tolerance was probably the result of insulin resistance (p. 101). Figure 11.14 shows that, in contrast, high intakes of protein and fat in the Scottish men and women

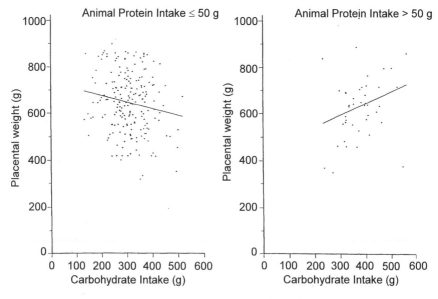

Fig. 11.13 Placental weight according to mothers' intake of animal protein and carbohydrate in Aberdeen.

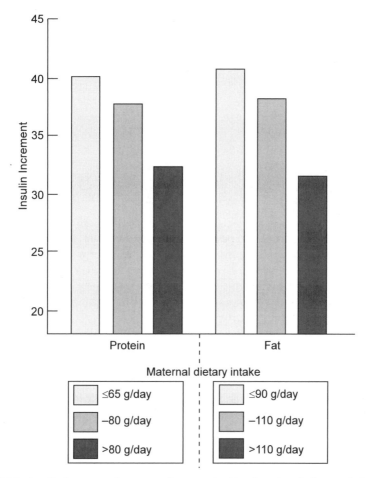

Fig. 11.14 Insulin increment in men and women in Aberdeen in relation to their mothers' protein and fat intakes in pregnancy.

were associated with a sharply reduced insulin increment, that is with insulin deficiency (unpublished). This association is independent of maternal body mass, size at birth or placental weight. It may be relevant to the untoward effects of protein supplementation on fetal growth (p. 139). Supplements with a higher percentage of calories derived from protein are associated with low birthweight.[72, 73] The existence of long-term effects of mother's protein intake on glucose-insulin metabolism in the offspring is consistent with the observation that mother's intakes of protein and carbohydrate during pregnancy alter the concentration of insulin in cord blood.[74]

The findings in Aberdeen point to the importance of protein in programming the fetus. Studies by Forrester and colleagues in Jamaica suggest that mother's protein metabolism changes early in pregnancy.[75] Jackson and colleagues have proposed that glycine becomes an essential amino acid during pregnancy because of the high demand for nucleic acid synthesis.[76] The availability of amino acids to the fetus will be determined by the mother's protein turnover. Larger mothers with a greater lean body mass will have a higher protein turnover, though this will be modified by dietary intake.[77] James has

Table 11.10 Mean difference in systolic pressure (mmHg) between children aged 5 to 9 years whose mothers received calcium during pregnancy and those who did not

Children's body mass index, kg/m^2	No. of children		Mean difference (95% CI) in systolic pressure, mmHg
	Calcium group	Placebo group	
≤14.4	61	65	0.5 (– 2.7 to 3.8)
–15.7	62	65	1.8 (– 1.2 to 4.8)
–17.5	63	69	– 3.2 (– 6.3 to – 0.1)
>17.5	68	60	– 5.8 (– 9.8 to – 1.7)
All	254	260	– 1.4 (– 3.3 to 0.5)

CI, confidence interval.

emphasised the probable importance of essential fatty acids in programming the fetus, though at present there is little information on this.[77] He suggests that since about 1% of maternal fat stores turn over each day, the fatty acid composition of the mother's diet during pregnancy may be of modest importance compared with the amount and composition of her body's fat stores.

Calcium may also be linked to in utero programming of blood pressure. The first evidence from a randomised control trial that nutritional intervention in pregnancy programs the offspring's blood pressure came from the WHO trial carried out in Argentina of calcium supplementation in the prevention of hypertensive disease in pregnancy.[78] Children whose mothers received calcium had lower blood pressures than those whose mothers were in the placebo group. Interestingly this effect was seen in children with a higher body mass (Table 11.10) and was unrelated to the mother's blood pressure.

TODAY'S BABIES

Law and colleagues[79] compared the size at birth of an unselected sample of more than 1000 babies born recently in Salisbury, a prosperous town in southern England, with that of a similar sample born in Burnley, one of the less affluent industrial towns in northern England. Burnley has had high perinatal mortality (stillbirth and early neonatal deaths) since the beginning of the century (Ch. 10). Its rates of coronary heart disease are above the national average while those in Salisbury are below. Burnley babies today are thinner, as measured by ponderal index and arm and abdominal circumferences, and have smaller head circumferences (Table 11.11). The thinness of Burnley babies is not the result of a shorter period of gestation. Nor is it explained by differences in ethnicity, social class, maternal smoking, height, age, or parity, although these account for much of the difference in head circumference. Figure 11.15 shows that the lower mean ponderal index in Burnley reflects a different distribution of the measurements throughout the population and is not simply the result of an excess of very small, thin babies. The same applies to abdominal circumference.[790]

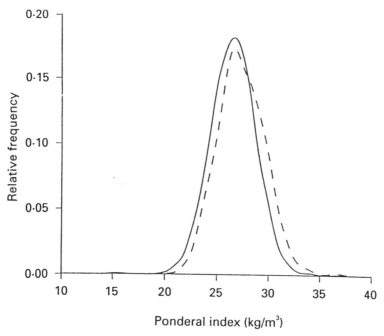

Fig. 11.15 Distribution of ponderal index (weight/length³) in newborn babies. —, Burnley; ...., Salisbury.

Low ponderal index and reduced abdominal circumference at birth are followed by an increased risk of coronary heart disease. Table 6.9 showed the blood pressures of an unselected group of 4-year-old children born in Salisbury during 1984–85. Regardless of their current size, and of other influences such as their mothers' blood pressure or smoking habits, those who were thin at birth already had higher blood pressure. By the time they were 7 years old their ability to store and metabolise glucose was reduced.[80] Seemingly a predisposition to develop hypertension and non-insulin-dependent diabetes is already apparent in the next generation. The findings in Table 11.11 suggest that Burnley will continue to have higher rates of coronary heart disease than Salisbury into the next generation. This prediction of continuing worse health among people living in poor areas is consistent with the long-term forecasts of Osmond, based on statistical analyses of recent trends.[81] They suggest that there will be a large fall in deaths from coronary heart disease in England but a worsening in the differential between the north and south of the country.

Table 11.11 Average size of babies born in two English towns, 1991

	Burnley (n = 1544)	Salisbury (n = 1025)	Difference Burnley – Salisbury (95% CI)
Birthweight	3342	3458	– 166 (–154 to –77)
Crown–heel length, cm	50.0	50.1	– 0.1 (–0.3 to 0.04)
Ponderal index, kg/m³	26.6	27.4	– 0.8 (–1.0 to –0.6)
Head circumference, cm	34.8	35.1	– 0.3 (–0.4 to –0.2)
Upper abdominal circumference, cm	33.5	34.0	– 0.5 (–0.6 to –0.4)

CI, confidence

The findings described in this book have profound implications for current preventive health policies. This is now recognised in Britain.[82] The Chief Medical Officer for Scotland has written:[83]

At present we do not know whether it is more important to improve living conditions in adult life and try to persuade people to change their lifestyles, or to improve the health and nutrition of pregnant women and pre-school children. Obviously any sensible policy for improving Scotland's health must do both. But much depends on which is likely to yield greater long term benefits, and at present we do not know. We are equally ignorant about the interactions that almost certainly exist between the enduring metabolic sequelae of inadequate nutrition early in life and unhealthy eating, drinking and exercise patterns in middle age.

The thesis of this book is that great benefit will come from improving the health and nutrition of girls and young women, and mothers during pregnancy and lactation. This chapter has described how mothers who are thin, or short and overweight, may induce adaptations in their babies which increase their subsequent risk of coronary heart disease, hypertension and non-insulin-dependent diabetes. The balance of protein and carbohydrate in the mother's diet in late pregnancy, and the amounts of fat and protein in the diet, seem to be emerging as important influences on the later development of disease. They do so without exerting any important effect on birth size. Therefore to try to evaluate the long-term benefits of improved maternal nutrition by assessing its effects on birthweight is to miss the poin,[84] because birthweight is too crude a measure of fetal nutrition to be useful in such an evaluation. Conversely, whereas cessation of smoking in pregnancy is likely to increase birthweight it is of little detectable long-term benefit to the fetus (p. 132). If improving the body composition and diets of girls and young women is to be one of the new strategies for preventing coronary heart disease, another will be avoidance of childhood obesity. People who have low birthweight, or more importantly who are thin or short at birth, are a vulnerable group, vulnerable to the long-term effects of becoming obese (Fig. 11.12).

Developing countries face a different dilemma to that of western countries. High maternal and child mortality necessarily focus prevention on the mother and child rather than the lifestyles of middle-aged men and women. The dilemma is whether greater benefit will come from improving the nutrition of girls and young women than from improving the nutrition of young children. Hitherto interest in the nutrition and health of young women before pregnancy has been subordinate to interest in young children. This book points clearly to the need to change this emphasis. In rural India and other developing countries girls are thin and undernourished, while in towns they are becoming overweight but remain short in stature. Children in many developing countries remain stunted but are now becoming obese. It is not known to what extent this reflects low lean body mass, low intakes of high energy foods or hormonal changes associated with stunting. The likely benefits of improving the body composition and nutrition of girls and young women in developing countries include both a reduction in the rising epidemics of coronary heart disease and non-insulin-dependent diabetes and, it seems, an improvement in immune status and consequent lessening of infectious disease (p. 31).[85]

THE FUTURE

Studies of programming in fetal life and infancy are now established in the agenda for medical research. They have refocused attention on maternal nutrition and fetal growth.[86] They have two goals: preventing disease in the next generation and treating disease in the present one. The search for the causes of coronary heart disease has hitherto been guided by a 'destructive' model. The causes to be identified act in adult life and accelerate destructive processes: the formation of atheroma, rise in blood pressure and loss of glucose tolerance. This book has proposed a new 'developmental' model. The causes to be identified act on the baby. In adapting to them the baby ensures its continued survival and growth at the expense of its longevity. Premature death from coronary heart disease may be viewed as the price of successful adaptations in utero. We need to know more about these adaptations: what they are; what genes underlie them; what induces them; how they leave a lasting mark on the body; and how this gives rise to the diseases of later life. Up to the present much of the research has been epidemiological. We now need to understand the cellular and molecular processes that underlie the epidemiological associations. Thomas Lewis wrote 'the deeper our understanding of a disease mechanism the greater are our chances of devising direct and decisive measure to prevent disease, or to turn it around before it is too late'.[87] Further research requires a strategy of interdependent clinical, animal and epidemiological studies.

Reference

1 Clark GA. New method for assessing changes in growth and sexual dimorphism in paleoepidemiology. *Am J Phys Anthropol* 1988; **77**: 105–116.

2 Clark GA, Hall NR, Armelagos GJ, Borkan GA, Panjabi MM, Wetzel FT. Poor growth prior to early childhood: decreased health and life-span in the adult. *Am J Phys Anthropol* 1986; **70**: 145–160.

3 Goodman AH, Armelagos GJ, Rose JC. The chronological distribution of enamel hypoplasia from prehistoric Dickson Mounds populations. *Am J Phys Anthropol* 1984; **65**: 259–266.

4 Kuh D, Davey Smith G. When is mortality risk determined? Historical insights into a current debate. *Social History of Medicine* 1993; **6**: 101–123.

5 Derrick VPA. Observations on (1) error on age on the Population Statistics of England and Wales and (2) the changes in mortality indicated by the National Records. *Journal of the Institute of Actuaries* 1927; **58**: 117–159.

6 Kermack WO, McKendrick AG, McKinlay PL. Death-rates in Great Britain and Sweden. Some general regularities and their significance. *Lancet* 1934; **i**: 698–703.

7 Watt GCM, Ecob R. Mortality in Glasgow and Edinburgh: a paradigm of inequality in health. *J Epidemiol Community Health* 1992; **46**: 498–505.

8 Watt GCM. The chief scientist reports. Making research make a difference. *Health Bulletin* 1993; **51**: 187–195.

9 McKeown T, Lowe CR. *An introduction to social medicine.* Oxford: Blackwell, 1974.

10 Barker DJP. Rise and fall of western diseases. *Nature* 1989; **338**: 371–372.

11 Registrar General. *Registrar General's statistical review of England Wales Part 1. Tables, medical.* London: 1880 and following years.

12 Acheson RM, Williams DRR. Epidemiology of cerebrovascular disease: some

unanswered questions. In: Rose FC, ed. *Clinical neuroepidemiology*. London: Pitman Medical, 1980; 88–104.

13 Barker DJP, Osmond C. Childhood respiratory infection and adult chronic bronchitis in England and Wales predicted by past infant mortality. *Br Med J* 1986; **293**: 1271–1275.

14 Osmond C. Time trends in infant mortality, ischaemic heart disease and stroke in England and Wales. In: Barker DJP, ed. *Fetal and infant origins of adult disease*. London: British Medical Journal Books, 1992; 119–129.

15 Martyn CN, Barker DJP, Osmond C. Mothers' pelvic size, fetal growth, and death from stroke and coronary heart disease in men in the UK. *Lancet* 1996; **348**: 1264–1268.

16 Lambert PM, Reid DD. Smoking, air pollution, and bronchitis in Britain. *Lancet* 1970; i: 853–857.

17 Michels KB, Trichopoulos D, Robins JM, Rosner BA, Manson JE, Hunter DJ, et al. Birthweight as a risk factor for breast cancer. *Lancet* 1996; **348**: 1542–1546.

18 Ekbom A, Trichopoulos D, Adami HO, Hsieh CC, Lan SJ. Evidence of prenatal influences on breast cancer risk. *Lancet* 1992; **340**: 1015–1018.

19 Sanderson M, Williams MA, Malone KE, Stanford JL, Emanuel I, White E, et al. Perinatal factors and risk of breast cancer. *Epidemiology* 1996; **7**: 34–37.

20 Barker DJP, Winter PD, Osmond C, Phillips DIW, Sultan HY. Weight gain in infancy and cancer of the ovary. *Lancet* 1995; **345**: 1087–1088.

21 Cresswell JL, Barker DJP, Osmond C, Egger P, Phillips DIW, Fraser RB. Fetal growth, length of gestation and polycystic ovaries in adult life. *Lancet* 1997; **350**: 1131–1135.

22 Cooper C, Kuh D, Egger P, Wadsworth M, Barker DJP. Childhood growth and age at menarche. *Br J Obstet Gynaecol* 1996; **103**: 814–817.

23 Rees M. Commentary: Menarche when and why? *Lancet* 1993; **342**: 1375–1376.

24 Cresswell JL, Egger P, Fall CHD, Osmond C, Fraser RB, Barker DJP. Is the age of menopause determined in-utero? *Early Hum Dev* 1997; **49**: 143–148.

25 Richardson SJ, Senikas V, Nelson JF. Follicular depletion during the menopause transition: evidence for accelerated loss and ultimate exhaustion. *J Clin Endocrinol Metab* 1987; **65**: 1231–1237.

26 Francois I, de Zegher F. Adrenarche and fetal growth. *Pediatr Res* 1997; **41**: 440–442.

27 Barker DJP, Osmond C, Golding J. Height and mortality in the counties of England and Wales. *Ann Human Biol* 1990; **17**: 1–6.

28 Tibblin G, Eriksson M, Cnattingius S, Ekbom A. High birthweight as a predictor of prostate cancer risk. *Epidemiology* 1995; **6**: 423–424.

29 Ekbom A, Hsieh CC, Lipworth L, Wolk A, Ponten J, Adami HO, et al. Perinatal characteristics in relation to incidence of and mortality from prostate cancer. *Br Med J* 1996; **313**: 337–341.

30 Francois I, de Zegher F, Spiessens C, D'Hooghe T, vanderSchueren D. Low birth weight and subsequent male subfertility. *Pediatr. Res* 1997; **42**: 899–901.

31 Sharpe RM, Shakkebaek NE. Are oestrogens involved in falling sperm counts and disorders of the male reproductive tract? *Lancet* 1993; **341**: 1392–1395.

32 Trowell HC, Burkitt DP. *Western diseases; their emergence and prevention*. London: Edward Arnold, 1981.

33 Phillips DIW, Barker DJP, Winter PD, Osmond C. Mortality from thyrotoxicosis in England and Wales and its association with the previous prevalence of endemic goitre. *J Epidemiol Community Health* 1983; **37**: 305–309.

34 Greaves JP, Hollingsworth DF. Trends in food consumption in the United Kingdom. *World Rev Nutr Diet* 1966; **6**: 34–89.

35 Barker DJP, Phillips DIW. Current incidence of thyrotoxicosis and past prevalence of goitre in 12 British towns. *Lancet* 1984; ii: 567–570.

36 Pisa Z, Uemura K. Trends of mortality from ischaemic heart disease and other cardiovascular diseases in 27 countries, 1968–1977. *World Health Stat Q* 1982; **35**: 11–47.

37 Kline J, Stein Z, Susser M. *Conception to birth – epidemiology of prenatal development*. New York: Oxford University Press, 1989.

38 Mohan M, Shiv Prasad SR, Chellani HK, Kapani V. Intrauterine growth curves in North Indian babies: weight, length, head circumference and ponderal index. *Indian Pediatrics* 1990; **27**: 43–51.

39 Woods DL. The constraint of maternal nutrition on the trajectory of fetal growth in

humans. In: Bruton MN, ed. *Alternative life-history styles of animals*. Dordrecht: Kluwer Academic, 1989; 459–464.

40 Forsen T, Eriksson JG, Tuomilehto J, Teramo K, Osmond C, Barker DJP. Mother's weight in pregnancy and coronary heart disease in a cohort of Finnish men: follow up study. *Br Med J* 1997; **315**: 837–840.

41 Godfrey KM, Barker DJP, Robinson S, Osmond C. Maternal birthweight and diet in pregnancy in relation to the infant's thinness at birth. *Br J Obstet Gynaecol* 1997; **104**: 663–667.

42 Ramachandran A. Epidemiology of diabetes in Indians. *Int J Diab Dev Countries* 1993; **13**: 65–67.

43 Jarrett RJ. Epidemiology and public health aspects of non-insulin dependent diabetes mellitus. *Epidemiol Rev* 1989; **11**: 151–171.

44 Dowse GK, Zimmett PZ, Finch CF, Collins VR. Decline in incidence of epidemic glucose intolerance in Nauruans: implications for the 'thrify genotype'. *Am J Epidemiol* 1991; **133**: 1093–1104.

45 Marshall BJ, McGechie DB, Rogers PA, Glancy RJ. Pyloric campylobacter infection and gastroduodenal disease. *Med J Aust* 1985; **142**: 439–444.

46 Hales CN, Barker DJP, Clark PMS, Cox LJ, Fall C, Osmond C, et al. Fetal and infant growth and impaired glucose tolerance at age 64. *Br Med J* 1991; **303**: 1019–1022.

47 Lithell HO, McKeigue PM, Berglund L, Mohsen R, Lithell UB, Leon DA. Relation of size at birth to non-insulin dependent diabetes and insulin concentrations in men aged 50–60 years. *Br Med J* 1996; **312**: 406–410.

48 Melton LJ, Chrischilles EA, Cooper C, Lane AW, Riggs BL. Perspective: How many women have osteoporosis? *J Bone Miner Res* 1992; **7**: 1005–1010.

49 Cummings SR, Nevitt MC, Browner WS, Stone K, Fox KM, Ensrud KE, et al. Risk factors for hip fracture in white women. Study of osteoporotic fractures research group. *N Engl J Med* 1995; **332**: 767–773.

50 Cooper C, Cawley M, Bhalla A, Egger P, Ring F, Morton L, et al. Childhood growth, physical activity, and peak bone mass in women. *J Bone Miner Res* 1995; **10**: 940–947.

51 Cooper C, Fall C, Egger P, Hobbs R, Eastell R, Barker DJP. Growth in infancy and bone mass in later life. *Ann Rheum Dis* 1997; **56**: 17–21.

52 Fall C, Hindmarsh P, Dennison E, Kellingray S, Barker DJP, Cooper C. Programming of growth hormone secretion and bone mineral density in elderly men: an hypothesis. *Clinical Endocrinol and Metab* 1998; (in press).

53 Weinberger DR. From neuropathology to neurodevelopment. *Lancet* 1995; **346**: 552–557.

54 Hultman CM, Ohman A, Cnattingius S, Wieselgren I, Lindstrom LH. Prenatal and neonatal risk factors for schizophrenia. *Br J Psychiat* 1997; **170**: 128–133.

55 Gunther-Genta F, Bovet P, Hohlfeld P. Obstetric complications and schizophrenia: a case-control study. *Br J Psychiatry* 1994; **164**: 165–170.

56 Jones P, Rodgers B, Murray R, Marmot M. Child developmental risk factors for adult schizophrenia in the British 1946 birth cohort. *Lancet* 1994; **344**: 1398–1402.

57 Mednick SA, Machon RA, Huttunen MO, Bonnett D. Adult schizophrenia following prenatal exposure to an influenza epidemic. *Arch Gen Psychiatry* 1988; **45**: 189–192.

58 Venables PH. Schizotypy and maternal exposure to influenza and to cold temperature: The Mauritius Study. *J Abnorm Psychol* 1996; **105**: 53–60.

59 Susser E, Neugebauer R, Hoeak W, Lin S, Brown A, Gorman J. Schizophrenia after prenatal exposure to famine. *Lancet* 1998; (in press).

60 Warner R. Time trends in schizophrenia: changes in obstetric risk factors with industrialization. *Schizophrenia Bulletin* 1995; **21**: 483–500.

61 Barker DJP, Osmond C, Rodin I, Fall CHD, Winter PD. Low weight gain in infancy and suicide in adult life. *Br Med J* 1995; **311**: 1203.

62 Checkley S. Neuroendocrinology. In: Paykel ES, ed. *Handbook of affective disorders*. Edinburgh: Churchill Livingstone, 1992.

63 Aihie Sayer A, Cooper C, Barker DJP. Is lifespan determined in utero? *Arch Dis Child* 1997; **77**: F161–F162.

64 Kirkwood TBL, Wolff SP. The biological basis of ageing. The Medical Research Council Research into Ageing Workshop 6 October 1993. *Age and Ageing* 1995; **24**: 167–171.

65 Yu CE, Oshima J, Fu YH, Wijsman EM, Hisama F, Alisch R, et al. Positional cloning of the Werner's syndrome gene. *Science* 1996; **272**: 258–262.

66 Godfrey KM, Forrester T, Barker DJP, Jackson AA, Landman JP, Hall J St E, et al. Maternal nutritional status in pregnancy and blood pressure in childhood. *Br J Obstet Gynaecol* 1994; **101**: 398–403.

67 Margetts BM, Rowland MGM, Foord FA, Cruddas AM, Cole TJ, Barker DJP. The relation of maternal weight to the blood pressures of Gambian children. *Int J Epidemiol* 1991; **20 (4)**: 938–943.

68 Clark PM, Atton C, Law CM, Shiell A, Godfrey K, Barker DJP. Weight gain in pregnancy, triceps skinfold thickness and blood pressure in the offspring. *Obstet Gynecol* 1998; (in press).

69 Langley SC, Jackson AA. Increased systolic blood pressure in adult rats induced by fetal exposure to maternal low protein diets. *Clin Sci* 1994; **86**: 217–222.

70 Clapp JF, Seaward BL, Sleamaker RH, Hiser J. Maternal physiologic adaptations to early human pregnancy. *Am J Obstet Gynecol* 1988; **159**: 1456–1460.

71 Campbell DM, Hall MH, Barker DJP, Cross J, Shiell AW, Godfrey KM. Diet in pregnancy and the offspring's blood pressure 40 years later. *Br J Obstet Gynaecol* 1996; **103**: 273–280.

72 Godfrey K, Robinson S, Barker DJP, Osmond C, Cox V. Maternal nutrition in early and late pregnancy in relation to placental and fetal growth. *Br Med J* 1996; **312**: 410–414.

73 Rush D. Effects of changes in maternal energy and protein intake during pregnancy, with special reference to fetal growth. In: Sharp F, Fraser RB, Milner RDG, eds. *Fetal Growth*. London: Royal College of Obstetricians and Gynaecologists. 1989; 203–233.

74 Godfrey KM, Robinson S, Hales CN, Barker DJP, Osmond C, Taylor KP. Nutrition in pregnancy and the concentrations of proinsulin, 32–33 split proinsulin, insulin, and C-peptide in cord plasma. *Diabet Med* 1996; **13**: 868–873.

75 Jackson AA, Persaud C, Werkmeister G, McClelland ISM, Badaloo A, Forrester T. Comparison of urinary 5-L-oxoproline (L-pyroglutamate) during normal pregnancy in women in England and Jamaica. *Br J Nutr* 1997; **77**: 183–196.

76 Child SC, Soares MJ, Reid M, Persaud C, Forrester T, Jackson AA. Urea kinetics varies in Jamaican women and men in relation to adiposity, lean body mass and protein intake. *Eur J Clin Nut* 1997; **51**: 107–115.

77 James WPT. Long-term fetal programming of body composition and longevity. *Nutr Rev* 1997; **55**: S41–S43.

78 Belizan JM, Villar J, Bergel E, del Pino A, Di Fulvio S, Galliano SV, et al. Long term effect of calcium supplementation during pregnancy on the blood pressure of offspring: follow up of a randomised controlled trial. *Br Med J* 1997; **315**: 281–285.

79 Law CM, Barker DJP, Richardson WW, Shiell AW, Grime LP, Armand-Smith NG, et al. Thinness at birth in a northern industrial town. *J Epidemiol Community Health* 1993; **47**: 255–259.

80 Law CM, Gordon GS, Shiell AW, Barker DJP, Hales CN. Thinness at birth and glucose tolerance in seven year old children. *Diabet Med* 1995; **12**: 24–29.

81 Osmond C, Barker DJP. Ischaemic heart disease in England and Wales around the year 2000. *J Epidemiol Community Health* 1991; **45**: 71–72.

82 Department of Health. *The health of the nation. A strategy for health in England*. London: HMSO, 1992.

83 Kendall R. From the Chief Medical Officer. *Health Bulletin* 1993; **51**: 351–352.

84 Joseph KS, Kramer M. Should we intervene to improve fetal growth? In: Kuh D, Ben-Shloma Y, eds. *A life course approach to chronic disease epidemiology*. Oxford: Oxford University Press, 1997.

85 Moore SE, Cole TJ, Poskitt EME, Sonko BJ, Whitehad RG, McGregor IA, et al. Season of birth predicts mortality in rural Gambia. *Nature* 1997; **388**: 434.

86 Goldberg GR, Prentice AM. Maternal and fetal determinants of adult diseases. *Nutr Rev* 1994; **52**: 191–200.

87 Lewis T. Medical lessons from history. In: *The Medusa and the Snail: more notes of a biology watcher*. New York: Viking Press, 1979; 158–175.

abdominal circumference 54
  LDL cholesterol and 82–3, 84, 85
Aberdeen diet in pregnancy study 203–5
Adelaide 67, 70
adipocytes 22
adrenarche 188
affluence, diseases of 185–9
Africa 109, 156
ageing 21, 201
air pollution 119, 185
air temperature 119
alcohol consumption 55, 65, 84
allergy 31
altitude, high 142
alveoli 24
amino acids 27, 134, 135
amniotic fluid 24
androgens 30, 31
anaemia in pregnancy 142
Anglesey 155
animal programming experiments 14,
    20–31
  blood pressure 22–3
  endocrine systems 27–31
  immune system 31
  maturation and ageing 21
  metabolism 26–7
  obesity 22
  organ growth 23–6
apolipoprotein 82, 88
appendicitis, acute 196, 197
  diet and 153–4
  geography of, 153
  hygiene hypothesis 154–6
  social class and 153
  time trends of 151–2
asthma 156
atheroma 81, 89
atopic disease 19, 31, 156
Australia
  Paget's disease of bone in 157, 159

bile acids 26, 27
birds 20
birth place 10
birth records from Jessop Hospital,
    Sheffield 51–2
birthweight 50, 52
  age of menarche and 187
  atopic disease and 156
  blood pressure and 63–4
  cancer of breast and ovary and 185–6
  cardiovascular disease and 46–50, 60
  chronic bronchitis and 121–2, 123
  diabetes and 97–100
  diet in pregnancy and 138–9
  fetal nutrition and 192
  growth hormone and 29

immune system and 31
  LDL cholesterol and 85
  maternal effect on 129–30, 131–2
  maternal nutrition and 136–9, 139–41
  obesity and 111–12
  of fathers 139–40
  placental weight and 143
  polycystic ovary disease and 187
  see also body proportions
blood clotting 89–90
blood pressure 22–3
  amplification 72
  body proportions at birth and 52, 56
  calcium and 206
  childhood 72
  diet in pregnancy and 203–4
  fetal growth and adult 63–9
  fetal growth and childhood 69
  fingerprints and 75–6
  lifestyle and 76
  maternal influences on 71–2
  placental weight and 69–70, 143–4
  undernutrition and 29
body fat 136–7
bones 17, 18
bottle feeding 86, 89
body mass 65
  blood pressure and 76
  coronary heart disease and 193–4, 195,
    198
  in pregnancy 202–3
  LDL cholesterol and 84
body proportions 15–18
  at birth 52, 56, 139–41, 192, 206–7
  before pregnancy 136–7
  blood pressure and 66–7, 76
  cardiovascular disease and 50–5
brain
  blood flow and 134
  growth 23–4
breast cancer 185–6
breast feeding 27, 31, 119
  appendicitis and 155
  in Lancashire towns 167, 171
  serum cholesterol concentrations and 86,
    87, 88, 89
breast milk 24, 26, 81
bronchiolitis 117
bronchitis, chronic 184–5
  birthweight and 121–2, 123
  follow-up studies 120–1
  geography of 117–20
  infant mortality and 8
  lung growth and 124, 125
  mortality from 118, 119
Burnley, Lancashire 167–72
  birth size sample in 206–7
Burnside, Ethel Margaret 44, 45, 46

calcium 206
calorie intake in pregnancy 138, 139
cancer
  breast 185–6
  lung 120, 121, 184, 185
  ovarian 185–6
  prostate 188–9
Canada 110
carbohydrates 28, 132, 142
cardiovascular disease
  birthweight and 46–50, 56, 57
  body proportions at birth and 50–5
  early menopause and 188
  fetal growth and 60
  in London in the past 172
  infant feeding and 87–8
  maternal mortality and 8–10
  migrants and 10–11
cattle 131
cell
  clones 19
  numbers 18–19
  replication 15
change, diseases of 189–97
China
  body proportions at birth in 192–3
  fetal growth and blood pressure in 68–9
cholesterol, serum 26, 81–9, 92
  LDL 82–4
  triglycerides and HDL 84–5
cholestyramine 26
Clean Air Act (1956) 185
Colne, Lancashire 167–72
coronary heart disease 2–5, 27, 190–5, 197
  birthweight and 46–50
  body proportions and, 50–5
  childhood environment and 5–7
  cholesterol and 81, 89
  fetal growth and 3, 58–60
  fibrinogen and 89–90, 91
  geography of 3–5
  hazard ratios for death from 196, 197
  infant mortality and 7–8
  lifestyle and 2, 56
  liver growth in utero and 85–6
  long-term effect of fetal undernutrition
    and 144–5
  mortality rates for 191–2
  place of birth and 10
  ratio of placental weight to birthweight
    and 143
coronary thrombosis 89
corticosteroids 23, 29
cortisol 29, 73–4, 124
cotton industry 167, 171
Croatia 89

death rates in generations 181–2
Denmark, multiple sclerosis in 162
depression 200
Derbyshire 121, 123, 125
dexamethasone 29
DHEAS 188
diabetes see non-insulin dependent diabetes
diaphragmatic hernia 24

diarrhoea 6, 171
diet 2, 3, 4–5
  acute appendicits and 153–4
  famine and 101
  fetal growth and 131
  high carbohydrate 28, 142
  in industrial towns circa 1900 176, 179
  in pregnancy 138–9, 203–6, 208
  iodine intake 190
  placental growth and 142
  protein-deficient 131–2
Domestic Servants Society 176
domestic service 175–6
duodenal ulcer 196–7

eczema 31, 156
Edinburgh 182
elephant seals, breeding habits of 130
embryo, growth of 14, 16, 132–3
emphysema 118, 125
encephalitis lethargica 159
endocrine systems 27–31
  abnormalities of 187
  blood pressure and 73–4
  control of fetal growth 19–20
  see also hormones
environment
  childhood 5–7
  in utero 7–8
environmental change and diseases 197–9
Epstein-Barr virus 162
Ethiopian Jews 110
Europe 109
  Paget's disease of bone in 158
exercise 104, 131, 143
eye development 13

factor VII 90, 92, 93
family studies 129
  asthma and 156
  NIDD and 97, 110
famine 178
  birthweight and 138, 140–1
  diabetes and 100–2
  immune system and 31
fetal growth 15
  adult haemostatic factors and 90–3
  atopic disease and 156
  blood pressure and 63–9
  childhood blood·pressure and 69
  coronary heart disease and 3, 58–60
  endocrine control of 19–20
  famine and 101
  growth hormones and 28–9
  intergenerational constraints on 131–2
  maternal constraint of 131
  obesity and 58
  of twins 111
  retardation 73, 74, 124, 141
  serum cholesterol and 82–5
  see also birthweight
fetal undernutrition 57, 197, 201
  adaptations to 132–6
  coronary heart disease and 144–5
  insulin resistance and 107

fibre consumption 154
fibrinogen 89–93
fingerprints 75–6
Finland, coronary heart disease study in 6, 50
  hazard ratios 197–8, 199, 203
  mortality ratios 53, 193–4
  obesity 57
  placental weight 55
  stroke 183
forced expiratory volume in 1 second (FEV$_1$) 121–2, 123, 124, 125
forced vital capacity (FVC) 122, 123
Framingham study 91
France 75, 157

Gambia 31, 71, 139
generations
  death rates in 181–2
  diet and 131–2
genes
  fetal adaptations and 135–6
  maternal fetal conflict 130
  NIDD and 110–1
geography 3–5
  migrant studies and 109–10
  of acute appendicitis 153
  of chronic bronchitis 117–20
  of Paget's disease of bone 157–8
  of stroke 9
Germany 89, 138
gestation, cardiovascular disease and length of, 54–5
Glasgow 182
glucocorticoids 29–30, 104
glucose
  concentrations 28, 135
  tolerance 56, 97–8
goitre, toxic nodular 190
gonadotrophins 20, 30, 186, 187
growth
  body form and 15–18
  disproportionate 18, 82, 192
  linear 24
  retardation 18, 141, 192
  tracking 16
  trajectory 16
  see also fetal growth
guinea pigs 23, 24, 26, 139

haemoglobin concentrations 142
hay fever 156
head circumference at birth 52, 53, 54, 85
height
  cancer and 188
  cardiovascular disease and 92–3
  fetal growth and mother's 132
hepatitis B virus 162
Hertfordshire studies 57
  ageing 201
  birthweight 54, 73–4, 75, 84, 90–1, 165
  blood pressure 63, 64
  chronic bronchitis 121
  diabetes 97–9, 100
  growth hormone 200

infant feeding 86–7, 88, 89, 92
  Miss Burnside's records 43–5
  mortality ratios 46–7
  obesity 111
hip width and blood pressure 202–3
HMG-CoA reductase 18, 26
Holland, famine in
  birthweight and 138, 140–1
  NIDD and 100–1, 111
  schizophrenia and 200
Hong Kong 155
hormones 14, 30–1, 104, 130
  brain development and 23
  cancer and 185–6, 188, 189
  fetal 19–20, 134
  growth 28–9, 104, 144, 200
  sex 137
  thyroid 30, 88
horses and ponies 131
housing conditions in Lancashire towns 171
hot water systems 155, 197
Hull 176–7
hygiene 178, 198
  appendicitis and 154–6, 197
hypertension 25, 64, 65, 72, 73, 74
hypogonadism 188
hypothalmus 20

IGF-1 28, 29, 74, 134
immune system 31
India 28, 50, 56, 74, 76
  body proportions at birth in 192, 193
  chronic bronchitis in 122
  coronary heart disease and fetal growth in 58–60
  NIDD in 105–6, 107, 108, 194
infant feeding 86–9
infant growth
  adult haemostatic factors and 90–3
infant mortality 3–5, 6, 7
  from bronchitis and pneumonia 119
  in Lancashire towns 169, 170, 171
infant weight at one year 47, 48
  chronic bronchitis and 121–2
insulin 25, 27–8, 97, 132
  deficiency 105–6, 144
  diet in pregnancy and 204–5
  fetal 134
  resistance 98, 102–5, 108–9
intestine growth 26
iodine 190
iron deficiency 136

Jamaica 71, 85, 205
Japan 71
Jessop Hospital, Sheffield 48, 82
  see also Sheffield studies

kidney 25, 73

Lancashire towns 167–72, 178
Leningrad 101, 138
lifestyle
  blood pressure and 76

lifestyle (*contd.*)
  coronary heart disease and 2, 56–7
  NIDD and 110
lipid metabolism 24, 26–7
lipoproteins 81
liver 27, 81
  growth and development 24–5, 85–6, 92, 93
London 92, 93, 110
  mortality 172, 173
  socioeconomic conditions in the past 172–7, 178
lung
  cancer 120, 121, 184, 185
  growth 24, 124
  sex differences in early growth 125

macrosomia 106
maternal-fetal conflict 130
maternal mortality 8–10
maternal nutrition 8–10, 56
  birthweight and 136–9
  body proportions at birth and 139–41
  placenta and 141–4
  thymus and 31
  undernutrition 194
maturation 21
measles virus 158
menarche, age of 187–8
menopause 91, 187, 188
metabolic syndrome 104, 144
metabolism 26–7
migrants
  cardiovascular disease and 10–11, 58
  chronic bronchitis and 117
  diet and 198
  multiple sclerosis and 160–1
  NIDD and 109–10
  Paget's disease of bone and 157
  to London from rural areas 175, 178
motor neuron disease 160, 161
multiple sclerosis 160–2
myocardial infarction 89

Naples, Italy 155
Naurua 109
  diabetes in 110, 195
Nelson, Lancashire 167–72
nephrons 25, 73
nervous system and blood pressure 75
neurological disease 159–62
New York 139
New Zealand 156, 157
non-insulin-dependent diabetes (NIDD) 56, 57, 59, 144, 195–6, 197
  famine and 100–2
  genetic effects and 110–11
  geography of 109–10
  high birthweight and 100
  in India 105–6
  insulin deficiency and 105–6
  insulin resistance and 102
  low birthweight and 97–9
  studies of children and young adults 107–8
  'thrifty phenotype' 108–9

North America 109
Northern Ireland 155
Northwick Park Heart Study 89
Norway 5, 93, 117
nurses' health study in USA 57–8, 64, 185, 186
nutrition *see* maternal nutrition; pregnancy; undernutrition

obesity 22, 63, 208
  fetal growth and 58
  NIDD and 97, 105, 111–12
oestrogens 30, 137, 185
oligohydramnios 24
organ growth 23–6
osteoporosis 188, 199–200
ovarian cancer 185–6
ovum donation and birthweight 129

Paget's disease of bone 157–9
pancreas 19, 25, 27–8
Papua, New Guinea 109
paramyxoviruses 158
Parkinson's disease 159–60
Peking Union Medical College Hospital 68, 103
PEPCK 25
pigs
  growth of 15, 16, 18
  undernutrition of 133
Pima Indians 100
placenta 72, 110, 135
  maternal nutrition and 141–4
placental weight 29, 55, 131
  blood pressure and 69–70, 73
  diet and 203, 204
pneumonia 117, 118, 119, 123, 125
poliomyelitis 160, 189, 196
polycystic ovary disease 187
ponderal index 131
  birthweight of parents and 139–40
  coronary heart disease and 52, 192, 194
  NIDD and 104, 106
poverty 9
  diseases of 182–5
pregnancy
  body mass in 202–3
  body size before 136–7
  diabetes in 100–1, 106
  diet in 138–9, 203–6, 208
  nutrition in 130, 140
  undernutrition in early 134–5
  undernutrition in late 135
  undernutrition in mid 135
  weight gain and diet in 137–9
Preston studies
  blood pressure 65, 66, 67, 69–70, 75
  cotton industry in 167, 168
  fibrinogen analysis 91
  NIDD 99, 100, 105
preventive health policies 208
programming 14
  animal experiments 20–31
  mechanisms of 18–20
  placenta and 72

prostate cancer 188–9
protein
  deficiency 19
  intake 140, 204
  maternal restriction of 29–30
  metabolism 27

rats
  blood pressure experiments in 22–3, 29
  diet and fetal growth in 131
  insulin and 28
  intestine growth in 26
  obesity in 22
  sex hormones and 30
  undernutrition of 16–17, 18, 19, 21, 24, 25, 56–7, 144
  weaning of 27
renal structure 73
renin-angiotensin system 73
reproductive physiololgy 187–8
respiratory infections, infant 117, 119–21, 123–4
  sex differences and 125
respiratory syncytial virus 158
rheumatic heart disease 2

Saliisbury, UK 70, 73, 74, 107, 108
  birth size sample 206–7
salt 76
schizophrenia 200
Scotland 89, 157
sensitive periods in development 14–15
sex determination of reptiles 14
sex differences in early lung growth 125
sexual maturation 21
sexual physiology 23
sheep
  androgens and 31
  undernutrition of 17–18, 24, 70, 130, 133, 135, 139, 142
Sheffield studies on coronary heart disease 82
  blood pressure 65, 66, 67, 73, 74
  body proportions 50–2, 188
  fetal growth 91
  infant growth 92
  liver growth 85, 144
  mortality ratios 55
skinfold thickness 137, 139, 202
smoking 2, 4, 56, 58, 197
  blood pressure and 71, 72
  chronic bronchitis and 119, 120, 184
  fetal growth and 132, 143
  fetal lung development and 124, 125
  FEV1 and 122
  fibrinogen and 90
  LDL cholesterol and 84, 88
social class
  acute appendicitis and 153
  infant feeding and 88
socioeconomic conditions 57
  in Lancashire 169–72, 178
  in London 172, 173–7, 178
sodium intake 76
sperm count 188–9

streptozotocin 28
stroke 90, 91, 144,
  age-specific mortality 183–4
  birthweight and 46–7, 48, 49
  body proportions and 55
  infant mortality and 7, 8
  place of birth and 10
stunting at birth 50–4, 60, 67, 139
sweat glands 13
Swedish studies
  blood pressure 63, 65, 66
  body proportions at birth 192
  coronary heart disease 50, 54, 56
  NIDD 99, 100, 105
  prostate cancer 188

teeth 181
temperature
  air 119
  incubation 14
testosterone 20, 30–1
thinness
  at birth 50–3, 104, 112, 139, 140, 194
  of mothers 201–2
thrombosis 89
thyrotoxicosis 189–90
thymus 19, 31
thyroid-stimulating hormone 20, 30
thyroxine 30
time trends in acute appendicitis 151–2
trends in disease 182
triglycerides 81, 84–5
twin studies 97, 110

undernutrition 29,178
  animal 21
  brain and 23
  gestational 15, 16–18
  in Hull in 1913 177
  programming mechanisms of 18–20
  thymus and 31
  see also fetal undernutrition; pregnancy
USA 117
  coronary heart disease in 6, 10, 48, 49
  diabetes in 99, 100
  motor neuron disease in 160
  nurses' health study 57–8, 64, 185
  obesity in 111
  Paget's disease of bone in 157, 158
  Parkinson's disease in 159–60
  stroke in 10

vascular structure and blood pressure 74–5
viruses 158, 159, 160, 161, 162
vitamins 88, 89, 136

waist-hip ratio 91
Wales 50, 56, 58
weaning 27, 31. 86
weight gain in pregnancy 137–9
  see also body mass
Western diseases 197–9

X-linked genes and blood pressure 71

zinc deficiency 136